THE
NATURAL
FAMILY
DOCTOR

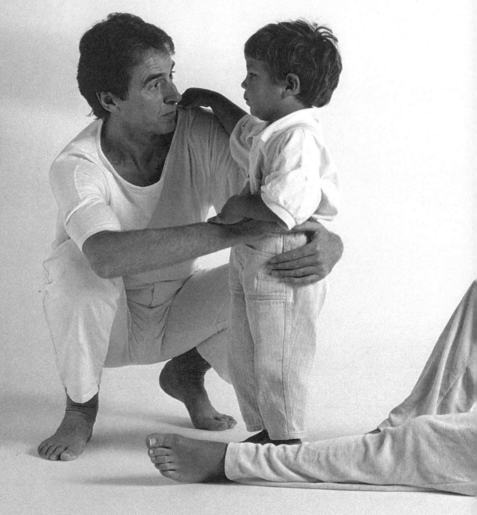

A Fireside Book
Published by Simon & Schuster, Inc.
New York

THE
NATURAL
FAMILY
DOCTOR

The comprehensive self-help guide
to health and natural medicine

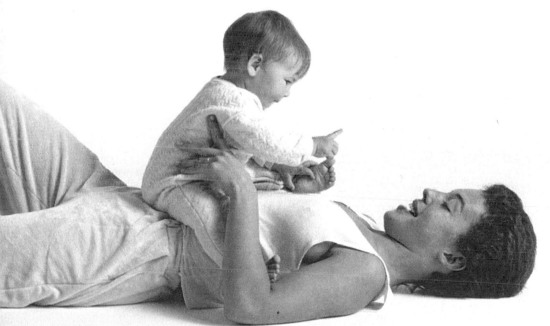

By Dr Andrew Stanway, MB, MRCP
with Richard Grossman, PhD

A GAIA ORIGINAL

From an idea by Lucy Lidell

Direction	Joss Pearson
	Lucy Lidell
Production	David Pearson
Photography	Fausto Dorelli
Photographic reference	Peter Warren
Project editor	Roslin Mair
Editorial and research	Hetty Einzig
	Jonathan Hilton
	Joanna Jellinek
	Anna Kruger
	Susan McKeever
Project designer	Jerry Burman
Design	Peter Barney
	Lucy Oliver
	David Whelan
	Rita Wuhtrich

A FIRESIDE BOOK
published by Simon & Schuster, Inc.,
Simon & Schuster Building, Rockefeller Center,
1230 Avenue of the Americas, New York, N.Y. 10020

FIRESIDE and colophon are registered
trademarks of Simon & Schuster, Inc.

First published by Century Hutchinson, London
Printed and bound in Great Britain

First printing 1987
1 2 3 4 5 6 7 8 9 10

Library of Congress Cataloguing-in-Publication Data
Stanway, Andrew.
    The natural family doctor
    "A Fireside Book"
    Bibliography: p.
    Includes index.
    1. Naturopathy. 2. Self-care, Health. I. Grossman, Richard L.
    (Richard Lee), 1921-   . II. Title
RZ440.S73 1987b   615.5'35   86–26941
ISBN 0-671-61966-7 (pbk)

Typesetting by Bookworm Typesetting, Manchester, UK
Reproduction by F.E. Burman Ltd, London
Printed by Purnell Book Production Limited,
Member of the BPCC Group

Contents

Garlic, lemon, essential oils and
Bach flower remedies – natural
medicinal treatments

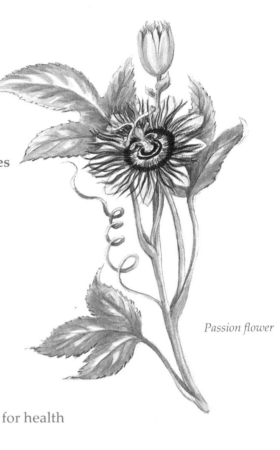

Passion flower

Foreword

To the patients and staff
of The Valentine Lane Family Practice

In the past twenty-five years, perhaps no idea has seized the public imagination so compellingly as the notion that human beings can participate more fully in controlling their own health. The new and vigorous emphasis on the prevention of illness and disease through self-designed and self-managed changes in lifestyle habits and behavior has caused a significant shift away from the old-time dependency on the prescriptions and injunctions of the classical medical establishment.

Just as masses of people have come to demand alternatives to thoughtless methods of disposing of hazardous waste materials, or dangerous ways of disinfecting crops or generating energy, so have they begun to question and reject the heavily drug-based therapies that dominate the standard medical strategy. The nagging worries about the unpleasant, even damaging side-effects of many drugs have been transformed into overt resistance to synthetic medicines, coupled with an expanding interest in alternatives to therapeutics that have become two-edged swords.

Along with the expanding consciousness of the risks of powerful medications there has been an equally growing awareness that attempts to treat or cure disease and disability must do more than only minister to symptoms. As the lay public has become better informed about health and illness, it has likewise understood that the *causes* of human distress deserve every bit as much attention as temporary relief or short-term "cures". As a result, both ancient and modern systems that lie outside what is thought of as "scientific" medicine are capturing the interest of people all over the world, particularly when such systems are based on a deep understanding of how human emotions and the powers of the human mind can be as important as physical conditions in determining whole health.

These factors – the heightened sense that individuals must take increased responsibility for their health, the widespread turning away from exclusive reliance on drug-based therapies, the realization that the root causes of illness and disease must be given as much importance as the mere alleviation of symptoms, the near universal acceptance of the interdependent relationships of body, mind, feelings, and spirit – all these have combined to foster the rise of the "natural" therapies, medical systems that are safe, effective, relatively inexpensive, and often self-administered. And as we learn more about such systems – some from the eastern traditions, some from the western perspective, some old and some modern, some sophisticated and some almost primitive – it becomes increasingly clear that those who wish to benefit from *all* the best and most relevant medical knowledge need reliable guidance and helpful assistance to assure that an integrated medical approach is readily available, one that makes the optimum use of the best of *every* medical tradition and technique devoted to the relief of human suffering.

THE NATURAL FAMILY DOCTOR is a book comprehensively and explicitly dedicated to that goal.

Richard Grossman

Introduction

Over the last five years there has been a dramatic shift in public opinion in favor of natural medicine. A growing number of people now realize the importance of health and fitness and are looking to take more responsibility for their own health. Health food stores and exercise studios abound in every town and even neighborhood supermarkets are being forced to satisfy the public's increasing demand for healthier products. In fact, natural medicine has been called the fastest growing industry, second only to computers. For while no one would deny the immense contribution of modern medicine, nor its crucial role in emergencies, many have grown disenchanted with its shortcomings and are seeking alternative ways of understanding and dealing with ill health.

Health begins in childhood, and today more and more of us are conscious of the importance of giving our children the best possible start in life. In order to take responsibility for our own health, however, we need to stop thinking of ourselves as "patients" who turn to "doctors" to solve our health problems, and to recognize instead that for everyday purposes we ourselves are in the best position to monitor our health and minister to our own needs and those of our family. Each one of us is born with a doctor of unparalleled wisdom in our own being, given the body's inbuilt mechanisms of defence and self-healing (see pp.32-3). If we can learn to assist these natural healing powers, through discovering the fundamentals of a healthy lifestyle and learning how to use safe natural remedies in times of need, then our bodies have the best chance of rewarding us with vibrant good health. In this book, therefore, we look in Part One at the essential elements of preventive health care. In Part Two we present some of the most popular natural therapies available, both for self-medication and professional treatment.

"Health is a state of complete physical, mental and social well-being and not merely the absence of disease or infirmity."
WHO

Prevention and personal responsibility

Today it is hardly a matter of debate that good food, fresh air, plenty of exercise, sufficient sleep and so on are the basics of health. But even though prevention is a much-applauded concept, few people actually live their lives as if it were a reality, despite abundant evidence that proves beyond doubt that preventive health care pays. This is partly because we in the

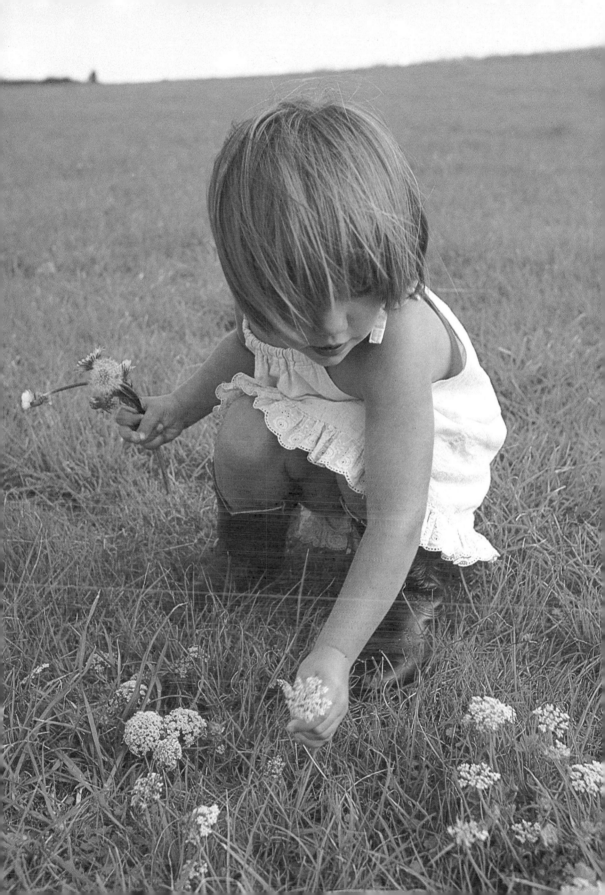

West don't have a strong tradition of preventive medicine, apart from the public health measures, such as safe water supplies and improved sanitation, which were largely responsible for the dramatic decline of infectious diseases like typhoid and cholera in the 19th century. The Chinese system of medicine, by contrast, has always emphasized preventive measures. In fact, the Chinese physicians of the past were said to be paid only when their patients were well, not when they were ill, thus giving them a greater incentive to maintain their patient's health.

Many of us look after our cars better than we care for ourselves. We snatch hurried meals, often of "convenience" foods, sleep fitfully, without being properly relaxed, travel stressfully in crowded trains or buses, our lives ruled by the clock. We accept excessive demands from home and work, incessantly neglecting our real needs. But eventually the constant strain of living out of tune with ourselves begins to take its toll. We may become irritable and overtired and fall prey to a host of minor infections, aches and pains. Sadly, however, few of us stop to ask why, few of us recognize our ills as a consequence of our own self-neglect. At best we may take a few days off work or simply go to the doctor or to a pharmacy, hoping to have the inconvenience removed quickly, so that we can return promptly to our busy lives, without pausing to look at why we become unwell.

This book, therefore, is aimed at teaching you to be aware of and to honor your own needs, both physically and psychologically, so that you can avoid some of the drains on your resources of health and energy that 20th-century living can entail. We look first at the nature of the body you inhabit, at how the different parts work together to maintain the whole and at how you can best look after them. This is followed by an extensive section on personal health care, with advice on all the ingredients of a healthy lifestyle, the means at your disposal to keep yourself and your family in the best of health, physically, mentally, and emotionally. Here you will find how to keep your energy up by eating well; how to maintain a balance of exercise and relaxation; how to increase your vitality through breathing more effectively; and how to combat stress and increase your mental and emotional well-being – for happiness is known to be important to health.

"Sages do not treat those who are already ill; they rather instruct those who are not yet ill . . . The superior physician helps before the early budding of disease. The inferior physician begins to help when the disease has already developed."
The Yellow Emperor
from the Nei Ching

The origins of traditional medicine

Given the incredible rise of complementary therapies in recent times, it is tempting to think of natural medicine as a modern phenomenon. But in fact, until the start of the 19th century, most medical practice was "traditional" and even those therapies that came into being in the last hundred years are largely derived from ancient practices. As you can see on the time chart (p.15), several of the therapies described in this book date back to prehistoric times – herbal prescriptions, such as the Ebers papyrus, still survive from 6,000 years ago, and evidence suggests that acupuncture may have already been in practice around the same time, using needles made of bone.

For thousands of years, sickness was blamed largely on the displeasure of the gods or on demons. Then, around 2,500 years ago, both in the ancient Chinese and Indian worlds of the East and in the Greek civilization of the West, the supernatural view was displaced by the belief in health as resulting from a balance of natural forces in the body, and in disease as evidence of a disturbance of this balance. But while the Chinese and Indian medical systems based on this view have survived virtually intact, the idea of harmony gradually disappeared from the West, especially with the rise of scientific medicine.

While the scientific approach has brought remarkable improvements in the treatment of injuries and infectious diseases, orthodox medicine has proved less effective in the treatment of chronic degenerative diseases and psychosomatic conditions. And many people have grown cautious of using over-the-counter drugs for common everyday ailments, concerned about the possibility of side-effects.

Today it is precisely in those countries with a long history of orthodox medicine that most of the newer natural therapies have originated, as shown by the map (p.14), and it is there that interest in the possible alternatives is most widespread. In the UK, for example, according to a report by the Research Council for Complementary Medicine in 1985, around 10 percent of all medical consultations are now with complementary practitioners. In the Netherlands, a survey of over a thousand members of the public in 1979 showed that 75 percent were in favor of complementary medicine being included in their national health system.

"The cure of the part should not be attempted without the treatment of the whole. No atttempt should be made to cure the body without the soul and, if the head and body are to be healthy, you must begin by curing the mind."
Plato
The Republic

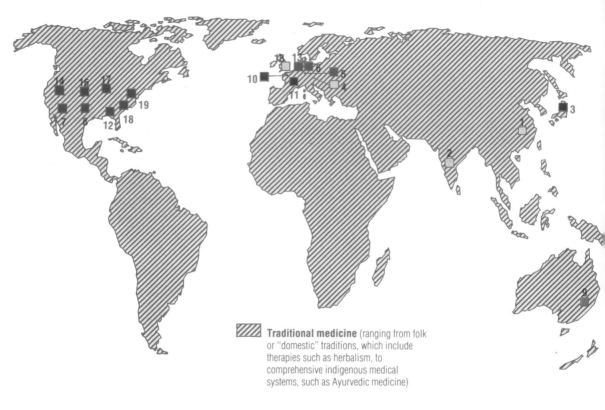

Traditional medicine (ranging from folk or "domestic" traditions, which include therapies such as herbalism, to comprehensive indigenous medical systems, such as Ayurvedic medicine)

The common bonds of complementary medicine

Natural medicine is known by many names, including "unorthodox", "unconventional" and "alternative". In many ways the best description for the therapies contained in this book is "complementary", for they are intended to add to rather than replace what orthodox medicine has to offer. So in what ways is complementary or natural medicine different from orthodox medicine? And what characteristics do the natural therapies have in common?

The term "natural medicine" covers a wide range of different therapies and medical practices. It includes complete medical systems, such as homeopathy, as well as manipulative therapies, like osteopathy or Rolfing, that work primarily on the musculoskeletal system, and therapies such as the Bach flower remedies, that are directed toward correcting negative states of mind. Nevertheless there are many areas of agreement among the different disciplines.

First, they tend to be more holistic in approach than does the orthodox system. This means that in treating a patient they tend to look at the whole person, body, mind, and spirit, rather than simply

Origins
Most ancient therapies are practically universal in their origins – notably herbal medicine, meditation, healing, massage, and hydrotherapy. Some forms of medicine which developed in the East, in particular acupuncture, have made an enormous impact on the West; and a few western concepts, such as homeopathy, have taken firm root in the East. "Modern" therapies, such as Rolfing, tend to remain centred in areas of westernized health care.

1970s **(19) Therapeutic touch** A secular version of healing used by nurses and lay
1960s people, developed by Dr Dolores Krieger, Professor of Nursing at New York University.

1940s **(16) Rolfing** A manipulative therapy developed by Dr Ida Rolf, designed to re-form the body and liberate it from distortions.

1930s **(15) Bach flower remedies** A therapy created by Dr Edward Bach, that counters negative emotional states through the use of the healing powers in common plants.

1920s **(12) Reflexology** A touch technique in which the whole body can be treated by working on reflex zones in the feet and hands. The therapy is of ancient origins, but it was researched and developed by Dr William Fitzgerald and Eunice Ingham
1900 in the 1920s and 30s.

1890s **(8) Chiropractic** A technique specializing in manipulation of the spine and joints,
1870s developed by the US healer and osteopath, D.D. Palmer.

1850s **(6) Naturopathy** A combination of various therapies centering on dietary treatment and hydrotherapy.

1700s

1740s **(4) Hypnotherapy** The use of trance-like states to influence mind and body, demonstrated by the Austrian Franz Anton Mesmer in the 1740s and later applied for therapeutic purposes.

(18) Touch for health A health-enhancing programme, which includes muscle testing and working on the meridians, developed from applied kinesiology by Dr John F. Thie specifically for lay people.

(14) Biofeedback A monitoring technique that uses a variety of instruments to measure bodily changes. It is used especially to control stress reactions.

(11) Aromatherapy A therapy based on the use of essential oils – first explored scientifically in the 1920s, although essential oils have been used medicinally since ancient times.

(9) Alexander technique F.M. Alexander's body-mind therapy, which treats and prevents disorders through correcting the posture, and is designed to encourage a more economical and less stressful "use of the self".

(5) Homeopathy A comprehensive system of medicine developed in Leipzig in the late 18th century by Dr Samuel Hahnemann, based on the belief that "like cures like".

(17) Applied kinesiology A method of diagnosis and treatment based on the testing and correcting of muscle imbalances, invented by Dr George Goodheart in Detroit, USA.

(13) Autogenics A method of deep relaxation based on auto-suggestion, pioneered by Dr Johannes Schultz in Berlin in the 1920s.

(10) Radiesthesia A distant healing technique, developed by Abbé Mermet in the 1920s. The technique is closely related to radionics, which uses pendulums, diagnostic charts and other equipment to diagnose and heal illness, usually at a distance.

(7) Osteopathy A method of manipulating joints and muscles in order to correct musculoskeletal and other disorders, discovered by Dr Andrew Still in Missouri, USA.

BC **(3) Shiatsu** A Japanese therapy, developed from acupuncture and ancient Japanese massage, mainly involving the use of finger or thumb pressure.

(1) Acupuncture A system of treatment rooted in ancient Chinese thought, which seeks to rebalance energy by inserting needles in points on the body's meridians (energy channels).

Healing The channeling and directing of energy to restore health – usually by the laying-on-of-hands or by prayer. Healing has prehistoric roots in tribal religions all over the world.

(2) Yoga A comprehensive discipline embracing meditation, physical exercises, and breathing practices, developed in India at least 4,000 years ago.

Herbalism The use of herbs for medicinal purposes dates back at least 5,000 years, according to ancient Chinese and Egyptian records.

Massage A systematic form of touch given to promote health and relaxation. The earliest known massage techniques include Amna from Japan, and foot massage from Egypt, Africa, and China.

Hydrotherapy The use of water's healing powers, including the medicinal use of mineralized waters, and the application of heat and cold, amongst other treatments.

Meditation A method of stilling the mind and bringing the mental processes under control, encompassing a variety of techniques, both spiritual and secular. Its practice dates back as far as recorded history.

dealing with the ailment he or she reports. The practitioners of natural medicine recognize that health depends on a great variety of factors – on the emotional climate of our lives as well as physical causes. To treat someone successfully, they argue, all these factors need to be considered both in diagnosis and treatment, and counseling or advice on preventive care given if necessary. Thus if you go to a natural medicine practitioner suffering from, say, high blood pressure, all aspects of your health, both physical and mental, as well as your lifestyle, will be taken into consideration. Where orthodox medicine focuses on the disease, natural medicine treats the whole person.

Second, most natural remedies are safe and non-toxic and are thus far more suitable for self-medication than orthodox medicines, which can have unpleasant side-effects. One criticism often levelled at complementary medicine by the orthodox medical profession is that their remedies are not only harmless but also useless and that patients get better because of the placebo effect. While there is no doubt that the placebo effect applies to many patients of both natural and orthodox medicine, the argument collapses when, for example, you consider homeopathy's eminently successful track record in veterinary medicine.

It is important to understand, however, that taking responsibility for your own health through the use of natural medicines is not a matter simply of substituting a herb or a homeopathic remedy, say , for an aspirin. It involves recognizing the need for preventive care, looking at the causes of illness as well as the symptoms and, above all, understanding the philosophy behind whichever therapy you are using as a means of self-help. Ideally you should consult a professional practitioner in any therapy you use regularly to treat yourself or your family, in order to learn more.

Third, most natural therapies stress the body's innate capacity for self-healing (p.33) and many natural remedies are directed at strengthening the body's own healing mechanisms and rebalancing its energy flow rather than at fighting disease or curing symptoms as such. Natural medicine practitioners generally encourage their patients to understand as much as possible about why they are ill and to take an

"Traditional wisdom . . . sees illness as a disorder of the whole person, involving not only the patient's body, but his mind, his self-image, his dependence on the physical and social environment, as well as his relation to the cosmos . . ."
Fritjof Capra
The Turning Point

"It is our natures that are the physicians of our diseases."
Hippocrates

active part in their own recovery process, whether through diet, special exercises, or relaxation. This more instructional approach is facilitated by the length of time a natural therapist generally spends with his or her patient. It has been estimated that the average natural therapist takes at least eight times as long over a consultation as the average orthodox health professional.

Natural health

It is perhaps in their views of health and disease that orthodox and natural medicine practitioners diverge most widely, however. Orthodox medicine is based on the concept of the body as a machine, and of illness as the breakdown or malfunctioning of parts of the machine. In this view health is seen mainly as the opposite of disease. To the natural medicine practitioner, by contrast, health is a vibrant positive state of wholeness and harmony, a dynamic evolving process which allows us to adapt to change. Disease is seen to result less from germs, which are always present, than from disharmony in the body, caused by too much stress, for example, or an excess of toxins, which lowers our resistance. Symptoms of disease, such as fever, headaches, or nausea are seen as the body's attempts to deal with imbalance through adapting to change or fighting infection, or as useful guides to the nature of a patient's imbalance, rather than as indications of illness to be eliminated or suppressed. Though a few natural therapies treat symptoms during a patient's consultation, most gear their treatment to strengthening the body's defences, aiding its self-healing, and unblocking its energy flow, or eliminating toxins. As the patient's energy or balance returns, symptoms disappear naturally and the body restores its own health.

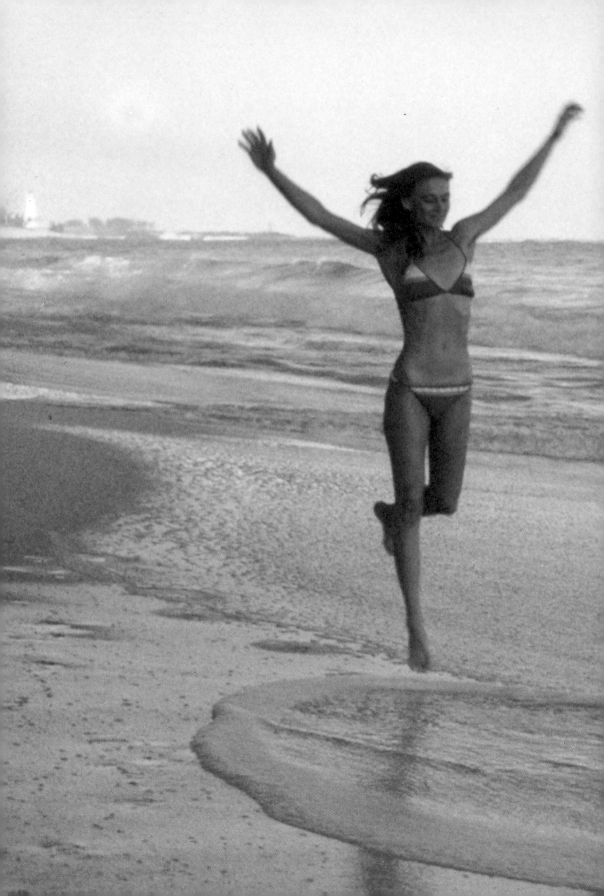

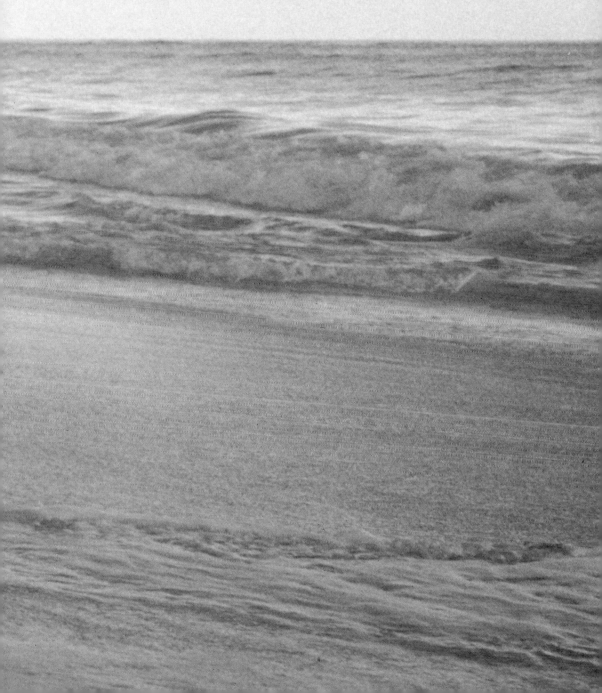

Part One: HEALTH

CHAPTER ONE
The living body

Our closest friend for life is our own body–a constant, enduring companion. Yet most of us treat it casually at best, cruelly at worst, subjecting it to mal-treatment and neglect we would balk from imposing on another. We tend to lead unhealthy lives, ignoring routine maintenance, and turning a blind eye to warning signals of disrepair. And if something goes wrong, we often assume that outside medical help will be able to solve years of abuse. Although we are familiar with our bodies, in fact we live as strangers in them, ignorant of how we work, or why they go wrong. Surely we should know and care for our bodies, so they can serve us well.

This chapter describes the workings of the living body. It takes you on a guided tour of its remarkable capacities – from energy supply and waste dispos-al to action and awareness, control and homeostasis, defence and repair – and considers the interplay of body with mind, and their powers of health and self-healing. It also includes essential points on preventive health care.

The human village
The body is much like a village – a collection of individual parts, all work-ing together to create a comfortable existence. This community organizes an efficient set of service systems to care for it, and ensure harmonious well-being. Many different maps can be drawn of a village. One might show its transport routes and service stations, another its climate, or flow of energy. Many different maps have been drawn, too, of the human village.

Western science has come to rely on "biomedical" maps – precise descrip-tions of the functions of organs such as the heart, liver, or pancreas, or of systems such as respiration or circula-tion, or the chemistry of cells – as though each operates separately, mechanically, without reference to the whole being. These very useful maps have undoubtedly helped medical adv-ances. But they have also narrowed our thinking. We go to the doctor to find out which bit of us has gone wrong, hoping to repair it, like a part in a machine.

But the body is not a machine. Machines do not grow, change, reorga-nize and repair themselves, adapt to new situations, or feel love or despair. The body is a living entity, and if it is disturbed or stressed, all its parts are involved in the "dis-ease" we suffer.

The body in harmony
Eastern traditions of medicine, far older than ours, have always concerned themselves with this holistic view. Their maps of the human village are con-cerned with the harmony and the dyna-mic balance of the system, and with flows of vital energy.

These ideas are difficult to reconcile with the western view. It may be widely accepted that acupuncture gives pain relief, but the energy channels which the acupuncturist manipulates are in-visible to a western anatomist. And the Chinese view that body organs are not simply service stations, but far-reaching influences on the whole system – the liver, for example "calms the emotions" – seems almost mystical to us in the West. Yet ancient eastern knowledge is increasingly being validated by western science. The liver does have a calming influence; among its functions is the removal of excess adrenalin, the stress hormone. And acupuncture points do show a higher electro-potential than nearby tissues. Traditional systems have much to teach us. Perhaps one of their greatest contributions is their understanding of subtle energy, the life force whose flow affects the health or disease of the whole body.

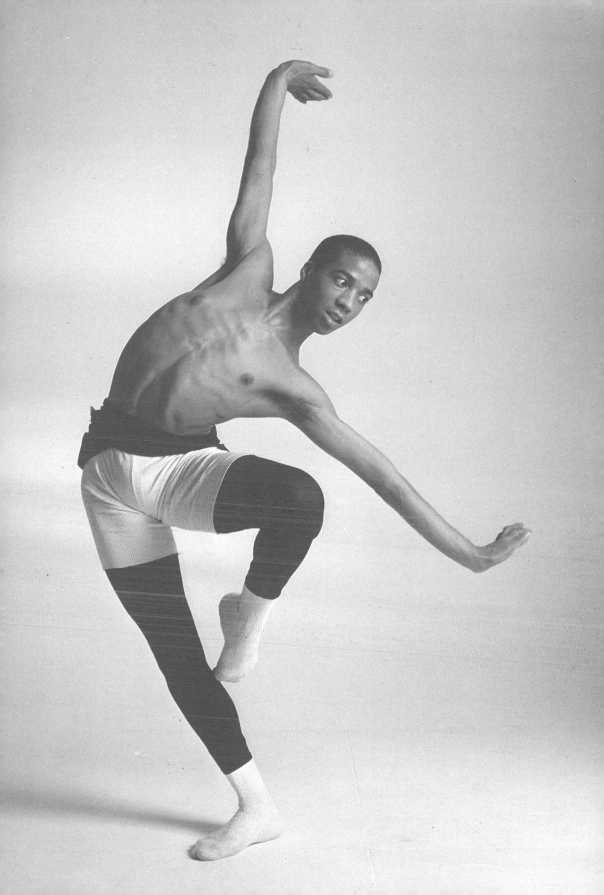

Energy

What is the life force – that vibrant energy that animates all living things, and seems to power our being, and our well-being? Such questions do not concern orthodox medicine, but the concept of life energy inspires eastern systems of medicine which have survived thousands of years, and it is the basis of many natural therapies too. All believe that flowing through and around the body are fields of subtle energy. If this flow is impeded, the body becomes ill; if it is balanced and free flowing, health is restored.

The Chinese call this force "chi". It is the stuff of the universe, animating all things, but it is not solely energy, nor is it solely matter. Chi flows through the body's meridians (channels), and it can be manipulated by acupuncture treatment. In yoga, the universal life force is called prana, and it flows through the body in nadis, radiating from energy centers or chakras. Prana can be seen by some people as a faint colored shadow around the body, an energy field that is also called the aura. The western science that comes nearest to describing yoga's subtle energy is high energy physics, where matter and energy are one, and the dance of particles and energy fields fills the universe, ourselves included. It is ecology, however, that best describes the energy patterns of life on earth.

The energy of the life force comes ultimately from the sun, but only plant life, through photosynthesis, can use it directly. Plants "breathe" carbon dioxide, release oxygen, and store solar energy in chemical form, which we use as food. We also use the oxygen to burn this fuel in our bodies (much as a car combusts fuel) and we release carbon dioxide and waste. And this harmonious cycle sustains all planetary life.

In our cells, the fires of life burn bright, as oxygen releases the stored sunlight once again – in a sense, we are all solar powered. This raw energy forms the heat of the body, the power of the muscles, the pulsing electrical activity of the brain. Physical energy is channeled through nerve, tissue, and blood supply, which after all is not dissimilar to the subtle energy of eastern thought.

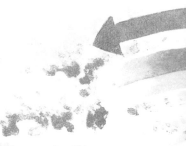

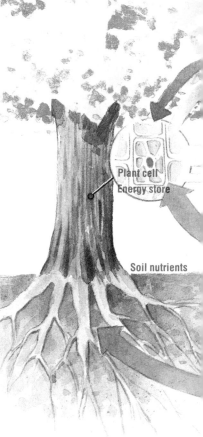

Energy for life
The sun powers all planetary life. Green plant cells tap its energy, and make sugars, starches and oils to store it, while releasing oxygen. Animal cells use oxygen to burn plant fuels and release their stored energy for use.

Plant cell
Energy store

Soil nutrients

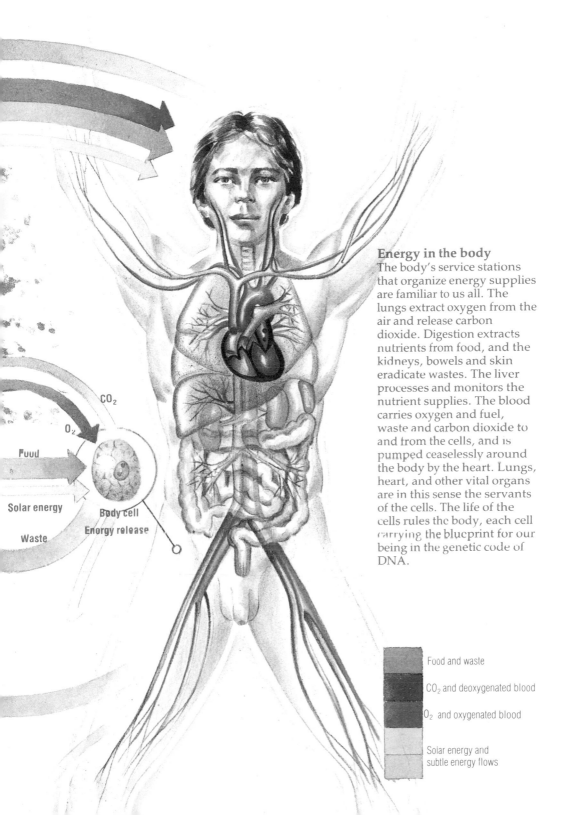

CO₂

O₂

Food

Solar energy

Waste

Body cell

Energy release

Energy in the body

The body's service stations that organize energy supplies are familiar to us all. The lungs extract oxygen from the air and release carbon dioxide. Digestion extracts nutrients from food, and the kidneys, bowels and skin eradicate wastes. The liver processes and monitors the nutrient supplies. The blood carries oxygen and fuel, waste and carbon dioxide to and from the cells, and is pumped ceaselessly around the body by the heart. Lungs, heart, and other vital organs are in this sense the servants of the cells. The life of the cells rules the body, each cell carrying the blueprint for our being in the genetic code of DNA.

Food and waste

CO₂ and deoxygenated blood

O₂ and oxygenated blood

Solar energy and subtle energy flows

The breath of life

Breathing is life's most natural act. You do it effortlessly 25,000 times a day. It is also essential because the body does not store oxygen. The lungs are a sophisticated oxygenation plant, filtering and exchanging gases at every breath via some 300 million tiny sponge-like cavities, or alveoli. Through their delicate membranes, oxygen enters the blood stream to combine with the hemoglobin of red blood cells, traveling first to the heart, then to the whole body.

The rhythm of life flows gently through the human village with each rise and fall of breath. If you need more oxygen to run, climb stairs, or meet any extra energy demand, the brain signals to increase the rate of respiration. Your emotions can trigger such signals too, especially under stress. Correspondingly, the conscious use of slow breathing can calm the body and mind (see Relaxed breathing, p.59, for example).

At each breath, we share with other creatures in the flowing life energy of our whole planet. But we also expose our vulnerable lungs to hazards in the outside environment. Rather than recklessly putting the breath of life at risk by smoking or creating pollution, we should care for our lungs, and for the air we breathe, all our lives.

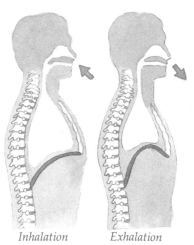

Inhalation   Exhalation

How we breathe

When we inhale, the diaphragm moves down and the ribs outward, enlarging the chest cavity. Like a bellows, the lungs suck in air. On exhaling, the muscles relax, the cavity shrinks, and air is expelled. Tension and poor physique can restrict breathing, which reduces our energy and well-being.

Breathing and subtle energy

Many eastern philosophies link breathing with the flow of subtle energy known also as chi or prana, in the body. In Chinese medicine (p.270), air is one of the three sources of chi. In yoga, more prana is drawn in by the practice of asanas (exercises) and pranayama (controlled breathing). Prana flows through energy channels, or nadis (right), which emanate from the chakras or energy centers (see also pp.285-6).

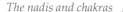

The nadis and chakras

Caring for your lungs

● Get plenty of fresh air and avoid pollution (p.72).

● Don't smoke (p.57).

● Practice breathing exercises (pp.58-9) and relaxation (p.63).

● Take aerobic exercise (p.53) for improved lung capacity.

● Correct your posture (p.296) to ensure that ribcage and diaphragm are allowed their full range of movement.

The heart of the system

All the machinery ever made fades to clumsy inadequacy compared to the heart, the powerhouse of the body. It is the master of a vast transport system that reaches every cell in the body, pumping up to 5,000 gallons of blood a day, under pressure, around the network of arteries, veins and capillaries. If you could clench and relax your fist 70 times in the next 60 seconds, you would become aware of the minimum effort your heart has been making, without pause, since long before you were born. So awe-inspiring is this performance that we should want just to sit for a moment listening to that pulsing, living rhythm, as it responds to our every mood, every demand. Unfortunately, what most of us are more likely to do – sooner or later – is to wreck it.

Arteries, which are elastic and responsive in youth, can become hardened and clogged with cholesterol, from a diet deficient in minerals and heavy with saturated fats. Blood pressure rises, straining the heart. Inactivity, stress and smoking make matters worse. Heart and arterial disease are endemic in the West, yet with a little forethought we can protect the heart and keep it strong.

How the heart works

The heart has two chambers on each side, an upper atrium and a lower ventricle. The atria relax, then contract to pump blood to the ventricles, which similarly relax and contract. This fourfold beat is triggered by a natural pacemaker. The right side of the heart receives blood from the body and pumps it to the lungs, the left receives blood from the lungs and pumps it to the body, and also to the heart itself via the coronary arteries. If these are scaly or obstructed, the cardiac muscle is starved and heart attacks may result.

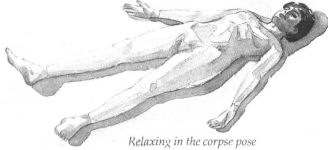

Relaxing in the corpse pose

Heart and mind

In Chinese medicine, the heart stores "shen", the human spirit or the consciousness. Western tradition sees the heart more as the home of the emotions – love, anger, or grief, and instead links consciousness with the mind. Medically, the link between conscious mind, emotions, and the health of the heart is clear – not least from the effects of stress on pulse and blood pressure. Many doctors now accept that relaxation and meditation protect the heart. Regularly practicing the yoga corpse pose, above (p.63), is known to counter raised blood pressure and hypertension.

Protecting your heart

• If you are a smoker, stop. Nicotine raises the pulse and blood pressure and, with carbon dioxide, adds to the risk of clotting.

• Change your diet to avoid fatty foods, sugar, and salt (pp.44-5), which are linked to arterial disease.

• Take regular exercise. It greatly improves the heart's performance (p.49).

• Keep your weight down, to prevent strain on your heart.

• Practice relaxation (pp.62-3) and therapies such as meditation, yoga, or autogenics, to combat stress.

• If you are in any doubt about your heart, consult your doctor. High blood pressure can be a signal that the heart is in danger.

The supply system

Food is a fundamental source of energy, and of building materials for the body. The intestine is the food production line of the human village, and from here the process of digestion and the transport systems of the blood must get the right supplies to the cells. These busy factories use up supplies depending on the rate of metabolism, but they can't work well with poor materials. And any of the various organs supplying them may suffer if we have a damaging diet. Our health largely depends on the quality and type of food we eat.

The state of our digestion also influences our moods and thoughts – the vital organs are intimately involved in the chemical climate of the whole body. Equally, our state of mind and emotions affect both our digestion, and our dietary habits. Anorexia, obesity, addiction to "junk" foods or alcohol are plain examples of the latter. Anxiety is known to upset digestion, and emotional disturbances are felt "in the guts" – we use such phrases as "I could not 'stomach' it" when life strikes us a blow.

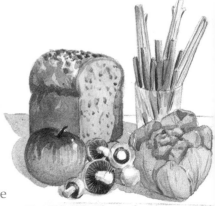

Food for body and spirit
In eastern thinking, food is a fundamental source of prana, or chi (p.24). This energy is present in its strongest form when foods are not "denatured" or polluted. A pure diet of fresh, whole foods brings vital life energy to body, mind and spirit. Yogic and macrobiotic diets (p.37), and naturopathic diets (pp.192-3) are based on this understanding.

Digestion and the liver
Gastric juices break down the food as it passes through the stomach to the small intestine. Here nutrients enter the blood, and go via the portal vein to the liver – the organ that the Chinese call "the general of the army". The liver rules the supply system, storing and assembling glucose and other nutrients to release them as needed, via the hepatic vein. It makes red blood cells, de-toxifies drugs and chemicals, breaks down excess protein, and removes adrenalin. In eastern medicine the liver is seen as harmonizing the body, and calming the emotions.

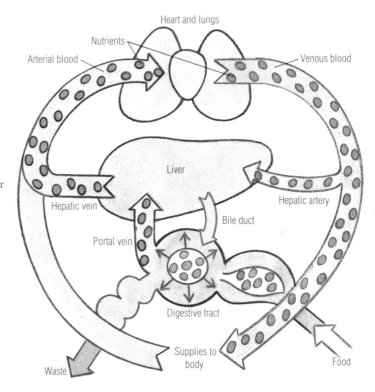

Heart and lungs

Nutrients

Arterial blood

Venous blood

Liver

Hepatic vein

Hepatic artery

Bile duct

Portal vein

Digestive tract

Supplies to body

Food

Waste

Waste disposal and the body environment

The body must have efficient sanitation if life is to be pleasant and healthy. Living tissues too need a harmonious environment, and the body has a set of disposal services which work ceaselessly to maintain it. Blood and lymph collect up the waste and toxic by-products of the cell factories, and clear them away. Blood is filtered by the kidneys (and the waste passed out in the urine), by the lungs for the removal of carbon dioxide, and by the skin – which removes about a quarter of all waste, in sweat. The bowels eliminate the remains of the food supply system; and the liver handles poisons, such as drugs and alcohol.

For most of our lives, the human village keeps itself spick and span without any fuss, handling whatever we care to throw at it. But as we get older, the effects of an unhealthy lifestyle begin to show. If one disposal station is overloaded, other organs have to take the strain, and the whole system is disturbed. Accumulated toxins clog up the tissues, and disease begins – as direct toxic effects like headaches, constipation, arthritis, and arteriosclerosis, or as infection attacking toxified tissues. Fortunately, we can prevent these serious consequences by taking better care, from the start.

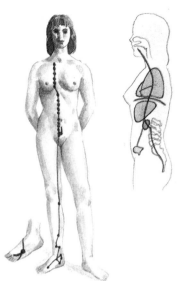

The kidney meridian

Organs and meridians
In oriental medicine, each vital organ has its own meridian (p.271). By working on the kidney meridian, above, the practitioner can treat disorders of the chest or digestive system, as well as of the kidneys.

The vital kidneys
The kidneys are among the hardest workers in the body, and vital to life. Without them, we would soon be poisoned by our own wastes. These little organs service all the circulating blood about every 5 minutes, clearing toxins and wastes through more than a million tiny filters or nephrons, and maintaining water, glucose, amino acid, and mineral content. In Chinese thought, the kidneys store "jing", the substance of organic life, and rule birth and maturation. They are "the root of life".

Caring for your system

• Eat fresh, raw, whole foods as often as you can, and take plenty of fiber.

• Reduce fat, sugar, and excess animal protein – they provoke digestive disorders.

• Avoid foods with hidden toxins – additives, factory-farmed, or sprayed products.

• Reduce alcohol, and avoid medicines and drugs if you can, to preserve the liver.

• Take exercise; it aids digestion and circulation and clears the tissues. Use stretching exercises (pp.54-5) to tone the organs.

• Relax – stress and anxiety interrupt digestion and can damage the system.

• Use natural therapies, whenever possible, and avoid powerful medicines, unless they are life-saving.

• Keep your skin healthy (pp.65-6) – it should be able to sweat freely.

• Drink plenty of fluids to keep kidneys healthy – 4 pints a day are recommended, preferably as water or watery drinks.

• Try an occasional fast to rest the system (pp.192-3).

Action and awareness

Throughout life, we depend for strength, mobility, and action on the body's dynamic frame – the interacting skeleton, muscles, ligaments, and skin, that both support and shelter the human body, and guard the vital organs, brain and major nerves. The health of this system inevitably affects our whole being, and vice versa. Bone and muscle are living tissue, with a remarkable capacity for self-repair and growth. We need to care for them, even from before birth. The right foods in pregnancy and infancy, the right habits from childhood of posture, breathing, exercise, and weight, all determine our future.

In childhood, the body is elastic and flexible – we rejoice in its freedom of movement, and our posture is natural and easy. In adulthood, the body frame begins to reflect the frictions of the mind: joints stiffen and wear, and our posture mirrors – and affects – our response to life. When we speak of feeling "tense" or "uptight" we literally describe the state of spine and muscles. Conversely, a fit and relaxed frame benefits both mind and body.

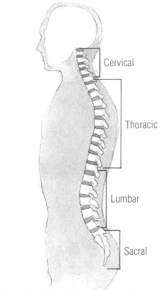

The natural curves of the spine

Healthy disc   Herniated disc

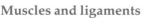

Muscles and ligaments
Muscles need oxygen and other fuel, a toxin-free environment, and regular use to keep healthy. Most voluntary muscles are paired, with opposing actions – one contracts while another relaxes, for example – thus keeping the body in dynamic balance. A muscle weak from under-use, or permanently tense, will affect the greater part of the system. So too will problems with the tendons, the ligaments which link bones, and the elastic fascia (p.266). We need gentle, stretching exercise (and perhaps, also, tension-releasing massage), to keep our bodies supple, relaxed, and strong.

The spine and body energy
The spine encapsulates the precious spinal cord, and houses the roots of the major motor and sensory nerves. It also anchors the voluntary musculature of the body. Its health is critical to the free flow of energy in the body. In yoga, the spinal cord corresponds to the main energy channel of the subtle body; the asanas keep its pathway clear and make the spine flexible. Some of the natural therapies, especially osteopathy and chiropractic, focus on the influence of the spine on body harmony and energy (pp.228-41).

Posture and health
The upright human posture requires a remarkable balancing feat from the spine, to support our weight yet allow full movement. If its natural curves – in the cervical, thoracic and sacral areas – become exaggerated, there are serious repercussions. Rounded shoulders, or a hollow back, increase the stress on particular vertebrae. A "slipped" or "herniated" disc occurs if the vertebrae become so compressed that the cushioning cartilage between them is displaced. Poor posture also puts stress on major weight-bearing joints, such as the knees, ankles, and pelvis.

Balance and perception

The grace of a dancer, the speed of an athlete – we delight in these feats of muscular co-ordination, but they are only made possible through the flow of information between body and brain. We are equipped with remarkable intelligence services.

As we move, spindle-shaped sensors in the muscles inform the brain of what each part is doing, and where it is – the brain has its own "map" of the body, drawn from this flood of sensations. With every action, we "resculpt" and redefine our own body shape, and re-orient it in space. Staying upright and balanced depends on the fixed reference provided by our eyes, and by the organs of the inner ear, which tell us what is up or down, near or far, and which way up the body is.

We use our "inner map" of the body to define who and where we are, our self-image, our intentions. If we are upset, we often feel "unbalanced", or that everything is "upside down". Our sense of stability, of ground under our feet, is mental and emotional as well as physical.

Inner and outer worlds

The sensations which inform us of our selves, our shape, our actions, are referred to as "proprioception" – as opposed to sensory awareness of the world outside, which is called "exteroception". Most sense organs perform both roles. The skin is a sensory sheath which signals external contact, and its own state; the ears and eyes tell of the outside, but also of our own orientation. In eastern medicine, this two-way role of the sense organs is more strongly stated – the eyes, for instance, mirror and map the health of the body, and are "windows of the soul".

Keeping a healthy frame

• Take regular aerobic exercise, graduated to your fitness (p.49 and 53).

• Keep flexible with stretching movements (pp.54-5).

• Learn body awareness, and improve your posture with body-mind therapies, such as the Alexander technique.

• Learn relaxation to free body and mind of conflict.

• Avoid positions that impose strain (p.243) and seek prompt attention for back or joint problems.

• From early youth, make sure your diet helps build a healthy frame (pp.38-41) and avoid excess red meat, acid foods, or toxins which may later affect joints.

Learning body awareness

The tension and unease which habit and mental stress inflict on our frame often go unnoticed, until damage and pain result. Try, for a moment, quietly attending to your body – feel how each limb is placed, where your weight falls, where you are unbalanced or stiff. One of the first steps in many body-mind therapies, such as Rolfing or the Alexander technique, is to reach this awareness. Only then can we learn how to relax and re-orient our frame, to recover ease and free movement.

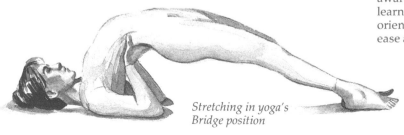

Stretching in yoga's Bridge position

Control and the body-mind

The human brain is the most complex and mysterious physical structure we know, its billions of nerve cells, or neurones, organized into uncounted corridors of power. It processes huge amounts of information, to keep life functioning in order and harmony, to tell us how we feel, and how to behave. The brain regulates many body rhythms, and has its own rhythms, too, associated with different states of body-mind – alpha waves with relaxation, beta with arousal, delta with sleep. Like all the vital organs, the brain needs freedom from toxins and stress – as do its servants, the nervous and endocrine systems.

Like a vast telephone exchange, the voluntary system of sensory and motor nerves handles our conscious affairs. Meantime, the autonomous system of sympathetic and parasympathetic nerves profoundly influences the body, adjusting and ordering our inner world, along with the circulating messenger chemicals, or hormones, released by the endocrine glands. The work of the glands is vital to every organ and function of the body, harmonizing cell chemistry, regulating blood sugar, determining sexual activity, and governing our moods and emotions.

In eastern philosophy, the endocrine glands also correspond to the subtle energy centers, which govern energy flow. Indeed, many natural therapies approach physical problems through the psyche and by harmonizing energy balance. The two major control systems – nervous and endocrine – are responsible for a process fundamental to life – homeostasis, the maintenance of normal levels of function, with variation allowed between safety limits. We know this best from our "fight or flight" response to stress or excitement (p.61). The sympathetic system arouses the body, adrenalin floods through it: heart rate, breathing, and muscle tone increase. The crisis passed, the parasympathetic system redresses the balance and adrenalin flow ceases: the body slows, and all functions normalize.

Balance through feedback
The endocrine and nervous systems each use dual feedback controls to rouse or calm the body. The pituitary gland triggers hormone production in other glands, and these circulating hormones signal a reduction in pituitary activity. Sympathetic nervous arousal is balanced by parasympathetic signals to relax and restore balance.

Endocrine system

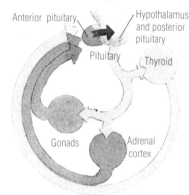

Anterior pituitary
Hypothalamus and posterior pituitary
Pituitary
Thyroid
Gonads
Adrenal cortex

Autonomic nervous system

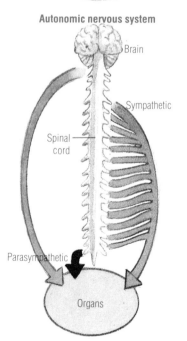

Brain
Sympathetic
Spinal cord
Parasympathetic
Organs

Chakras, glands and nerves

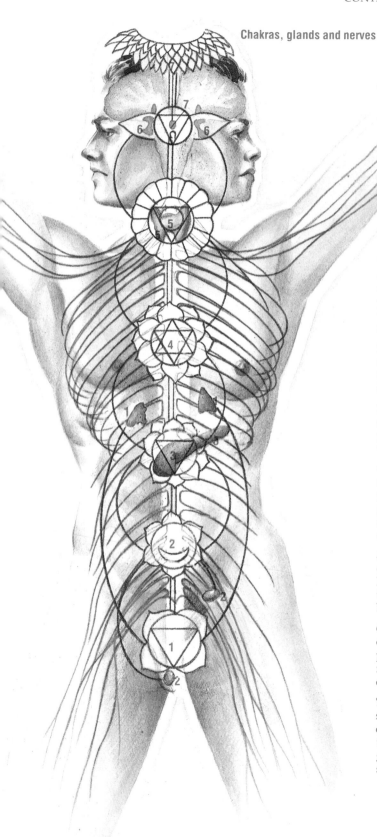

Chakras, glands, and nerves

The physical control centers of brain, nerve plexuses (relay stations along the spinal cord) and major glands show a remarkable correspondence with the chakras, the seven centers or staging posts of subtle energy as it flows up the body from base to crown. Each successive chakra represents a higher state of being.

1 *Muladhara*, the base chakra, seat of the will to live, corresponds to the **sacral plexus** and to the **adrenals**, which rouse the body to action.

2 *Swadhishthana* corresponds to the **prostatic plexus**, and the **gonads** which rule our sexual nature and activity.

3 *Manipura* stores prana, and corresponds to the **solar plexus**, and to the **pancreas** which regulates blood sugar.

4 *Anahata*, the heart chakra, corresponds to the **cardiac plexus** and the **thymus**, a gland (atrophied in infancy), a vital part of the immune system.

5 *Vishuddha*, the throat chakra, corresponds to the **laryngeal plexus** and to the **thyroid**, which governs the body's metabolic rate.

6 *Ajna*, the brow chakra, corresponds to the **cavernous plexus** and the **pituitary** – the master gland which rules the endocrine system.

7 *Sahasrara*, the crown chakra, seat of the highest consciousness, corresponds to the **pineal**, a mysterious gland thought to govern sleeping and waking.

Health and healing

Health of body and mind is an irreplaceable gift, and the living body is designed to defend and restore it throughout our lives, if we let it. The natural defenses of the body are formidable. Like a strongly fortified wall, the skin protects us from invaders, shock or damage, and shelters our inner world. Entrances are guarded with filters and traps, while vital supply lines are protected by the powerful reflexes of coughing and vomiting, which forcibly eject the culprit. Invaders that pass these physical defenses meet a range of chemical barriers – mucous linings to mouth, nose, and throat, and acid juices in the stomach. If, nonetheless, our outer defenses are breached, the body rushes into action – to repair the damage or detoxify the system, or to mobilize the army of the immune system against infection.

Repair and emergency
If tissues are damaged and blood starts to flow , the platelet cells carried in blood plasma start the clotting process, to seal the wound, and white cells start the fight against infection. Should the body be under major threat, say from loss of blood, it declares a state of emergency – withdrawing supplies from less essential areas (this is why the skin is cold and pale in shock) to rush them to the vital organs, and to the site of repair.

The immune system

The body's capacity to resist infection depends on a simple strategy – the ability of certain white cells to tell friend from foe. First the phagocytes – killer white cells that roam the body – recognize and destroy alien organisms in the blood. If this fails, B lymphocytes start to make antibodies tailored to the specific antigen; later, T lymphocytes destroy it with antibody-bearing cells. Lymphocytes reach all the tissues via the body's network of lymph channels, that work in conjunction with the blood vessels; the lymph glands which produce them are found particularly in the respiratory tract, armpits and groin. The battle of alien versus lymphocyte produces strong reactions, such as fever, swollen glands, and rashes.

Once a particular invader has roused the immune system, the body memorizes its defense strategy, and we are "immune" – at least to that particular organism. We are born with immunity to many infections, acquire immunities from skirmishes with invaders, and vaccination confers artificial immunity.

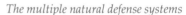

The multiple natural defense systems

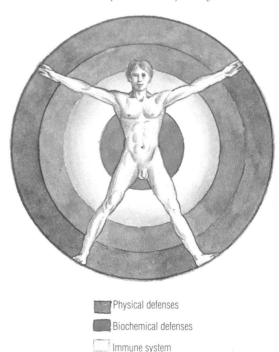

■ Physical defenses

■ Biochemical defenses

□ Immune system

■ Emergency controls

Self-healing

The natural state of the body is health, its natural tendency to restore this condition after any disturbance. It is as if every part of the human village has an"ideal" of wholeness and performance to work to, and instantly gives the alert when this model is challenged. The greater the threat, the more extreme the response; as the threat is reduced, the response too diminishes.

Through this homeostasis, we live in a dynamic balance with our inner and outer worlds – the body ever ready to rise to an emergency, yet seeking always to restore its wholeness, harmony and equilibrium, and return the vital functions such as heartbeat, blood pressure, temperature, and the chemical composition of the body's "inland sea" to within the "ideal" norms of health.

Beyond childhood, however, we rarely experience the exuberant well-being of full health. It is our habit to accept this as "wear and tear", yet in the view of natural therapies it is more the result of disharmony in the whole system. When we lead stressful lives, eat unhealthy diets, and ignore the needs of mind and spirit, we are like a person who chooses to live at a very high altitude – our system is constantly paying for keeping things normal, against the odds. And ultimately, if disease threatens, it has no spare capacity to produce the healing response we need.

When we do fall ill, we are accustomed to look for help from outside. Yet, already, the best doctor we could go to – our own body – is giving us full-time care. Surgeons would be helpless it blood did not clot, bones mend, tissue regenerate and our system adapt to loss of parts by reorganizing its work. Only the body can heal. Self-repair, and renewal of function and vitality, are powers of life and last as long as life itself. In this sense, we are our own natural physicians.

All too often, orthodox treatments either suppress natural healing, or create further stress on the body systems. The natural therapies, by contrast, are all concerned with stimulating the body to heal itself (see Homeopathy, p.145, for example) – by correcting imbalances, easing the disturbed inner climate, and most of all by unblocking channels to release the vital force, the recuperative power of our whole being.

Caring for yourself
The more you learn about the workings of the human village, the more you will be able to feel at peace within it, and offer help to its self-healing mechanisms. Listen to the language of the body – headaches or indigestion for example may warn of stress. Many common symptoms of illness are in fact signs of the body restoring health. Swollen glands are fighting alien organisms; while inflammation around a cut opens access to blood with oxygen, white cells and repair materials. A high temperature impedes a multiplying virus; sweating cools the body and eliminates toxins, and so on. Rather than suppressing such symptoms, you can help the body with rest, diet, and natural therapies that rebalance the system. Living in harmony with your body and mind enables you to take greater pleasure from life, and give more to it.

CHAPTER TWO

Looking after your health

The concept of preventive health is one that the great majority of people tend to ignore. Most of us are simply not tuned in to the idea of protecting ourselves from the possibility of illness. We tend to think of health as the absence of disease and when we become unwell we blame our illness on external factors, such as germs, extremes of weather, or crowded trains. We dissociate our health from the general pattern of our lifestyles and, once recovered from an illness, we carry on regardless , continuing to live as we have always done. Yet, with a little thought and forward planning, most of us could protect ourselves from a great number of "unnecessary" ailments. And, what is more, we could positively enhance our health and vitality.

This chapter concentrates on the fundamental elements of a healthy lifestyle, in particular on those areas of living that are within our direct control. The most obvious way of enhancing our well-being is by paying attention to our diet, but sufficent exercise and proper breathing and relaxation techniques are equally important. A responsible attitude to personal and sexual hygiene, and to the management of our home environment, is also essential – not only for our own health, but for the well-being of our families and friends too.

But physical elements such as diet and exercise are only a part of the story. Increasingly, attention is being paid to the role of mental and emotional health in the well-being of the whole person and to the contribution of spiritual practices. Taking care of your mind and your personal relationships is every bit as important as servicing your body.

Changing your lifestyle

The advice contained in this chapter does not demand major lifestyle changes – what it involves is an awareness of health in all areas of your life. The programs suggested here, such as the basic health diet and the aerobic fitness programs, allow for gradual change. Radical, sudden changes would undoubtedly be stressful – and probably wouldn't last.

Even small steps toward a healthier lifestyle can prove immensely rewarding. When you start a new exercise program, for instance, you may well find that your appetite is more easily regulated, and that you have less desire to smoke or drink (if these are problems for you). Regularly practicing a relaxation technique, too, though it may take only a few minutes each day, will reduce the need for stimulants, encourage better sleep and, by releasing the energy locked up in stress, increase your vitality.

The importance of preventive health

A good diet, a balance of activity and rest, and time to devote to your mental and emotional well-being – all these elements amount to a preventive health care strategy. Certainly, if the guidelines described in this chapter were to be followed by the majority of people, the global death rates from serious diseases would fall dramatically. To take a well-known example, if no one smoked, death from all cancers would fall by a third. Similarly, deaths from heart disease could be greatly reduced by dietary changes, non-smoking, and by alleviating stress through relaxation.

But it is not just at the most serious diseases that preventive health care is aimed. Taking responsibility for your own welfare includes the simplest of daily activities, such as brushing your teeth to prevent tooth decay or washing your hands before preparing food. On a calendar basis, it means regular health check-ups – having your blood pressure tested at intervals, for example. And finally, it means taking problems to a health professional promptly, when it is necessary. (See also pp.112-19.)

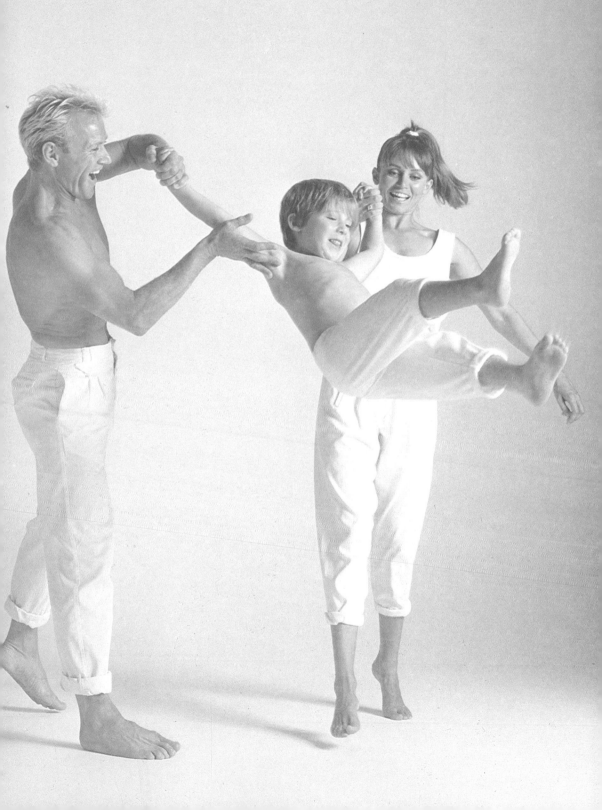

Diet

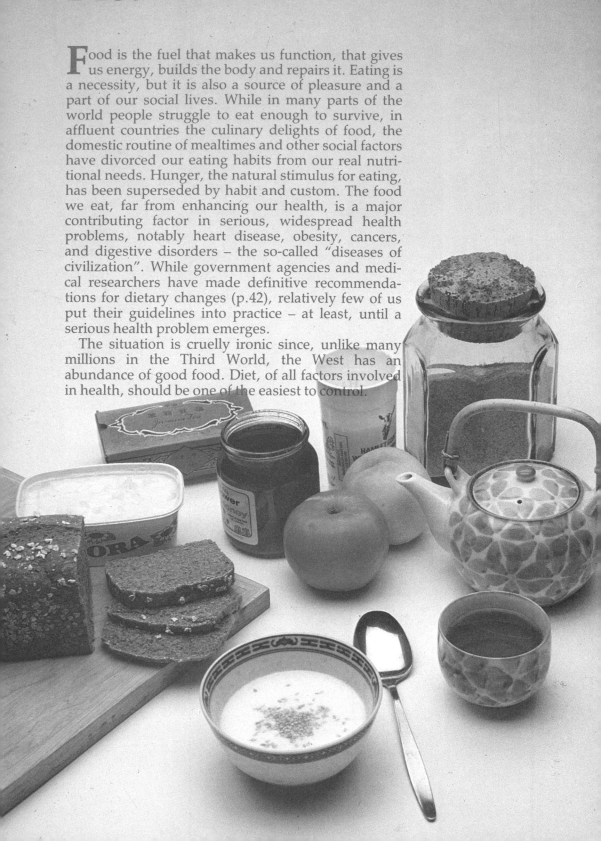

Food is the fuel that makes us function, that gives us energy, builds the body and repairs it. Eating is a necessity, but it is also a source of pleasure and a part of our social lives. While in many parts of the world people struggle to eat enough to survive, in affluent countries the culinary delights of food, the domestic routine of mealtimes and other social factors have divorced our eating habits from our real nutritional needs. Hunger, the natural stimulus for eating, has been superseded by habit and custom. The food we eat, far from enhancing our health, is a major contributing factor in serious, widespread health problems, notably heart disease, obesity, cancers, and digestive disorders – the so-called "diseases of civilization". While government agencies and medical researchers have made definitive recommendations for dietary changes (p.42), relatively few of us put their guidelines into practice – at least, until a serious health problem emerges.

The situation is cruelly ironic since, unlike many millions in the Third World, the West has an abundance of good food. Diet, of all factors involved in health, should be one of the easiest to control.

The malnutrition of overconsumption

The damaging pattern of the western diet is embedded in social and industrial development – since the turn of the century, greater wealth has led to increased consumption of processed, high-sugar and high-fat foods, foods that were once regarded as luxuries. There has been a correspondingly sharp decline in the consumption of plain nutritious staples. The general quality has altered too, with modernization in the food industry involving chemical additives and refining techniques which have "denatured" much of the stock in the supermarket.

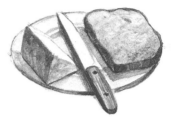

Wholemeal bread and cheese, and other combinations of vegetarian foods (p.43) provide complete protein for a well-balanced vegetarian diet.

Fortunately, the nutritional component in enhancing health and preventing, even curing illness is now widely recognized. It is well known that a poor diet can exacerbate stress, cause nervous disorders, and affect mental as well as physical development. There is also increasing concern about food allergies, and about the possibility of the potentially toxic cocktail of food additives reacting in the body. Obesity, too, is a matter of widespread anxiety. It is one of the most serious risk factors in many types of illness and although there is a genetic element, it is largely a result of poor dietary habits. In the natural therapies (notably naturopathy, pp.188-207, and herbalism, pp.160-75), dietary changes play an extremely important part in treating illness.

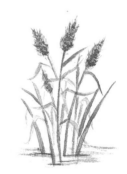

The macrobiotic diet involves a complex Yin/Yang balance of types of food. Cereals play a large part in the diet.

Choosing whole food for whole health

Changing to a good diet should not be a matter of making stressful adjustments, such as avoiding all sweet and fatty foods, and living on a monotonous fare of brown rice and vegetables. Fad diets are also not the answer either to ill health or to obesity. They can deprive the body of essential nutrients, and lower the body's metabolic rate. What counts most is establishing a good ratio of nutrients, choosing good quality foods, and being aware of special individual requirements (p.46). Within a sensible framework, such as the basic health diet shown on page 47, or some of the alternative diets shown right, there is scope for infinite variation, and occasional treats can be enjoyed without harm. You should also combine a balanced diet with a regular exercise program. But the simplest rule is to choose foods that are as close to their natural state as possible – they are most likely to yield the full range of nutrients that the body needs.

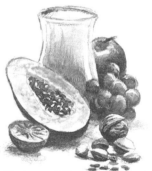

To the yogi "Sattvic" food, which includes whole foods, fresh fruit and vegetables, and dairy products, is ideal. It nourishes the body and calms the mind.

Raw materials for life

Food is the raw material from which the body derives its energy, builds, restores and maintains itself in good order. Our choice determines what the body receives. The basic nutrients provided by food are: carbohydrates; protein; fats; vitamins and minerals.

The charts below and on pp.40-1 give good food sources for each nutrient and a brief account of its special functions. Note that water soluble vitamins should be replaced on a daily basis.

Raw materials	Types	Sources	Functions
Sugars	Sucrose	Mainly from sugar cane and sugar beet, in form of white sugar, brown, castor, icing sugar, etc; added to most processed foods, both sweet and savory	Sugar gives short term energy. Molasses, the waste from the refining process, has a few nutrients, but refined sugar has none. It creates a nutrient debt by using up the body's store of vitamins and minerals in its digestion and absorption (see also p.44).
	Glucose (dextrose)	Grapes, honey; made in body from other sugars and starches	Also referred to as blood sugar. Quickly absorbed by the body and used for energy. In excess it has the same effects as sucrose.
	Fructose (levulose)	Fruit, honey	Fructose gives slow-release energy. In fresh fruit it contains extra nutrients.
	Lactose	All milk products	Nutritious sugar which requires the enzyme lactase for digestion. "Lactose intolerance" is very common: symptoms include nausea, sinus trouble, indigestion and diarrhea.
Carbohydrates	Starch	Fruits, vegetables, seeds, nuts, grains, pulses, beans, tubers	This is the storage form of carbohydrate in plants. Eaten in whole form, it is absorbed slowly into the body. It contains nutrients to aid digestion. Some complex carbohydrates, such as oats and beans, are known to reduce the risk of cardiovascular disease, perhaps due to their cholesterol-absorbing activity.
	Fiber	In all whole plant foods, whole grains, vegetables, and fruit, in the form of bran, cellulose, pectin, etc	The undigestible part of the plant, essential for healthy bowel function. Fibre helps protect against gallstones, reduces cholesterol levels and ensures all-round better health.

Raw materials	Types	Sources	Functions
Proteins	Animal protein	Meat, fish, eggs, all dairy products	Animal protein contains all the essential amino acids the body needs to construct body tissues, hormones, enzymes, blood, etc, and to repair and regenerate cells. Lack of protein causes fatigue, lack-luster skin and hair and a weak immune system, with a lack of resistance to disease and infection. Excess animal protein is associated with many other disorders (p.45).
	Vegetable protein	All grains, beans, legumes, nuts, seeds, sprouted seeds	Vegetable protein is used in precisely the same way as animal, but few plant sources contain all the essential amino acids. Different vegetarian foods should be combined to get the full complement (p.43).
Fats	Saturated fats	Dairy products, meat, processed fats (many margarines, cooking fats, some oils, cakes, biscuits, pies, sausages etc), coconut oil and palm oil	These give concentrated energy, but they are linked to serious diseases and a host of minor ailments (p.45).
	Mono-unsaturated fats	In peanut, olive, and fish oils	Neutral in terms of health. Nations that eat large quantities of olive oil have good records on heart disease and other fat associated problems.
	Poly-unsaturated fats	Corn, sesame, soya, sunflower, olive, and nut oils. Margarines labelled "polyunsaturated". Fish, seeds, nuts, vegetables	Good sources of energy. Fresh polyunsaturated oils are essential for health (see Essential fats, below). Polyunsaturates may help to reduce cholesterol in the blood
	Essential fats (vitamin F) (linoleic acid, linolenic acid)	Polyunsaturated oils, fatty fish and offal, game, grains and all whole foods	These are not just good for us, they are essential to health and life itself; part of every cell structure. They nourish the skin and normalize blood consistency. The body uses linoleic and linolenic acid to make arachidonic and other acids.
	Cholesterol	Manufactured in the body. Found in animal fats, including eggs	Needed for body tissues, to form sex and adrenal hormones, vitamin D and bile (for digestion of fats). Too much cholesterol damages health (p.45).

Raw materials	Types	Sources	Functions
Vitamins	Vitamin A (fat soluble)	Liver, kidneys, fish oils, carrots, beet, broccoli, milk products	Protects from infections; helps growth and repair of tissues; good for healthy eyes.
	Vitamin B1 (thiamin) (water soluble)	Vegetables, brewers' yeast, oatmeal, whole grains, milk, meats, nuts	Promotes growth, improves mental and nerve function. Essential in metabolism of carbohydrates.
	Vitamin B2 (riboflavin) (water soluble)	Fish, eggs, milk, yeast	Aids growth and reproduction; healthy eyes, skin, nails, and hair.
	Vitamin B3 (niacin) (water soluble)	Body makes its own. Poultry, nuts, grains, fish, eggs, liver, yeast	Regulates blood sugar and cholesterol. (Used in treating a variety of mental conditions.)
	Vitamin B5 (pantothenic acid) (water soluble)	Grains, yeast, eggs, green vegetables, liver, legumes, dairy products	Aids adrenal gland function (essential for body under stress). Needed for energy production. Aids immune system.
	Vitamin B6 (pyridoxine) (water soluble)	Fruit, wheatgerm, eggs, liver, kidneys, milk, yeast, green vegetables	Essential for protein manufacture and production of red blood cells and antibodies. Aids manufacture of hormones and enzymes.
	Vitamin B12 (water soluble)	Body can make its own. Eggs, meat, fish, milk	Essential for cell life, healthy nervous system; important for iron metabolism.
	Folic acid (Vitamin H) (water soluble)	Green leafy vegetables, avocados, apricots, whole grains, egg yolks	Important in construction of proteins and DNA and for healthy cell life. Prevents anemia.
	Vitamin C (ascorbic acid) (water soluble)	Green leafy vegetables, potatoes, tomatoes, fruits, berries	Vital for many body functions, including wound and disease healing. More needed when ill or under stress or smoking.
	Vitamin D (fat soluble)	Made by body from sunlight. Fish, dairy foods	Enables proper use of calcium and phosphorus to build healthy bones.
	Vitamin E (fat soluble)	Vegetable oils, nuts, dark green vegetables, whole grains, eggs	Protects circulatory system, cells, and retards ageing process.
	Vitamin K (fat soluble)	Green leafy vegetables, egg yolks, yoghurt	Vital for blood clotting.

Raw materials	Types	Sources	Functions
Minerals and trace elements	Calcium	Spinach, milk, cheese, yoghurt, sesame seeds, fish, cereals	Important for function of muscles, nerves, and heart, strong bones and teeth, normal clotting of blood, and enzyme activities. Aids sleep.
	Iron	Dark green vegetables, legumes, poultry, cereals, meat, wheatgerm	Promotes growth and helps protein metabolism. Used in hemoglobin production, vital for oxygen transport in blood.
	Sodium	Most vegetables; table salt	Helps to maintain normal fluid levels of cells, and normal nerve and muscle function.
	Magnesium	Most vegetables and whole grains	Important for protein metabolism, cell, muscle and nerve function.
	Potassium	Fruit and vegetables, milk, legumes, seafood	Essential for functioning of heart muscles, kidneys, nerves, and blood circulation.
	Zinc	Legumes, whole grains, seeds, oysters, meat	A part of many vital enzymes. Required for normal wound healing, the growth process, insulin activity, and healthy liver function.
	Iodine	Vegetables, fruit (if soil has iodine); seafood	Essential part of the thyroid hormones which control metabolism, energy and growth.
	Chromium	Liver, shellfish, yeast, cheese	Increases the effectiveness of insulin and acts with enzymes in metabolism of energy.
	Chlorine	Seaweed, salt, olives	Maintains fluid balance. Aids digestion.
	Copper	Dried beans, peas, whole wheat, liver, seafood	Co-factor for red blood cells and many enzymes. Essential for the use of vitamin C, and iron absorption.
	Manganese	Green leafy vegetables, whole grains, egg yolks, nuts	Enzyme activator. Essential in carbohydrate and fat metabolism, normal body development and sex hormones.
	Selenium	Vegetables, onions, garlic, wheatgerm, organ meats, shellfish, yeast, grains	Essential role in sex hormones. Essential for tissue elasticity and liver function. Protective against cancer and heart disease.
	Sulphur	Legumes, cabbage, garlic, eggs, fish, lean beef	Essential for hair, nails and skin. Important for brain function. Helps liver secrete bile.
	Phosphorus	Whole grains, seeds, nuts, eggs, fish, meat, all high-protein foods	Essential for bone structure and heart and kidney function. Nerve impulses depend upon it, and some vitamins can't function without it.

Good eating guidelines

The ideal eating pattern can be either a balanced vegetarian or non-vegetarian diet. It should include three meals a day, as suggested in the basic health diet, page 47. The general guidelines given below include those of the US Senate Select Committee on Nutrition and Human Needs, 1977, and the British National Advisory Committee on Nutrition Education (NACNE), 1983.

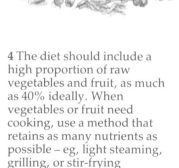

1 Refined carbohydrate foods should be minimized and replaced with complex carbohydrates, such as wholemeal bread, unpolished rice, and potatoes. Starches should make up at least 50% of dietary intake (Senate Committee).

2 Fats should be reduced to no more than 30% of the food eaten, less if possible (Senate Committee and NACNE). The Senate suggests an equal amount of polyunsaturated and saturated fats. Low-fat meats, such as chicken and game, and offal, such as kidneys and liver should be preferred to high-fat meat. Try to choose oils that are fresh and "cold-pressed".

3 Protein should provide about 12% of the daily intake of calories (Senate Committee), and this should come as much as possible from fish, and vegetable sources, such as legumes, whole grains, seeds and nuts.

4 The diet should include a high proportion of raw vegetables and fruit, as much as 40% ideally. When vegetables or fruit need cooking, use a method that retains as many nutrients as possible – eg, light steaming, grilling, or stir-frying (quickly, with a little oil).

5 Refined sugar and sugary processed foods should be kept to a minimum.

6 Salt intake should be greatly reduced. (NACNE recommends a maximum of about 5 grams per day).

7 Processed and chemicalized foods should be minimized.

8 Caffeine-containing foods should be avoided – at least on a regular basis.

9 Alcohol limits should be observed carefully (p.105).

10 Plain, clean water should be drunk in quantity. This is the best health drink to take with a good diet. But tap water tends to contain an unhealthy level of pollutants, particularly in urban districts, where it is likely to have been reprocessed several times (see also p.73), so it is a good idea to fit a filter to your drinking tap, buy a filter jug, or drink bottled water when possible.

Good foods

The selection of foods shown here include the basic ingredients which vegetarians need to combine for complete vegetable protein (whole grains, legumes, and dairy products). Further sources of good nutrients, and supplements, are described on pages 338-41. The good eating guidelines (p.42) and the basic health diet (p.47) suggest a balanced framework.

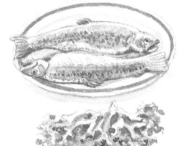

Whole grains Grains contain starch, fiber, vitamins and minerals, and give excellent vegetable protein (when combined with dairy products or with legumes).

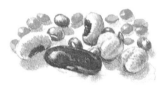

Legumes These give good nutrient value. Most need to be eaten with grains to provide complete protein. Soya beans are exceptional in having all the amino acids which make protein.

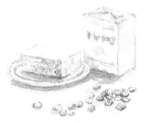

Soya bean products Soya is the one plant source that has complete protein. It is also low in fat. Its products include: tofu, a bean curd with many culinary uses; fermented soya sauces, and soya milk, an excellent substitute for cows' milk.

Fish Fish figures high in the nutrient ranks – it provides essential fats, vitamins and minerals, and it doesn't contain saturated fats. Fish oils are exceptionally healthy (see Glossary pp.338-41).

Sea vegetables Most seaweeds, such as kombu and carrageen, are rich in minerals, such as iodine, and they are one of the few non-meat sources of vitamin B12.

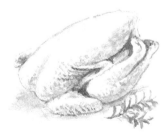

Low-fat meat Poultry, game and "offal" tend to be lean and relatively high in nutrients.

Low-fat dairy products Skimmed milk is widely available, and yoghurt is high in protein and aids digestion. Other good low-fat products include quark (a soft cheese), and smetana (a low-fat soured cream).

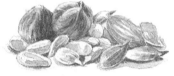

Nuts and seeds These should be eaten sparingly, since they are rich in fattening oils, but they are very nutritious – containing fiber, protein, vitamins and minerals. Some seeds, such as alfalfa, can be sprouted to provide fresh salad ingredients.

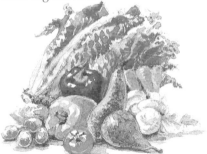

Raw fruit and vegetables Many fruit and vegetables are much better for health when eaten raw. Raw food retains nutrients that are often destroyed in cooking.

Damaging diets

In different parts of the world, people's bodies have adapted, over hundreds of years, to a variety of diets. But the alterations in the western diet have been so rapid that the body has been unable to adapt fast enough. For example, in 1815, average consumption of sugar per head in the UK was 15 lb (7 kg) a year. It is now in excess of 100 lb (45 kg). US trends are improving, but meat, fat, and alcohol consumption have generally vastly increased.

Sugar Refined sugar supplies only "empty" calories, ie, no nutrients, only energy. It is the major cause of tooth decay and it is a principal factor in diabetes, obesity, and certain other disorders. It makes us hungry by creating a "roller coaster" effect in our blood sugar levels: blood sugar soars, the pancreas reacts by secreting more insulin, then levels rapidly plummet, making us tired, hungry and depressed. (This is the low blood sugar syndrome hypoglycemia.)

Animal protein Although animal flesh, eggs, dairy produce, etc, provide the complete protein that is necessary to health, in excess it can be harmful. People who live on a high animal protein diet are thought to be more disposed to bowel cancer, hypertension, diverticulosis and atherosclerosis. Vegetarian foods provide complete protein when they are properly combined (p.43).

Refined foods The inevitable result of a diet high in refined starches is a decrease in the the consumption of fiber. Without fiber, food can take up to 70-80 hours to pass through the digestive tract. Lack of fiber in the diet is responsible for sluggish bowels, constipation, and more serious disorders such as diverticulosis and possible cancer of the colon. A whole food diet, with plenty of fresh fruit and vegetables, provides sufficient fiber.

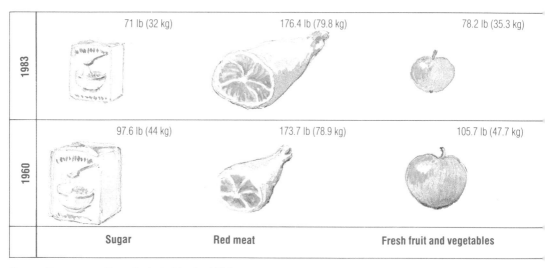

	Sugar	Red meat	Fresh fruit and vegetables
1983	71 lb (32 kg)	176.4 lb (79.8 kg)	78.2 lb (35.3 kg)
1960	97.6 lb (44 kg)	173.7 lb (78.9 kg)	105.7 lb (47.7 kg)

Per capita consumption of selected foods, USA

Salt Salt is a taste easily cultivated. Most of us eat too much – a little is necessary to health, and this occurs naturally in many foods. Excess salt is implicated in high blood pressure and related diseases, in arthritis, and other disorders. In the form of cured or pickled foods, salt has also been implicated in some cancers.

Saturated fats Excess saturated fat is implicated in cancers, obesity, cardiac disease, and a host of other disorders. Too much saturated fat makes too much cholesterol, which may build up on the arterial walls, from childhood onward, resulting in atherosclerosis (hardened arteries from fatty deposits).

Dairy products and fatty meats are major culprits; wild game has more polyunsaturated fat, and contains a substance that is thought to protect against atherosclerosis.

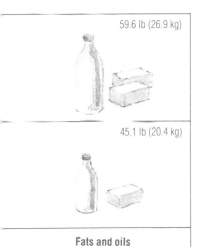

59.6 lb (26.9 kg)

45.1 lb (20.4 kg)

Fats and oils

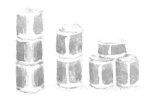

1980 $750 million

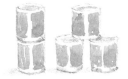

1970 $500 million

Sales of food additives to food processers, USA

Additives To "enhance" the flavor and appearance of processed and packaged foods, and to ensure a long shelf life in the supermarket, food manufacturers add a wide range of chemicals to their products. Over 3,000 are currently used. A large number have been removed from the "permitted" list, but the long-term effects of those that remain have not yet been fully evaluated. Additives have been blamed for hyperactivity in children, for decalcification of the bone, and for some cancers. Meat, fruit and vegetables may have unwanted ingredients too – residues of artificial fertilizers and pesticides, and hormones and antibiotics given to animals.

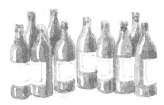

1979   10.3 litres

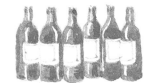

1950   6.3 litres

Average annual consumption of pure alcohol in population aged 15 and over, UK

Alcohol Like sugar, alcohol gives a false stimulus to the system and is rapidly followed by sedation and depression of certain body functions. It depletes the levels of vitamins, most notably the B group, and C, and minerals, such as zinc, magnesium, and potassium. Eventually, alcohol takes a heavy toll on health, causing cirrhosis of the liver, gastric troubles, heart disease, muscle disorders, nervous system problems, sexual impotence, etc.

Caffeine Coffee and caffeine-rich foods, like chocolate, tea, and cola drinks, produce a release of the body's stored sugar to combat the influx of what is essentially a poison. Like alcohol it provokes hypertension and nervous symptoms. Cholesterol levels go up and B vitamins and some minerals are depleted. Excess caffeine may also be involved in breast and prostate problems.

Special needs

The general rule for good eating is to eat a balanced diet with as little damaging food as possible, but it is also important to be aware that your nutritional needs may change. For example, medication, especially the Pill, will increase the body's need for certain nutrients, notably B6 and folic acid, vitamins C and E, zinc and chromium. And dietary adjustments are often necessary during illness (see Caring for the Sick, p.119, and Naturopathy, pp.192-3).

Life stages	Extra requirements
Fertility	Vitamin B complex, vitamins A, C, and E, zinc and iodine, selenium. These are all important for normal functioning of the hormone-producing glands, as well as sperm production.
Infancy, childhood	Energy foods (complex carbohydrates and fats), and vitamins A, C, D, calcium and zinc. Optimum nutritional support is essential.
Adolescence	Energy foods, protein, vitamin C, calcium, phosphorus, zinc. Surveys show a notable lack of calcium in this age group on "modern" diets.
Menstruation	Vitamin B complex (especially folic acid), vitamins A and C, iron, iodine. These nutrients are particularly helpful if menstrual or premenstrual problems occur.
Pregnancy	Protein, vitamin B complex, vitamins C, E, and K, zinc, calcium, iron. All these are required in greater quantities than normal. Protein is vital. Birth defects may be related directly to nutrient deficits.
Lactation	Energy foods, vitamins B1, B2, B3, C and D, and iron. All nutrient needs increase at this time.
Menopause	The danger of decalcification of bone is high. Vitamins D, E, and calcium. The anti-ageing aspects of E and C are helpful.
Ageing	Vitamin B complex, vitamins A, E, and C, calcium and iron. Adequate protein is important. Nutrients tend to be less well absorbed so supplements may be needed.

The basic health diet

The basic health diet comprises a foundation for all-round health. Sometimes, simply changing to this plan increases energy, cleanses the skin, and reduces chronic complaints, such as constipation and congestion. The diet is used in conjunction with other natural methods of treatment in naturopathy (pp.188-207).

If your current eating habits are very different, introduce changes gradually. Add more raw food at the start of the meal, or follow the main meal suggestions twice a week, then three times, and so on until you are close to the recommended pattern.

This diet has a number of alternative suggestions, and you can vary it further with any number of different fruits, vegetables and whole foods.

1 On rising Pure fruit juice, herb tea, or apple cider vinegar (a dessertspoon in a glass of hot water, with half a teaspoon of honey).

2 Breakfast Muesli with yoghurt and tahini, or whole grain cereal, eg shredded wheat with skimmed milk, or soya milk, or porridge, or fresh fruit with wheat germ and yoghurt. One or two slices toasted wholemeal bread with sunflower margarine and honey or savory spread.

Herb tea; cereal coffee substitute; or pure fruit juice.

3 Mid-morning Fruit juice; herb tea; or cereal coffee substitute. Wholemeal biscuit; or snack made with natural ingredients, eg, nuts, sunflower or sesame seeds.

6 Evening Choose a different suggestion from the lunch menu, eg, follow a mixed salad and yoghurt dessert lunch with a vegetarian savory and tofu dessert supper.

5 Mid-afternoon As for mid-morning.

4 Lunch Vegetarian savory made with egg, cheese, nuts or grains and legumes, with a selection of vegetables in season; or lean meat with vegetables; or fish with vegetables; or mixed vegetable salad with baked jacket potato or baked onion.

For dessert: soaked dried fruit; baked apple; fresh fruit; muesli; yoghurt; natural fruit jelly; or tofu dessert (tofu eaten with dried fruit, fresh fruit, or honey).

Exercise

Our bodies were made for activity. Movement is one of the definitions of life itself, and the human body is especially endowed for it in terms of strength, agility, flexibility, and precision. To remain in good health, strong and supple, with a sound circulatory and respiratory system (pp.20-33), each of us must exercise regularly. This is as crucial in childhood as it is in later years. In simple terms, what we don't use we lose – unstretched muscles grow permanently tense or, with inactivity, degenerate; immobile bones decalcify, and ligaments tighten.

Assessing individual needs

Fitness is not just to do with regular strenuous activity, such as jogging or work-outs. Any exercise program should include relaxation and stretching movements as well, and take individual needs into account. Among the factors involved are your body type, age, level of health and temperament. For example, a tendency to put on weight may suggest that you need prolonged, steady types of exercise, such as golf, swimming, or walking, which don't put an extreme burden on the joints. Older people have

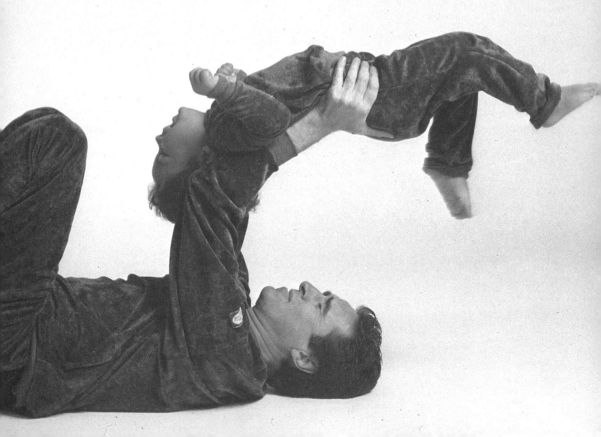

to take special care to avoid sudden, jarring move-ments that might impose excessive strain. And competitive, over-active personalities who may be inclined toward vigorous sports will benefit most from time spent on gentler exercise forms, such as leisurely swimming or yoga.

Your level of personal health can be a particularly decisive factor. Some conditions, such as high blood pressure or serious obesity, may preclude very vigorous exercise. If long-term postural abuse or any other problem has resulted in generally restricted mobility and stiffness, exercises which encourage flexibility are advisable (pp.54-5). Rolfing and the Alexander technique are particularly helpful if poor posture is deeply ingrained (p.267 and p.297). Specific disabilities or handicaps may call for specially adapted exercise programs – physiotherapists, hydrotherapists, and some yoga teachers, can tailor exercises to benefit individual conditions.

The medical benefits of exercise

The importance of regular exercise for good health is now firmly supported by medical evidence. Trials which involved groups of middle-aged men and women following a ten-week fitness program showed lower levels of blood sugar, fats and cholesterol, and also gains in strength, flexibility and stamina. Longer programs resulted in even greater benefits – reducing tension, improving res-piratory capacity, lowering body fat, and increasing general well-being. Another trial found that, out of the 15 variables which are known to affect the risk of heart disease (including uric acid levels, weight, mood, etc), all but the factor of heredity could be positively influenced by 25 minutes of vigorous exercise a day.

A wide range of disorders, from anxiety, depres-sion, and insomnia to obesity, cigarette and alcohol addiction, diabetes, and osteoporosis (thinning of the bones), improve with regular exercise. The metabolic rate increases, the digestive system and circulation improve, heart muscles grow stronger, and the skin takes on a healthy glow. The converse is also true: inactivity makes illness more likely, and those who drop out of exercise programs rapidly demons-trate negative factors, such as muscle weakness, loss of calcium and a general decline in well-being.

Exercise values

Any exercise which calls for constant effort pays dividends in health terms, if practiced regularly. This is the way to protect yourself from coronary disease, improve your circulation, reduce fat, control your appetite, combat stress, and improve your sleep.

Some exercises rank highly in developing stamina – running, and cycling, for example. These are aerobic or endurance activities, which can be maintained at just below maximum effort for a sustained period (not less than 10 minutes) using a steady supply of oxygen. Practiced regularly, aerobic exercise increases oxygen uptake and strengthens the heart.

The comparative table below gives a selection of sports and everyday activities, with an approximate rating of their special benefits. (The Feldenkrais method is a movement awareness technique.) Certain exercise categories, such as strength or stamina, may appeal to you more than others, but a sound body needs to be comprehensively trained. Posture – the way you stand, sit and move your whole body – co-ordination and flexibility are just as important.

	Stamina	Strength	Flexibility	Posture	Co-ordination
Badminton	ΔΔ	ΔΔ	ΔΔ		ΔΔ
Cycling	ΔΔΔ	ΔΔ	Δ		
Dance	ΔΔ	ΔΔ	ΔΔΔ	ΔΔ	ΔΔ
Feldenkrais method			ΔΔΔ	ΔΔΔ	ΔΔΔ
Football	ΔΔ	ΔΔ	ΔΔ		ΔΔ
Gymnastics	ΔΔ	ΔΔ	ΔΔΔ	Δ	Δ
Hockey	ΔΔ	ΔΔ	ΔΔ		ΔΔ
Rowing	ΔΔΔ	ΔΔΔ	Δ		Δ
Running	ΔΔΔ	ΔΔ	Δ		
Skiing (cross country)	ΔΔΔ	ΔΔΔ	ΔΔ		Δ
Skiing (downhill)	ΔΔ	ΔΔ	ΔΔ		ΔΔ
Squash	ΔΔ	ΔΔ	ΔΔ		ΔΔ
Swimming	ΔΔΔ	ΔΔΔ	ΔΔΔ	Δ	Δ
T'ai chi	Δ	Δ	ΔΔΔ	ΔΔΔ	ΔΔ
Tennis	ΔΔ	ΔΔ	ΔΔ	Δ	ΔΔ
Walking	ΔΔΔ	Δ	Δ	Δ	
Weight training	Δ	ΔΔΔ	Δ	Δ	
Yoga	Δ	ΔΔ	ΔΔΔ	ΔΔΔ	ΔΔ

Fair Δ   Good ΔΔ   Excellent ΔΔΔ

Testing for fitness

Anybody who is about to embark on a training program for fitness – whether they choose walking, running or any other exercise – should first gauge their fitness carefully. The pulse test, flexibility and abdominal strength tests described below can be carried out by all age groups. The walking test (p.52) is a tougher fitness check based on distance covered when walking briskly.

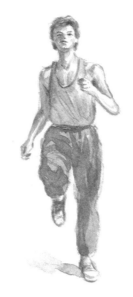

1 Testing your pulse

Whichever exercise form you choose, measuring your pulse rate during activity is a good way of testing fitness. It is especially useful for monitoring your progress in the course of aerobic training (p.53). You should take your pulse once or twice during activity, using the maximum pulse rate formula described below. Your pulse rate should not rise much above this safe limit, and it should drop down quickly.
If you are going beyond your safe limit, you are doing too much for your present level of fitness. Modify your activity, but keep training regularly. As you get fitter, your pulse rate during exercise will not rise so much, so you'll need to work harder to raise it to the safe limit. If you are not getting near the safe limit then you are not doing enough to stretch yourself.

Caution Your pulse rate is not the only criterion of safety. If you feel severe pain or dizziness, you should stop your exercise, and rest. If these symptoms continue, seek professional advice.

Maximum pulse rate formula

During vigorous exercise your pulse rate may rise steeply, according to how hard you work and to your level of fitness. The following rough formula gives you the safe limit for your age during vigorous exercise. From 220 deduct your age, then reduce this number by one quarter. For example, if you are 40 years old: $220 - 40 = 180 \times \frac{3}{4} = 135$. In this case your safe limit during activity is 135.

Recovery rate It is important that your pulse rate should drop down quickly after exercise, as shown below. If your pulse stays high you should take it easy. Try a gentler form of exercise, and build up your fitness more gradually

Pulse counting

All you need is a watch with which you can count seconds. Hold it in your left hand while, with the first two fingers of the right hand, you search for the pulse in your left wrist. You can usually find it a little below the base of the left thumb. (Reverse hands if you are left-handed.) Start by counting the number of beats of the pulse per 60 seconds. When you can do this easily, you can proceed to a quick assessment, counting for just 10 seconds multiplying by 6.

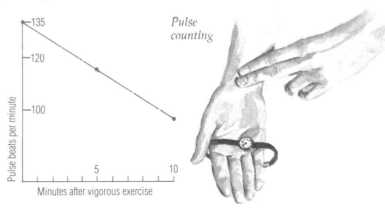

Pulse counting

Pulse beats per minute

135
120
100

5   10

Minutes after vigorous exercise

2 Testing for flexibility

Sit on the floor, as shown right (1) and stretch forward to touch your toes (2). If you can reach them without difficulty there is adequate flexibility of the spine and shoulders. If you only reach the mid-shin area you should take up an exercise type that rates high on flexibility (p.50). The salute to the sun (pp.54-5) is an excellent all-round stretching exercise.

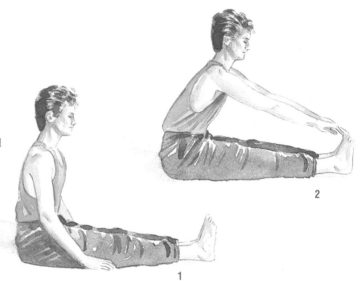

3 Testing abdominal tone

The abdominal muscles deserve special attention, since chronic weakness here exacerbates many common ailments (p.234).

To assess your abdominal strength, lie down on the floor and fold your arms across your chest, as shown below (1). Then try to raise the upper part of your body, without any jerking movements (2). Your back should be relaxed, not held stiffly, and your legs should remain on the floor.

If you can do this easily, your abdominal muscles are in good shape. If it is a bit of a struggle, or all you can do is lift your head, then you need to develop them. Try the abdominal tone exercises on p.198 and pp.234-5.

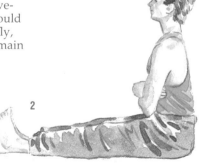

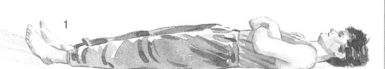

General fitness test

The test below, devised by Dr Kenneth Cooper, assesses fitness according to the distance covered in 12 minutes when walking fast. It is designed for anyone who is under 35 years of age, or for anyone over that age who has been exercising regularly at least 3 times a week for at least 6 weeks beforehand. If this excludes you, it is safest to categorize yourself as "poor" or "very poor". The ideal fitness program for anyone who rates fair, poor or very poor, is aerobic walking, shown opposite.

Rating	Distance covered in 12 minutes
Excellent	Over 2 miles (3.2 km)
Good	1½-2 miles (2.4-3.2 km)
Fair	1¼-1½ miles (2-2.4 km)
Poor	1-1¼ miles (1.6-2 km)
Very poor	Under 1 mile (1.6 km)

Planning a balanced program

To achieve complete fitness you should design yourself a varied exercise program, combining three distinct elements. Firstly, to stimulate your circulatory and respiratory systems and increase their capacity, you need a form of aerobic exercise. This can be tailored to your own fitness level, and should be practised for about 25 minutes every other day – longer if you choose a gentle type like walking. Secondly, you need some form of daily stretching and loosening exercise. And thirdly, you should choose a regular relaxation technique to refresh and restore you (pp.54-5).

The 3-point program

In these pages we suggest a three-point program suited to any age and level of fitness: aerobic walking; yoga's salute to the sun, and a relaxation routine (the relaxation exercise practised after a yoga session).

1 Aerobic walking

The following program, devised by Dr Kenneth Cooper, is designed for a low level of fitness. It is a progressive 16-week program that entails taking 5 walks a week, gradually increasing your time and the distance you cover. All you need is a stopwatch, comfortable, loose clothes, and sensible low-heeled walking shoes.

Weeks	Distance covered in each of 5 walks	Time
1	1 mile (1.6 km)	15 minutes
2	1 mile (1.6 km)	14 m
3	1 mile (1.6 km)	13 m 45 seconds
4	1½ miles (2.4 km)	21 m 30 s
5	1½ miles (2.4 km)	21 m 30 s
6	1½ miles (2.4 km)	21 m 30 s
7	2 miles (3.2 km)	28 m
8	2 miles (3.2 km)	27 m 45 s
9	2 miles (3.2 km)	27 m 30 s
10	2 miles (3.2 km)	27 m 30 s
11	2½ miles (4 km)	35 m
12	2½ miles (4 km)	34 m 30 s
13	3 miles (4.8 km)	42 m
14	3 miles (4.8 km)	42 m
15	3 miles (4.8 km)	42 m
16	4 miles (6.4 km)	56 m

2 Salute to the sun

In yoga the salute to the sun is performed several times a day as a warming-up, body-toning exercise. It energizes the body and is also an excellent breath control exercise. Do not force yourself into the positions – all movements should be relaxed and rhythmical. Practice it for 5 minutes daily to achieve the best results. (A further yoga sequence is shown on pp.288-9.)

1 Stand erect, feet together, and palms together in front of your chest. Keep your feet grounded, pushing steadily into the floor as your neck stretches upward. Exhale.

2 Breathe in deeply as you raise your arms high, hands still together, and bend backward from the waist.

3 Breathe out slowly as you bend forward from the hips. Place your hands flat on the floor at the side of the feet, if possible, with your face close to your legs. (Bend your knees if necessary.)

4 Breathing in, stretch your left leg backward, so that it rests on the knee and the toes; at the same time bend the right knee, and raise the head so that you look up.

5 Holding the breath, bring your right foot backward beside the left one. Your body should make a straight line, supported on the hands and toes.

6 Exhaling, lower your knees, chest and forehead to the floor, but keep your stomach and pelvis up.

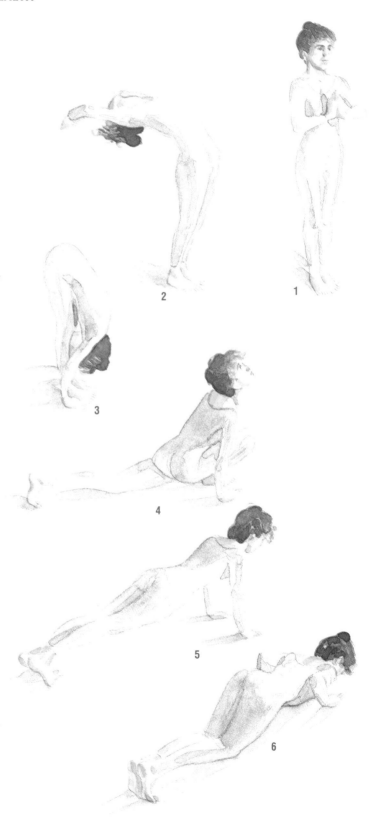

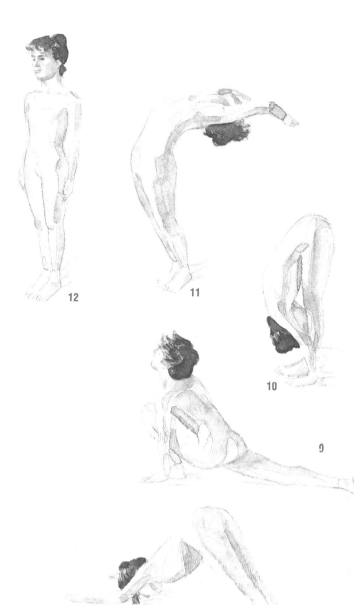

7 Breathe in as you raise the upper body by extending the arms. Look upward.

8 Keeping your hands flat on the floor, exhale as you curl your toes under and push your buttocks upward and back. Press your heels and head down toward the floor.

9 Inhaling, bring your left foot forward beneath your chest. Your right leg is extended backward, the knee resting on the floor.

10 Breathe out as you bring your right leg alongside the left, raising your buttocks, placing your face close to your legs.

11 Breathe in as you straighten upward, extending the arms up, hands together, then arching yourself backward.

12 Return to your standing position and exhale. Repeat the sequence, leading with the right leg, so that the stretching action on the body is balanced.

Relaxation

Practicing the Tense and relax routine (p.63) enhances the benefits of vigorous exercise. By tensing and then relaxing each part of the body in turn you can learn to recognize tension in particular muscles, and thus to gain conscious control of each area. And deep relaxation, even for a few minutes, does much to refresh a tired body.

Breathing

Most of us take the process of breathing for granted, seeing it as a largely automatic act, in which air is inhaled and exhaled, bringing in oxygen and expelling carbon dioxide. In fact the process of breathing is far more complex than this, and it affects all the other body systems. Good breathing can cure stress-related ailments, depression and fatigue, reduce the ill-effects of respiratory diseases, and enhance well-being and vitality (pp.58-9). Conversely, if anything interferes with the mechanism – such as disease, incorrect breathing habits or poor posture – there may be serious repercussions. What we breathe is equally important. Anything inhaled by the body travels to the bloodstream – there is far less filtering involved than with the digestive system, for example. Obviously, avoiding airborne pollutants (p.72), notably tobacco smoke, is a priority for everybody.

Correct breathing plays an important part in several of the natural therapies. In yoga, for instance, breathing exercises revitalize the body, and create clarity of mind. Since breathing can be consciously controlled, it is a key area of self-help for all-round good health.

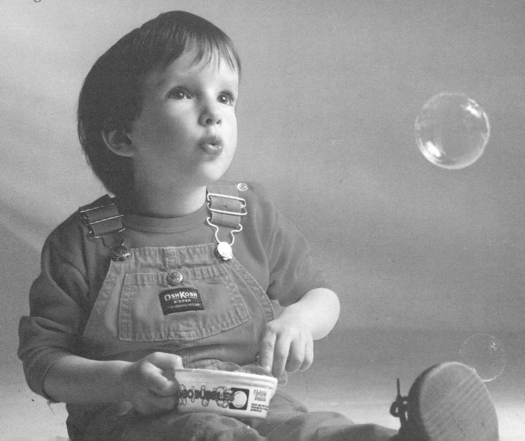

Giving up smoking

Inhaled smoke deposits tar in the lungs, and yields nicotine, a poisonous and addictive drug, plus carbon monoxide. The three main diseases associated with smoking, lung cancer, chronic bronchitis/ emphysema, and coronary heart disease, claim millions of lives each year. Smoking also aggravates high blood pressure, and, during pregnancy, puts mother and baby at risk. Passive smoking (being subjected to smoke from other people) can be almost as dangerous. If you are a smoker, consider giving up – or at least drastically cutting down.

Helping yourself give up

● Prepare to give up by keeping a daily count of how much you smoke and when you feel the need to smoke most. Use this either to reduce consumption gradually, or to set yourself a deadline for giving up completely.

● Motivation is crucial. In the first stages it may help to promise yourself rewards. Keep your original motives clearly in mind.

● Take regular exercise. It speeds up metabolism, reduces stress, and makes you feel fit, reinforcing your desire to give up.

● Try to introduce new patterns to your day. Going on vacation is an ideal time to give up.

● Adjust your diet to rid your body of toxic residues. Give yourself extra protein snacks. Don't worry if this affects your weight initially; you can attend to weight problems when you have conquered your craving for cigarettes.

● As a short-term measure, try anti-smoking tablets or nicotine chewing gum.

Therapeutic help

● Try "self-image thinking" to reinforce your motivation (p.313), or autogenics (pp.318-19) – these techniques can help to control addiction. Alternatively, consult a hypnotherapist (pp.310-13)

● Practice meditation (pp.314-17) and/or a relaxation routine (p.63) every day to reduce stress.

● Take up yoga (pp.284-93). A recent survey of 3,000 yoga subjects showed that a substantial number of smokers amongst them gave up smoking some months after starting regular yoga.

● Some acupuncturists claim over 50% success in treating tobacco addicts (pp.268-73).

Cigarette smoking in the USA, 1970-80
A recent survey of smoking in the US population, 17 years old and over, has shown that the smoking habit is on the wane, and more people are giving up.

	1970	1980	Overall trend
Non-smokers	44.8%	46.1%	up 3%
Former smokers	17.9%	20.6%	up 15%
Smokers	36.6%	32.6%	down 11%

Breathing exercises

The following routines teach you how to breathe to your full capacity, first by means of stretching exercises designed to open your rib cage and free your spine, then by learning consciously to control the three main areas involved in breathing fully.

These exercises will enhance your vitality and help you to feel more relaxed. In addition, there is a specific breathing method for relaxation for those with a tendency to hyperventilate. All your breathing should be through the nose, using a silent count of about three seconds for each inhalation and four for each exhalation. You can perform the stretching exercises either sitting down, or standing up.

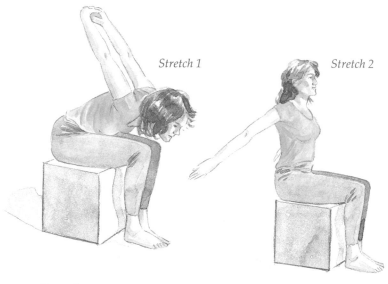

Stretch 1

Stretch 2

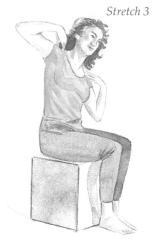

Stretch 3

Stretch 1

Sit up straight on a hard stool, feet together, hands clasped behind your back. Bend forward from the waist with the arms stretching back and up. Breathe in deeply in this position, then sit up straight as you breathe out. Repeat 5 to 10 times. This separates your ribs at the back and stretches the muscles of the lower back.

Stretch 2

Sit up straight with feet together and hands extended sideways, palms upward. As you breathe in, pull the arms back so that the shoulder-blades come together. As you breathe out, relax your arms so that they come forward. Repeat 5 to 10 times. This stretches and opens the front of the ribcage.

Stretch 3

Repeat Stretch 2, but this time place the tips of your fingers on your shoulder joints. As you breathe in, bend to one side, so that one elbow points to the ceiling, the other to the floor. As you breathe out, come back to an upright position. Repeat 5 to 10 times, on alternate sides.

Upper chest breathing
Lie down on a firm surface, with a pillow under your head and your knees slightly bent or supported by a pillow. Place your fingertips on the upper chest. Breathe in slowly, and feel your fingers being pushed up. Exhale, squeezing the air out by contracting the upper chest muscles. Repeat the in- and out-breaths 5 times.

Abdominal breathing
Still lying down, place your hands on your abdomen, just below the lower ribs. As you inhale, feel your abdomen rise. As you exhale, feel it return to normal. Use an extra effort from the abdominal muscles to squeeze out the last breath. Repeat 5 times.

Lateral chest breathing
Put your hands on the sides of the lower chest, fingers pointing inward. Breathe in slowly, feeling your hands separate as the ribs expand sideways. Exhale, squeezing the last air out by contracting the muscles under your hands. Repeat 5 times.

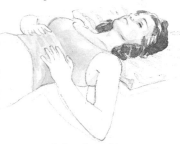

Lateral chest breathing

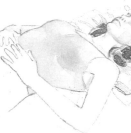

Abdominal breathing

Upper chest breathing

Complete breathing cycle
After practicing the previous exercises for a few weeks you can incorporate them in this advanced cycle.

Lie down on a firm surface. Rest your hands on your abdomen or by your sides. Fill your lower lungs, so that the abdomen rises and the lower ribs expand. Then fill the upper chest. Pause with the lungs full, then slowly exhale until the upper chest is completely emptied of air. Inhale for from 3 to 6 seconds, exhale for a little longer. Practice this full cycle 5 times, then rest a minute as you may feel light-headed.

Relaxed breathing

Breathing to ease stress
Hyperventilation (over-breathing) is a common stress-related disorder. It involves breathing rapidly from the upper chest only, so that too much carbon dioxide is breathed out and too much oxygen taken in, disrupting normal blood chemistry. Among the alarming symptoms this can produce are a pounding heart and dizziness. Use the relaxed breathing technique, right, when you first notice the symptoms. Even severe stress dis-orders, such as agoraphobia, can be helped in this way.

Relaxed breathing Lie down and place one hand on your abdomen and the other on your chest. On breathing in, you should feel the hand on your abdomen move markedly toward the ceiling, and the other hand move only slightly. You cannot hyper-ventilate if you breathe into the abdomen. Aim for about 8 in-and-out breaths per minute initially, and a slower rhythm in the long term.

Relaxation

Relaxation is not a matter of flopping down in front of the television, collapsing into an easy chair with a stiff drink, or falling into an exhausted sleep. While all these responses to tension and over-tiredness may fulfil an important role, they are quite different in quality and effect from conscious relaxation. Relaxation is a state of alert but passive awareness, a state in which our bodies are at rest while our minds are awake. To be relaxed in action is the ideal and natural state of a healthy creature; watch a baby or a young animal move and look and learn to walk, falling with soft limbs and starting again. When we are relaxed in action we bring the appropriate energy and attention to everything we do. And we feel a sense of healthy tiredness at the end of the day – rather than exhaustion.

But in today's fast-moving, competitive world we tend to live in a permanently stressed state, gradually wearing down our body's ability to cope. True relaxation is something we may have to rediscover consciously. To do this we must first understand the meaning of stress, its causes and symptoms, and then find appropriate ways to amend our stressful lifestyle.

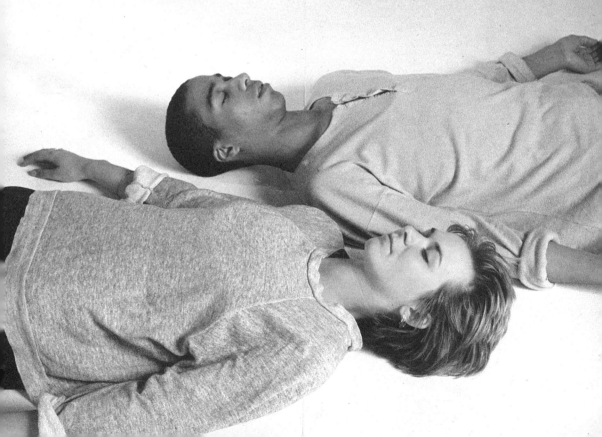

What is stress?

Stress is the body's physical, mental, and emotional response to any stimulus. Anything that excites, surprises, frightens, angers, or endangers us calls upon us to adapt or respond. In itself, stress is not bad. Our natural reactions are entirely appropriate to ensure our survival. But modern life presents us constantly with stressful situations, with little scope for immediate release through action. Unless we learn to discharge the stress and to relax, most of us begin to show signs of chronic tension – perhaps by drinking or smoking excessively. And if we don't heed these warning signals, serious illnesses, such as ulcers or heart problems, can occur. The first step toward successful stress management lies in recognizing our individual stressors.

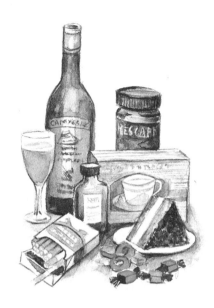

The "fight or flight" response

When we prepare for "fight or flight", the sympathetic nervous system is dominant – hormones are released, primarily adrenalin, blood sugar is mobilized to feed the muscles, muscles tense, heartbeat and breathing quicken, and metabolism increases. In a state of true relaxation, our muscles relax, heartbeat and breathing slow down, and metabolism decreases – the parasympathetic system is encouraged to regenerate the body's energies. The ability to concentrate without tension is heightened.

Intrinsic stressors

These are the factors that make up our internal stress response – attitudes, emotions or certain personality traits, such as competitiveness or anxiety, that in the view of many healthcare professionals contribute most to stress-related diseases. They are the key to the way we perceive or react to the extrinsic stressors but, unlike the latter, they can be changed or modified. Intrinsic stressors include: fear, anger, guilt and other highly emotional states; inability to express feelings; lack of assertion skills; preoccupation with your own thoughts; feeling guilty at relaxing; needing to control people or events.

A regular relaxation routine (p.63) or meditation will help, as well as several of the natural therapies, or a form of psychotherapy if necessary (p.83).

Chemical stressors

These are substances that are known to stimulate the body, using up its energy resources. These we can cut down or even cut out. They include: nicotine; alcohol; caffeine; sugar; additives; drugs; toxins (from air, water and food pollution)

Extrinsic stressors

These are potential stress factors that are generally beyond our control. All we can do is to find ways to reduce those that are within our control, plan to avoid undergoing too much at one time, and learn to react differently to those that are not events we can. Examples include: birth of a child; bereavement or separation; financial hardship; work pressures; exams; difficult relationships; environmental noise, pollution, crowds, traffic jams or glaring lights; isolation; inactivity; accidents; illness.

De-stressing your lifestyle

The major part of any good stress management regime should be geared to learning to live in a more relaxed way. There are a number of strategies you can adopt. First, try to remove those stressors over which you have some control. Modify your diet, your home environment, and your work patterns, for example. Take more and better balanced exercise (pp.53-5) and learn to breathe correctly (pp.58-9). Find a way to discharge any tension you may have built up during the day. You may be the sort of person who can go straight in to a session of relaxation, as described opposite, in order to calm and regenerate yourself. Or you may find you need first the thorough physical release of an evening run or a dance class, or even a good yell from the top of a hill.

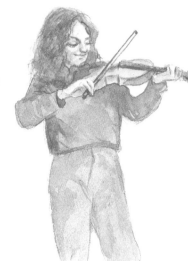

Playing music is one of the simplest ways of taking your mind off stressful thoughts.

Eating to relax

Sound nutrition (p.47) is a key factor in learning to be more relaxed. Eat at regular times of day, allowing adequate time for meals. Become aware of how stimulants affect you and try to cut them out.

Your ability to cope with both physical and mental stress will be severely reduced if your diet is deficient in vitamins and minerals. The following are particularly important: vitamin C, the B group, and the minerals calcium, magnesium, manganese, potassium, zinc, chromium, lithium, iron and selenium, (see pp.40-1 for food sources) as well as the amino acids tryptophan and phenylalanine.

Leisure and personal space

Make time for yourself, not only at weekends, but during your working week too, for reading, listening to music, sport, yoga, or for any creative, absorbing hobby such as gardening, which is non-competitive. Treat yourself to a warm bath, a massage or a workout in a gym. Try to reserve one room or area in your home where you can relax or pursue your interests freely, without being disturbed and without having to clear your things out of the way to make space for other people.

Other aids to relaxation

It is important to tackle the root causes of long-term stress. But some of the following aids can help you on a daily basis:

- Ionizers to purify the air (p.72)

- Tapes or videos of relaxation techniques or restful music

- Warm baths (hot ones can be enervating, see p.211)

- Showers, and high-powered water massage

- Aromatic essential oils for baths and massage (pp.176-81)

- Soothing herb teas or infusions (pp.160-75)

- Lambswool fleece or pure cotton underblankets.

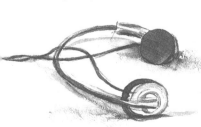

Relaxation techniques

Practicing a short session of relaxation once or twice a day is a wonderful way to unwind. Meditation, autogenics, and biofeedback (pp.314-21) are also excellent for relaxation but here we describe two simple techniques which you can practice straight away in your own home, without having to learn a special skill first.

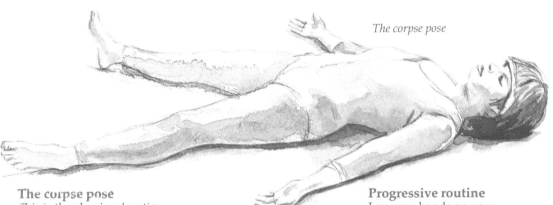

The corpse pose

The corpse pose

This is the classic relaxation pose practiced in yoga. First find a quiet place where you will not be disturbed. Wear loose, comfortable clothes, take off your shoes, and undo any belts or tight buttons. Now simply lie down on your back, feet about 18 inches (45 cm) apart, hands palms upward and about 6 inches (15 cm) from your sides. Allow your legs and feet to roll outward. Check that your body feels symmetrical. Now close your eyes and relax, centering your awareness on the rise and fall of your abdomen.

In this position, follow whichever of the two routines below suits you best – or do them both, one after the other.

"Tense and relax" routine

Some people don't realise how tense their bodies are until they experience how different relaxation feels. This routine enables you to really feel the contrast between tension and full relaxation.

First settle yourself in the corpse pose. Now working up from the feet, first tense, then relax each part of the body in turn – feet, legs, buttocks, stomach, back, chest, shoulders, arms and hands, head, and face. Tense the parts as hard as you can, lifting them a few inches off the floor, if you wish, then relax, dropping them down.

Progressive routine

Lay your hands on your abdomen and breathe in deeply, filling your belly first, (see Relaxed breathing p.59). Sigh as you breathe out, feeling any tension release with the breath. Repeat a few times, letting go more with each out-breath.

Now let your breathing continue at its own pace and depth and, as you breathe out, release any tension first in the feet then, with the next out-breath, the ankles, then the calves, and so on up the body. Try to really contact each part of the body with your mind and release it completely before moving on. It may help to silently repeat to yourself: "my feet are completely relaxed" and so on, with each out-breath, ending with: "my whole body is completely relaxed".

Body servicing

Personal hygiene and cleanliness play a vital role in good preventive health care. A balanced diet, regular exercise, rest, and fresh air are, of course, fundamental to looking and feeling good, to a clear skin, healthy hair, and strong teeth and gums. But we need to take care of the body externally too – not just to keep up a healthy appearance, but to cleanse it and protect it from infections, irritations, allergies and environmental conditions, using safe, mild, non-toxic soaps and cleansers. Just as we take care of our homes, keeping them clean and free of dirt and grime, so we need to regularly "service" our bodies. With proper skin, hair and dental care and a high standard of personal hygiene, our bodies will repay us by enhancing our self-confidence as well as by improving our resistance to disease.

Personal hygiene is important not only at an individual level, however, but in our contact with others too. Many diseases can be avoided by a responsible approach to hygiene. Given the prevalence of food poisoning and other bacterial infections and the alarming rise in sexually transmitted diseases, none of us can afford to neglect the basic rules.

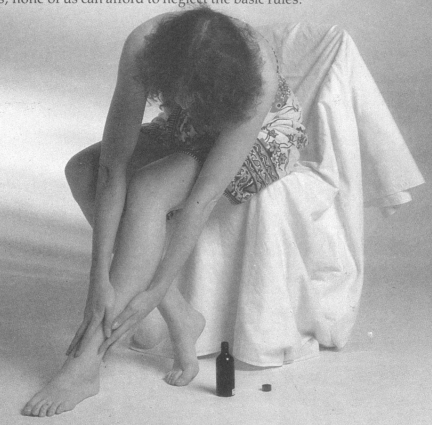

Personal hygiene

Washing doesn't have to mean always using soap – in most cases, water and gentle friction will do just as well. Use a loofah, brush, or friction glove to stimulate circulation and help wash away dead skin. Always rinse and dry thoroughly after washing.

Hair Wash hair at least once a week, more often if it's short or greasy. Use only one application of a mild shampoo, and rinse well. Wash brush and comb at the same time.

Teeth Brush your teeth morning and evening after meals, and after lunch too if you can. Follow a standard routine (p.67). If you wear dentures, remove them every night, clean well, and keep them moist.

Hands Dirty hands and nails can contaminate food and transmit disease. Always wash your hands after going to the lavatory, before preparing or eating food, as well as whenever they feel or look dirty. Keep your nails scrupulously clean with a nailbrush or a blunt-ended orange stick.

Feet Feet need regular washing and careful drying, particularly between the toes. Keep your toenails short, cutting them straight across rather than in a curve, to avoid ingrowing toenails. Buy well-fitting shoes of porous, not synthetic materials, that allow the feet to "breathe". Wear socks of natural fibers too, and be sure to change them daily.

Ears The outer ear may be carefully sponged, but the inner ear is very delicate. Use cotton buds to clean them if necessary. Never poke about inside the ear.

Armpits Most people sweat quite heavily under the arms and, since the armpits get little air, bacteria may grow, causing body odor. Wash frequently, and use antiperspirants sparingly.

Genital areas Wash daily, front and back, and dry thoroughly. Avoid strong soaps, and scents; sensitive skin is easily irritated. Use cotton underwear, and don't wear tight trousers.
Women: Because the anus is close to the vaginal opening and urethra, women need to take special care to wipe themselves from front to back after bowel movements. During menstruation, wash, and change towels or tampons frequently.
Men: Wash the penis daily. If you are uncircumcized, gently pull back the foreskin, wash, and dry carefully.

Natural skin and hair care

The skin is a permeable membrane. In order to "breathe" well, it needs washing to strip off excess grease and old cells, and to remove the toxins excreted in sweat. But just as what you take in to your body affects it externally, so what you apply to the outside affects it internally. Harsh chemicals, such as some hair dyes and depilatories, are best avoided. Hypoallergenic cleansers tend to be expensive, so it's worth trying out traditional natural cleansers which can be prepared at home without the use of chemical additives. Skin also needs protection from extremes of temperature, and strong winds. Use protective suncreams or oils, wrap up well in cold weather, and avoid very hot or cold water. The same goes for skin care during housework or manual jobs. Wear rubber gloves or use barrier creams to protect the hands.

Natural cleansers for healthy skin and hair

Soaps and cleansers

Most soaps are made from fats of animal origin, and caustic soda. Highly alkaline, they temporarily change the skin's natural acidity (pH), and strip it of oils. Instead, use the milder soaps based on vegetable products, such as palm kernel and coconut oil, or try soapless cleansing bars, which use synthetic ingredients to help keep the pH in balance.

If your skin is irritated or spotty, try herbal treatments (p.170), or use lanolin-based creams, or oatmeal soaps and ointments. Fine oatmeal also makes a soothing face pack, but test for possible allergic reactions first.

Bath solutions

Naturopaths advise a range of soothing solutions for the bath, using bran, hay-flowers, sodium bicarbonate or Epsom salts (p.195). For a relaxing bath with a luxurious aroma, try a few drops of an essential oil, such as lavender or chamomile (pp.176-81).

Anti-perspirants

Most of these are based on zinc or aluminium salts; they work by closing the sweat ducts, preventing the excretion of toxins. If you find them necessary, use those based on plant extracts, or try refreshing the armpits with lavender water.

Shampoos and rinses

Healthy, glossy hair needs a well-balanced diet. Strong shampoos, and some commercial hair dyes, can damage the hair and scalp. Some "medicated" shampoos may also cause irritation. Choose mild shampoos containing herbal extracts, and make your own natural rinses at home. For dandruff, try rinsing with an infusion of rosemary (p.223), and massage the scalp to improve circulation. Rinse fair hair in an infusion of chamomile flowers (p.164). To restore the scalp's natural acidity, add a tablespoon of cider vinegar or lemon juice to the final rinsing water.

Protecting teeth and eyes

Tooth decay and gum disease are caused by a build-up of plaque, a sticky film of bacteria which eats away at the enamel of the tooth. The best way of preventing tooth and gum problems is to avoid sugary foods and, above all, to brush your teeth regularly. Disclosing tablets are particularly useful when teaching children to clean their teeth thoroughly. Make sure that you go for a regular dental check-up every 6 months.

Eyes can be damaged by pollutants and dust and may also suffer in strong light or through over-use in poor light. Always use protective goggles for hazardous jobs. Wear sunglasses in strong sunshine and, if your eyes are especially sensitive, goggles when swimming. Vary your gaze and focus regularly. If your eyes are irritated or swollen, bathe them in cool, clean water, or an eyebright solution (p.171). Have your eyes tested every 2 years – more often if you are over 40, if poor sight demands it, or if you suffer from repeated headaches.

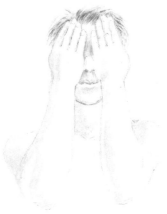

Palming the eyes

Gentle cleansers for teeth and gums

Toothpastes and gargles

Nearly all commercial toothpastes – and, indeed, many health store brands – contain the detergent sodium lauryl sulphate, and many contain bleaching agents, sweeteners, and artificial colorings. Some of these ingredients can cause allergic reactions – symptoms are tenderness, bleeding, and receding gums. Sodium bicarbonate with water is a good substitute, but it is not to everybody's taste.

For mouth ulcers and inflamed gums, try a soothing gargle with myrrh or red sage (p.169). Gargles can also help bad breath (p.181). If your mouth ulcers could be caused by ill-fitting dentures, you should consult your dentist.

Cleaning your teeth

Brush downward on your upper teeth, upward on your lower teeth, brushing from gum to tooth. Take care to reach all the back teeth, and the back surface of the front teeth. Brush the upper edges of the big back teeth with a rotating action.

Before or after brushing, use a length of waxed dental floss to remove particles of food from between the teeth or between teeth and gums.

Bates' eye exercises

Dr Bates' exercises have found many advocates, including the writer Aldous Huxley. Here are a few examples:

● Blink frequently, about 15 times per minute

● In the morning, splash your closed eyes 20 times with warm water, then 20 times with cold. Before bed, repeat, reversing the sequence

● "Palm" your eyes for a few minutes, at intervals during the day, by placing the palms of your hands over the eyes with the base of the little fingers on the bridge of the nose. This rests your eyes completely.

Sexual hygiene

In recent years, the incidence of sexually transmitted diseases (STDs) has escalated enormously, making a responsible attitude toward sexual hygiene a matter of great importance. Also called genito-urinary infections, because they may affect the urethra and bladder as well as the genitals, STDs are normally (though not always) passed through sexual activity.

There are at least 25 different kinds of STDs, ranging from the more serious, like syphilis or AIDS, to herpes and crabs. Although most of these can be dealt with swiftly and effectively by prompt medical attention, some can seriously damage health if left untreated. If you feel you may have an infection, check for the warning signs (see below), and go for a medical check-up.

Raspberry leaf tea (p.225) strengthens the female reproductive system.

General preventive measures

• Limit your sexual partners.

• Don't have sex if you or your partner has any inflammation, sores or an unusual discharge around the genital area. Avoid oral sex and don't kiss if you or your partner has a cold sore around the mouth, or sores in the genital area.

• Use a sheath or diaphragm (p.101) – barrier methods of contraception have been found to give some protection against both STDs and cervical cancer.

• Pass urine, and wash your genitals, as soon as possible after making love. This helps to avoid cystitis and urethritis.

• Tell your partner if you even think you have an infection.

• Keep yourself clean, especially genitals and hands (p.65).

• Don't share towels or wash cloths.

• To strengthen resistance to all infections, eat well, get plenty of sleep, and avoid constant stress. Women should be especially alert to the risk of vaginal yeast infections if pregnant, taking the pill, diabetic, anemic, or taking antibiotics. Try adding a little vinegar to the bath water every now and then, to help prevent or cure mild infections.

Warning signs

If you have any of the following symptoms, make sure you get prompt medical attention from your doctor or a special clinic:

• An unusual discharge from the vagina

• Any discharge from the penis

• Sores or blisters near the vagina, penis or anus

• Irritation around the vagina, penis or anus

• Pain or burning sensation on passing urine

• Passing urine more frequently than usual

• Pain during intercourse.

Herpes

There are two types of Herpes Simplex virus. Herpes 1 causes cold sores around the mouth and nose, Herpes 2 produces sores in the genital region. Both types are related; the virus can be passed from mouth to genitals during oral sex, or from mouth to hands to genitals. Don't panic if you get herpes. The attack may be a single occurrence, and future attacks, if they do occur, may be milder.

Symptoms

● Stinging, tingling or itching

● Small blisters which burst, leaving red ulcers

● General flu-like feeling, perhaps with a temperature

● Pain on passing urine.

Remedies

An attack can be treated with medication from your doctor or a specialist clinic. You can ease and heal the sores by bathing the area in a salt solution (about 1 teaspoon per pint (560 ml) of warm water). Ice packs will reduce the pain (p.212). Applying a little distilled witch hazel and exposing the sores to the air helps to dry them out. Wear loose, airy cotton clothing.

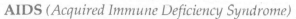

Witch hazel is a classic herbal astringent and antiseptic, a remedy for sores and other skin infections (see above, and p.169), and for cuts and bruises, burns, and sprains (pp.324-7).

AIDS *(Acquired Immune Deficiency Syndrome)*

Because so much is still unknown about this devastating disease, we strongly recommend that you contact your doctor or local AIDS hotline for the most current information regarding possible modes of transmission and the latest preventative measures. It is currently thought that while certain kinds of condoms *when used properly* provide some protection, abstinence is the only sure method of preventing *sexual* transmission. Again, we recommend that you consult your doctor or local AIDS hotline before making any assumptions about preventative measures or your own susceptibility.

The healthy home

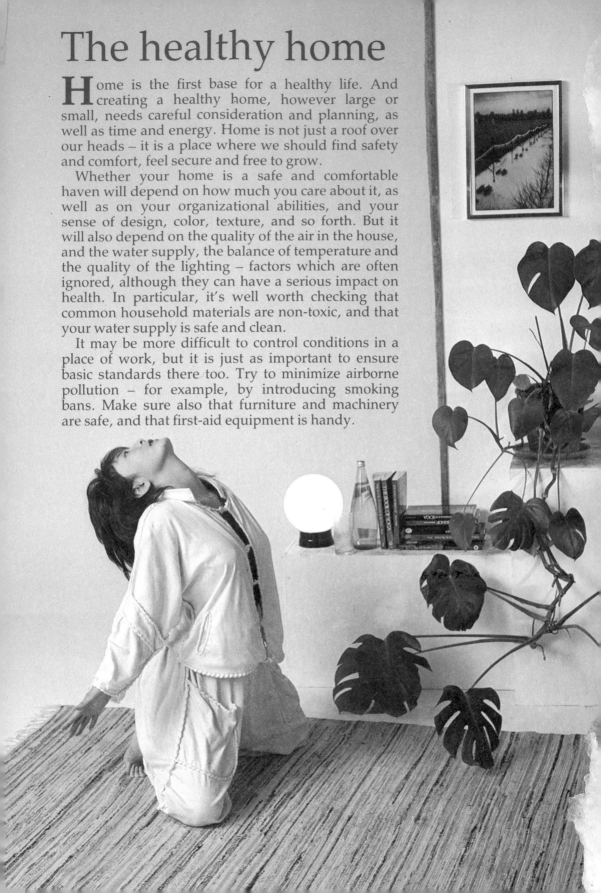

Home is the first base for a healthy life. And creating a healthy home, however large or small, needs careful consideration and planning, as well as time and energy. Home is not just a roof over our heads – it is a place where we should find safety and comfort, feel secure and free to grow.

Whether your home is a safe and comfortable haven will depend on how much you care about it, as well as on your organizational abilities, and your sense of design, color, texture, and so forth. But it will also depend on the quality of the air in the house, and the water supply, the balance of temperature and the quality of the lighting – factors which are often ignored, although they can have a serious impact on health. In particular, it's well worth checking that common household materials are non-toxic, and that your water supply is safe and clean.

It may be more difficult to control conditions in a place of work, but it is just as important to ensure basic standards there too. Try to minimize airborne pollution – for example, by introducing smoking bans. Make sure also that furniture and machinery are safe, and that first-aid equipment is handy.

Furnishing the healthy home

In the West, a distinctive style of furniture has become standard to nearly all households. We rarely consider its effect on our health, even though poor posture and back problems are endemic. It isn't necessary to slump in a sofa, hunch over a desk, or sleep on soft, yielding mattresses. Sitting cross-legged on the floor is good for you, and so is sleeping on a firm surface. Furniture should be designed to protect the body's structural balance, to allow for reasonable circulation of air, and it should not present a hazard. Try to avoid materials that produce asphyxiating fumes when they burn, such as foam rubber. Be sure that furniture is strong, and free from protruding nails or splintering wood.

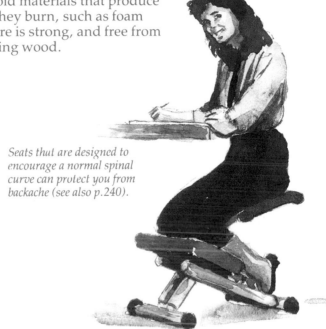

Worktops and chairs

Work surfaces such as desks and kitchen worktops must be at a reasonable height for the user, with chairs that can be adjusted to ensure correct posture. Straight-backed chairs are best, or those with adjustable backs which support your lower back. Alternatively, try placing a small cushion to support your lower back.

It's well worth exploring the range of "therapeutic" designs of chairs and stools. In the long term they may save much unnecessary pain and discomfort.

Seats that are designed to encourage a normal spinal curve can protect you from backache (see also p.240).

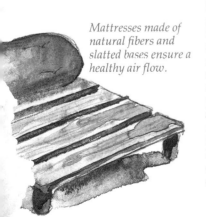

Mattresses made of natural fibers and slatted bases ensure a healthy air flow.

Beds and bedding

Mattresses should be firm (orthopedic mattresses are ideal), and the base of the bed should allow for air flow – slatted wooden bases are excellent. Bedding materials can exacerbate respiratory problems, and provoke allergic reactions. Quilts make good bedding, since they gather less dust than heavy blankets, but watch out that the filling isn't causing a problem (duck down, for instance, may cause allergies). Brightly colored sheets can be fun, but some people are allergic to their dyes.

Babies and small children should have cots with sides. Don't give them pillows (to avoid smothering). If a child is restless, try using a fleecy underblanket for extra warmth and comfort.

Fresh air and temperature control

The more clean, oxygenated air we breathe, the greater our potential for health. Outdoor pollution, from car exhausts, factory fumes, agricultural chemicals, and many other contaminants, is widely recognized as a serious health hazard – but indoor pollution is a reality too. Various building materials, notably asbestos, materials containing formaldehyde (such as chipboard), and wood that has been treated with toxic preservatives, give off dust and fumes that have been shown to be harmful. Central heating and air-conditioning systems can produce their own "exhausts", and ill-ventilated rooms compound the situation. Check that these systems are well maintained, and that your home is not polluted by toxic materials. Try to keep the indoor atmosphere as fresh and well aired as you can.

Pollutants

Many common airborne substances are known to damage health. Some can be avoided altogether. Try not to use any polishes, fresheners, and cleansers that come in sprays, and beware of harsh chemicals and biological detergents – they may taint the atmosphere. Major pollutants in the home include: paints and aerosols; tobacco smoke; cooking smells; smoke from burning garbage; glues; and fumes from rubber, plastic, or other synthetic materials (which will be worse if they are near a heat source).

Fresh air is a key factor in the healthy home

Humidifiers

Heating and cooling systems can make air uncomfortably dry – provoking headaches, drying the skin and irritating the throat. A simple water-filled container, or an electrically powered humidifier helps to adjust humidity.

Ionizers and purifiers

Ionizers make us sleep well and feel better. They counter the positive ions produced by air conditioning, central heating, tobacco smoke, and electrical equipment. An excess of positive ions – which occurs naturally in pre-storm weather or with certain winds – may produce feelings of lethargy and depression, headaches and respiratory problems.

It may also be necessary to use an air purifier, to remove pollutants. It helps to keep plenty of houseplants, which act as natural air purifiers.

Temperature control

Lack of adequate heating can produce hypothermia, a condition where normal body temperature drops from 98.6°F (37°C) to 95°F (35°C) or even less. This in turn can lead to lower resistance to infection, and may be fatal.

Thermostat-controlled heating, or air conditioning, may be efficient, but there are disadvantages. It's easy to get used to overheating, making yourself vulnerable to colds and sore throats. Most adults would do better to wrap up more warmly, and have a lower background heat.

Clean water, clear light

Household health can suffer from contaminated water and poor lighting. Taking a few simple precautions helps prevent accidents and illnesses.

Although much emphasis is placed on supplying clean water, the average drinking water in western countries is by no means pure. Water is often reprocessed several times, and contaminants, from industrial wastes or agricultural nitrate fertilizers, can find their way into the supply.

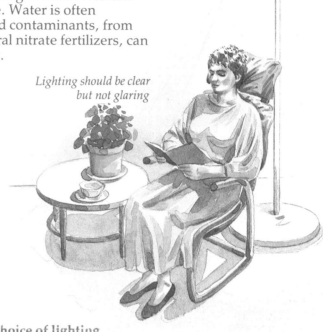

Lighting should be clear but not glaring

Ensuring clean water

Check that you don't have any lead pipes or other lead plumbing. If you do, you will have to filter the water or, a more radical step, replace the plumbing. If you are worried about the contents of your supply, arrange to have a sample analysed. It may be prudent to attach an additional filter system to your taps, or use a filtering jug for drinking water.

Whether you have lead pipes or not, always use the cold tap for drinking water, and run the tap for a few minutes in the morning to flush out stagnant water. And don't take short cuts by filling the kettle from the hot tap. Check the cold water tank at regular intervals to be sure that it is clean.

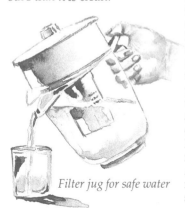

Filter jug for safe water

Choice of lighting

Lighting can influence the general atmosphere, as well as mental and emotional well-being. And recent research indicates that health can suffer through long-term lack of natural daylight. Make the most of the types of light available. Full-spectrum lighting simulates sunlight, compensating for lack of natural light. Try dimmers to vary the intensity of light and produce low, restful light when you need it. Select an appropriate type of light for each room or area. Fluorescent lighting is cool, muted, and bluish in tone. Although it is low glare, it may cause headaches in sensitive people. Tungsten lighting gives a warmer, yellowish light, closer to the natural light of a fire or candle. Tungsten halogen gives out an intense, bright light like the sun.

Safe lighting

Avoid accidents and eyestrain by positioning lights well, particularly on the stairs, in the kitchen, and over worktops. For reading, make sure the light source is behind you and to the side, preferably at shoulder height. Make sure the strength of the lighting is appropriate.

Natural home comforts

Don't underestimate the value of good design, and general comforts in the home. Pleasing sensory stimuli act as an antidote to noise, pollution, and other discomforts that assail us in the outside world. If there are conflicts of taste then it helps if each person has a personal space and, if musical tastes differ, a personal stereo system.

Personal space

A little privacy and peace are essential to everybody's health. This means both physical and emotional space. Try to ensure that every member of the household has some time for themselves, and a room or a corner of their own, in which to pursue an activity undisturbed, or perhaps to practice yoga, or meditate. Children and teenagers, in particular, need a room where they are not constantly invaded and supervised.

Color values

Colors affect moods and emotions (and therefore health); they can also give warmth and be used to "manipulate" space. Warm colors are ideal for rooms that tend to feel cold, cool colors for sunnier rooms. Light colors enhance space.

Some natural therapies use color to treat illnesses. Healers, for example, may use blue to calm disturbed body energies; red is said to stimulate, green is restful.

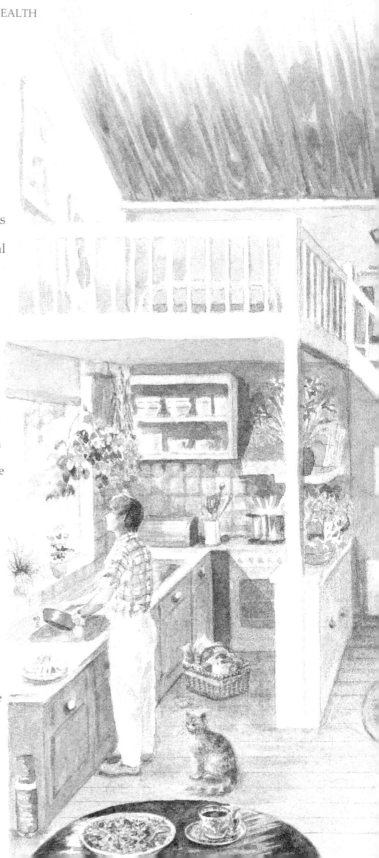

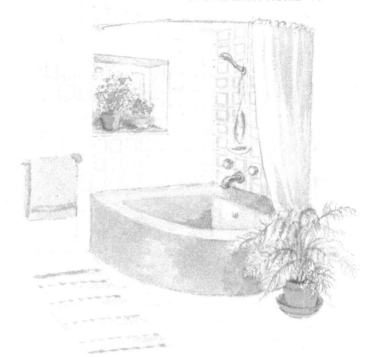

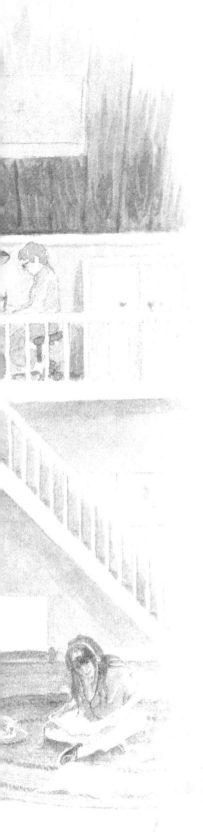

Natural scents and air fresheners

Natural air fresheners are less hazardous than commercial sprays. Living plants can absorb smells and destroy some airborne pollutants. Herbs have been used for freshening houses for centuries, often contained in a pot-pourri. Basil smells refreshing, and is said to keep flies away. Rosemary acts as a moth repellent. Juniper, hyssop, and thyme sweeten stale air. Spices are also used. Pomanders made with oranges and dried cloves, for example, keep closets and blanket boxes smelling sweet.

Try growing sweet-smelling herbs indoors. Or use essential oils in an incensor or vaporizer – there are many scents (pp.176-81).

Bathroom comforts

Baths and showers are for cleanliness, but they also relax us, and ease aches and pains. Showers in particular pay excellent dividends in health care. If you don't have one, consider the benefits: showers make more sense than baths, since you rinse the body of all dirty water; they don't raise your blood pressure in the way that a hot bath does (see Baths, showers, sitz baths, p.211); they're quicker when you're in a hurry; the action on the skin stimulates circulation; they use less water and so are cheaper to run; and a well-powered shower provides a refreshing hydro-massage. Baths, however, are the obvious choice if you want to use essential oils, or healing solutions (p.195).

Safe haven

Domestic accidents account for an alarmingly high number of injuries and fatalities every year. The very young and elderly are particularly susceptible, and the kitchen, living room, and garden are the highest risk areas. Prevention may well involve careful planning, and a regular calendar of safety checks. It is essential to make sure too that children as well as adults understand the potential dangers of fire, electricity, gas, and water.

Hazard	Area	Precaution
Fire	Whole house	Keep fire extinguishers in working order; use fire guards on fire places; keep fire blankets handy; don't smoke in bedrooms; use non-flammable furnishings; check all electrical appliances for loose connections, etc; check house wiring; make sure that gas appliances are regularly checked; take great care when lighting gas with matches; never leave heating fat or oil unattended; never block sources of heat with drying clothes; place "open" heaters, like kerosene stoves, away from walls, furniture, coats, etc.
Accidents	Kitchen	Keep pot handles turned in; don't let children handle kettles or fill hotwater bottles; don't run several appliances off one socket; don't fish for trapped toast in the toaster with a metal implement; take extra care when handling sharp knives; store sharp knives safely in covers, blocks, or drawers; don't store heavy objects and cans on high shelves as they may fall on you; keep bleach and other potential toxins safely stored.
	Bathroom	Water near electricity is a major hazard – all lights must have pull cords, and there shouldn't be any electrical outlets, except for small razor sockets; if the bathroom has no window it must have a ventilating fan in working order; have non-slip mats in the bath and shower; put all razors, scissors, chemicals, shampoos, dyes, etc, out of reach of children; keep medicines in childproof containers and locked away; keep a well-stocked medicine and first-aid supply closet.
	Hall and stairs	Make sure stair carpets are well fixed; don't make floors slippery with a glossy polish; have clear, bright light at every landing; don't use "open" forms of heating, eg, kerosene or gas heaters, in these areas. Protect small children from accidental falls by installing a simple child-proof gate at the top of the stairs.

Hazard	Area	Precaution
Accidents continued	**Sitting room**	Avoid trailing wires, which people can trip over; unplug the television when it is not in use; make sure the room is well ventilated; use fire guards on fire places.
	Garden	Never leave a power mower unattended when it is running, nor attempt to adjust it unless it is switched off; clear stones, twigs, etc, before mowing; don't throw aerosols or cans or other synthetic or explosive material on the bonfire; keep septic tanks well covered; don't leave garden tools lying around; lock away all pesticides, paints, etc, and mark them clearly; put a safety net around ponds. If you are planting a garden, and there are small children in your family, avoid poisonous plants such as poinsettia, laburnum, and yew; if you do have poisonous plants in the garden (or the house), teach children to recognize and avoid them.
Food poisoning and pollution	**Kitchen**	Keep waste well away from food in securely lidded containers; cleanliness in preparing and handling food is essential – always wash hands before preparing food; be extra careful if you have a cut or sore, a skin, nose or throat infection; cover any cuts with waterproof dressing, and don't sneeze or cough over food. Wash dishes and other equipment thoroughly, and rinse off detergents carefully. Don't touch cooked meat after handling raw meat, without washing your hands in between, and don't store cooked meat near raw meat – this is a prime cause of food poisoning; if you are defrosting frozen food, be sure to defrost it completely (especially meat and meat products); don't leave hot cooked food for any length of time in a cooling oven or other warm place – this encourages bacteria; if you are reheating cooked foods, do so thoroughly – use a high temperature to destroy potentially harmful organisms. Make sure that the kitchen is well ventilated – ventilating fans with ducts which take fumes outside, or carbon filter extractors, help to combat cooking fumes. Bear in mind that aluminium cooking utensils may contaminate food with metallic toxins.
Pests	**Whole house**	Flies, fleas, wasps, mice, rats, and cockroaches all carry germs and present a threat to health; if you find any signs of infestation you should call in professional fumigators. Use natural insect repellents, eg, lavender or rosemary (see also Natural scents and air fresheners, p.75). Be extra hygienic in summer – don't leave food open; wrap scraps before putting them in the trash can; and check that drains are clear. Keep pets clean – don't allow them to lie on beds; make sure they are innoculated and dewormed regularly; during house training clean up with lots of disinfectant; don't let children sleep with pets or kiss them; and make sure pets have their own beds.

Mental and emotional health

There is no hard and fast way of defining mental and emotional health, nor is there a precise dividing line between mental health and illness. Most people, however, would accept a number of common factors as adding up to a state of psychological well-being. These include: feeling content with your sense of who you are, your work and your personal relationships; being able to express your feelings; not being at the mercy of your emotions; being able to accept growth and change without feeling unduly threatened; having a sense of humor and being able to laugh at yourself; and having a sense of purpose. Being able to keep your balance during times of stress is also commonly taken as a gauge of mental and emotional health.

Balancing your needs

Maintaining psychological well-being is something of a balancing act. Firstly, you need to strike a balance between getting your own personal needs met and meeting the demands of others, both at home, at work and in the wider context of society. Secondly, you need to distribute your time and energy well,

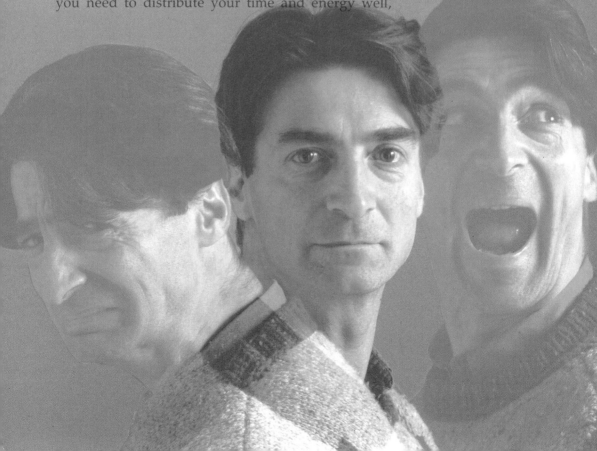

between, say, working and relaxing, or being alone and relating to others. If you devote too much time to one facet only, you not only become one-sided, but also run the risk of having no resources to fall back on in other areas when you need them. Thirdly, you have to maintain a balance between controlling and "letting go". Everyone needs to be able to make and put into effect conscious choices and to have at least one area in their lives where they feel responsible and in control. But it is equally important to come to terms with the fundamental insecurity of life, its constant changeability. To be able to say goodbye, to let go, to accept chaos and "not knowing" rather than wanting everything rigid, boxed and labelled, to be flexible and open to life and other people – these are the foundations of true peace of mind.

For many people, a belief in something larger than themselves is also an essential part of maintaining emotional balance, whether the belief is spiritual, philosophical or political. Certainly those of us whose belief structures are positive and those who find a meaning in life seem to be able to withstand its strains and stresses better.

Mind over matter

It is now becoming more widely accepted that the mind and emotions have a far greater influence on the body's state of health than was previously recognized in orthodox medicine. Most of us realize that if we feel worried or unhappy our bodies tend to feel sluggish and weary and we are more prone to aches and pains and to infections. But even those diseases which were once considered as having an exclusively "external" origin, such as cancer, rheumatism, or heart disease, are now generally acknowledged as having a considerable psychological component. Some complementary practitioners would go even further and claim that *all* disease originates in the mind – energy follows thought.

The way the body, mind and spirit interact for the well-being of the whole means that you can boost one area by positive action in another. So if you can maintain a positive, optimistic outlook, for instance, your physical health is likely to stay strong and, conversely, if you improve your sense of physical well-being through judicious exercise, diet and so on, your state of mind will certainly be enhanced.

"The body itself is like a garden, and the mind a gardener. Feelings of contentment and happiness promote balance and harmony in our inner ecology. The soil is made fertile for fruitful action. By contrast, feelings of distress and unhappiness drain the land of its energy and productive capacity."
Neville Hodgkinson,
Will to be Well

A sense of self

Central to mental and emotional well-being is self-esteem. Valuing yourself for who you are, acknowledging your own achievements, knowing your limitations, appreciating others for who they are, not for what you would like them to be, trusting your own judgment without constant reference to outside authority – these are the qualities of someone with good self-esteem. One of the foundations of self-esteem lies in having a strong sense of self – a sense of who you really are, rather than the roles you play in life. Getting in touch with this inner core enables you to see yourself as a potentially autonomous being, with the ability to shape your own life.

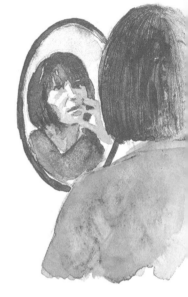

Self-esteem is something you learn, however, not something you are born with. You are more likely to have a positive self-image if you have had a loving, secure childhood, with parents who also had a good sense of themselves. But since many of us did not have a perfect childhood, our self-esteem often starts at a low ebb, and we need to build it up ourselves in adult life.

Building a sense of self

There are many ways you can improve your sense of self. First, define clearly what you want out of life. Aim high, imagining how you would like to live, thinking about what makes you happiest. Writing it down may help to make you clearer. Setting personal goals will enable you to focus and direct your energy, and your goals should help give you a sense of purpose and self-reliance.

Learn to listen to your inner voice and use it as a source of guidance and inspiration, cultivating it through regular sessions of quiet and stillness, and through meditation, yoga, or other relaxation techniques (pp.62-3). Set aside a time for this where you can be alone and undisturbed.

Be honest with yourself and others. This may involve some painful revelations but will also lead to some positive ones. Meditation may help you to recognize and accept parts of yourself you are trying to hide. The truth breeds clarity and strength, and encourages you to take responsibility for yourself and your actions.

Changing your beliefs

Beliefs are assumptions about reality that we hold as truths. They shape the way we act and how we feel about ourselves, but they also help to create our life experiences, since beliefs tend to be self-fulfilling – if you believe you're a loser, for example, people will tend to treat you as one.

Examine your own deep beliefs about yourself and your life, and start countering some of the negative ones with creative visualization (p.313) and positive affirmations (p.302). You will find you can alter your pattern of experience and increase your sense of self.

Relating to others

Building and nurturing good relationships with our family and friends is an essential part of emotional and physical well-being. Research studies have found that people with supportive relationships are less likely to become mentally or physically ill or suffer from accidents than those without, and that they recover more quickly from illnesses, and live longer.

We learn to relate to others from infancy onward, modelling ourselves mainly on our parents. If their relationships are fulfilling, we have a good blueprint, but relationship skills, like self-esteem, can be developed. Apart from learning to express our emotions and communicate better, see below, we can also improve how well we relate by being more tolerant; for example, by respecting one another's privacy and differences of opinion, and by developing a sense of humor.

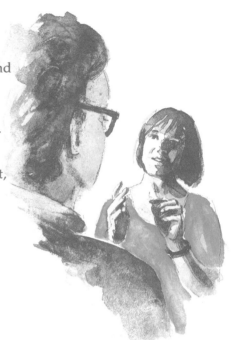

Expressing emotions

Acknowledging and expressing how we feel is healing, both for ourselves and our relationships. But sadly, many of us learn at an early age to suppress our tears or anger, or to rationalize away our strongest feelings. As adults we may then hold back, fearing that we will hurt or be rejected by others if we reveal our true feelings, or that we may be overwhelmed or lose control. In fact this generally makes matters worse, creating distance between us and our friends and partners or building up resentment. In the long run, the inability to express emotions is known to be a major cause of minor problems, such as headaches, as well as of serious illness.

If you tend to suppress your feelings.

● Learn to acknowledge to yourself how you feel, identifying the cause of your sadness, anger, etc. Try to express your feelings directly in relation to that cause.

● Try to say what's on your mind at the time, rather than bottling it up or coming out with it later.

● Share your feelings of sadness or fear with others, rather than denying them or keeping them to yourself.

● Find outlets for anger and aggression that do not harm others, eg, challenging physical exercise, or shouting from the top of a hill.

Communication skills

Communication can easily break down under stress as blame, criticism, defensiveness or impatience cloud what could be a clear interchange. To communicate more effectively:

● Listen carefully, giving the other person your full attention

● Tell the other person if you don't understand and ask him or her to re-phrase the point

● Don't interrupt. Allow the other person to finish speaking

● State your needs directly – don't drop hints or assume the other person knows what you want.

Understanding anxiety and depression

Anxiety is the brain's "alarm response" to a physical or psychological threat, real or imagined. Depression covers a complex range of conditions with a great variety of causes, both external and internal, varying from unexpressed anger or unfinished mourning to sheer physical exhaustion or illness.

If you are suffering from either severe depression or anxiety, seek professional help, to enable you both to uncover the root cause and to learn new coping skills. Try if you can to avoid relying on prescribed drugs, such as valium – they may help you to cope in the short term but in the long run they suppress or mask the problem and may create dependency.

For acute anxiety, proper breathing or a relaxation technique is invaluable (pp.59 and 63), and for depression, exercise. With depression, it is also important to consider food allergies. In either case, the support of family and friends is crucial and a nourishing diet and a good balance of rest and exercise are strongly advised.

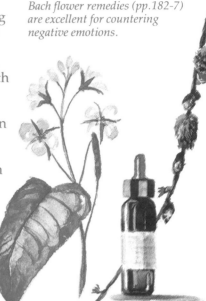

Bach flower remedies (pp.182-7) are excellent for countering negative emotions.

Positive self-help

In their early stages, both depression and anxiety may respond to a combination of positive thought and action.

● Sticking to regular mealtimes and doing mundane household chores encourages a sense of order at times when your inner life feels chaotic.

● Try to keep active rather than sit and brood. Physical activity, especially vigorous exercise, gets you back in touch with your body, and out of the habit of living in your head.

● Try to involve yourself wholeheartedly in whatever you are doing, whether it is cooking, writing a letter or making love. Learning to be fully in the present will give you more satisfaction and stop you worrying about the past or future.

● Treat yourself with kindness and compassion. Be tolerant and encouraging – don't keep putting yourself down. This may be easier if you imagine yourself as you were when young and realize that you still carry this child within you.

● Take a look at the roles you play in life – for example, mother, lover, meditative gardener, etc. Don't over-identify with any one of them, especially the "negative" ones. The more conscious you are of your roles, the more they can enrich your life without ruling it and the more clearly you can distinguish them from your real self.

● Choose natural remedies rather than drugs (see chart of ailments, p.132 and p.140).

Exploring psychotherapy

Many people shy away from the whole notion of therapy, because of its connection with mental illness. But you don't have to be "sick" to benefit from therapy. More and more people are choosing a form of psychotherapy simply to understand themselves better, or to find greater harmony.

There are many different psychological therapies available in both orthodox and complementary medicine. They range from psychoanalysis and individual counselling to group therapies, and from purely psychological approaches to those that involve bodywork. Some of the more common alternative therapies available are described below.

Since they deal with the whole person, all natural therapies affect both mental and physical health, but among them, six stand out as being especially valuable for psychological distress – meditation (pp.314-17), yoga, the Alexander technique (pp.284-97), hypnotherapy (pp.310-13), autogenics, and biofeedback (pp.318-21).

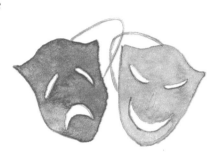

Bioenergetics

This body/mind therapy uses breathing techniques, body postures and other exercises. Many of the exercises place the body under stress, allowing you to become aware of and to release tension and suppressed emotions.

Transactional analysis (TA)

This is a group therapy, designed to enable you to understand and improve your "transactions" or communication with other people. It brings to light the "games" you play and the way you may switch between functioning as "parent", "adult" and "child".

Encounter

A form of group therapy, encounter helps you to discover yourself, by "encountering" and using feedback from other members of the group. It encourages direct expression of feelings and it teaches you to relate to people around you more honestly.

Psychosynthesis

This aims at synthesis of the psyche, helping you to integrate your personality and to contact and use your "transpersonal" self. Many techniques are involved in the process, including guided imagery, meditation, and journal-keeping.

Primal therapy and rebirthing

The goal of primal therapy is to help you to relive and integrate the traumatic experiences you may have had in the womb, during birth, or in infancy. Various techniques are used, including hypnosis and massage. Rebirthing encourages you to re-experience the birth trauma.

Co-counselling

This is a method of personal development in which, after training, two lay people take turns as "client" and "counsellor". The process encourages the re-evaluation and release of painful feelings, eg, inadequacy, loneliness, or anger.

Sex

Sex is central to our lives, as a means of expressing ourselves – emotionally, physically and spiritually. It is a way of communicating, and of giving and receiving pleasure at the most intimate level. Western people think of sex as a primarily physical activity, but in the East it has long been regarded as a powerful instrument to increase self-awareness.

Until recently, sex was regarded as something of a taboo in the West, but today, the advent of freely available contraception (pp.100-101), as well as a general broadening of views, have made it possible to separate sex from procreation and to encompass the view that people of all ages and persuasions have a right to express themselves sexually – married, single, old and young, homosexual and heterosexual.

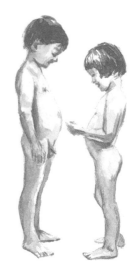

It is important not to discourage young children from learning about their bodies.

Is sex good for you?

Surprisingly, very little scientific evidence exists about the health-producing effects of sex. The only positive evidence comes from a study of middle-aged men which found that those who regularly enjoyed sex were less likely to have a heart attack than those who did not. Few of us, though, think of having sex for the good of our health. For most of us, sex answers a profound need for emotional acceptance and physical release and adds to our sense of well-being. Most people also claim that their self-esteem is higher when their sex lives are good.

What makes sex good?

A great many factors affect sexual activity, from age and physical fitness to mood and levels of stress. But above all it is your emotional well-being that affects your sex life – feeling good about yourself as well as your partner, and being able to communicate your needs. If you have not come to terms with your own sexuality, you are unlikely to enjoy a full sexual relationship with someone else. Real sexual sharing depends on openness and trust.

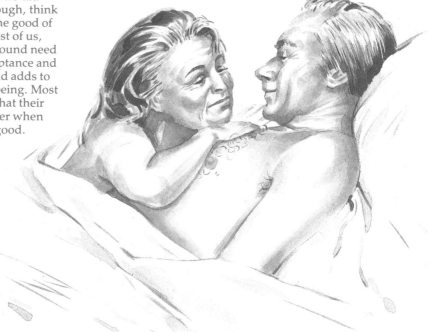

Why sex goes wrong

All of us experience times when our need for, or enjoyment of, sex drops – perhaps as a result of our general state of health, our work, or financial problems. But for some, sex is a continual source of anxiety or dissatisfaction. Ignorance of how our bodies work is responsible for many sexual problems and this is often compounded by an inability to talk about our likes and dislikes with one another. Since sexuality and ideas about sex are shaped in childhood, you may also need to unlearn a great deal that you have unconsciously absorbed. Other factors that may hinder free sexual expression are a lack of self-esteem, and fear – whether of rejection, pregnancy, or of looking foolish.

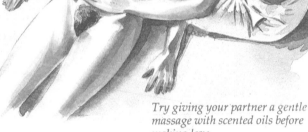

Try giving your partner a gentle massage with scented oils before making love.

Self-help measures

If you feel that you have never got the most out of sex – or certainly could get more – there are several ways you can help yourself. Since many problems are made worse by nervousness and tension, it may help to learn how to relax with relaxation exercises (p.63). Although sexual hang-ups are more often emotional than physical in origin, they are often easier resolved through working with the body. Taking up any form of regular physical exercise will not only give you more energy but also help you to feel more at ease with your body.

As a couple, there are many ways in which you can heighten your pleasure – perhaps by making love by candlelight or to your favorite music. Simply touching one another will help you to get to know your own and your partner's body and sensitivities better.

Getting professional help

While some problems can be overcome with a caring partner, others call for help from a sex therapist or psychosexual counsellor. But before consulting a therapist or counsellor, see your doctor, to confirm that there is nothing wrong with you physically.

Therapists treat both individuals and couples and help you to understand your fears about sex and communicate your needs. Many forms of sex therapy now incorporate a method called "sensate focus", in which couples learn about their own and their partner's responses through touching one another – initially avoiding genital contact, ultimately (after several weeks) progressing to intercourse when both partners feel ready.

Alternatively you could consider one of the body-mind therapies such as Rolfing (pp.264-7), which over time will help to dissolve your body "armor" and enable you to deal with emotional problems through releasing physical tensions.

Sleep and dreams

There are many different theories relating to the psychological and physiological roles of sleeping and dreaming, but what is generally agreed is that they play a crucial part in maintaining our mental and physical equilibrium. Good sleep does not need to last a set number of hours – some people wake up refreshed after only a few hours, while others rely on much more. More important than the quantity of sleep is its quality. If we are wound up when we go to bed, sleep with our bodies tense, or lose valuable dreaming time (see below), we are unlikely to feel relaxed when we wake up.

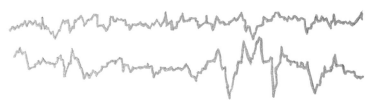

Brainwave traces in early sleep (left, above) show the same small irregularities as when we are awake. The traces during deep sleep (left, below) show large, slow, wave-like movements. Heart rate and breathing are slow and steady, and muscles have relaxed.

The patterns of sleep

An average night has a series of 4 or 5 sleep cycles, each lasting 1½ to 2 hours and consisting of a standard pattern of 5 stages. The first 4 stages in each cycle are known as "orthodox" sleep to distinguish them from the fifth stage, "dream sleep". During orthodox sleep, brain waves slow right down, and bodily functions, such as blood pressure, decrease. Eventually hormone production (from the pituitary gland) increases, and this has a restorative effect on the whole body.

Then in the fifth stage, REM (rapid eye movement) sleep, sleep lightens and vivid dreams begin; the eyes move rapidly under closed lids, as if you are watching something. The more REM sleep we have the better we function mentally.

To sleep, perchance to dream

Since the beginning of recorded history, dream interpretation has been a source of fascination. The ancient Greeks, for example, regarded dreams as having both a curative and a prophetic function. Freud, the great pioneer of dream study in the 20th century, was the first to perceive dreams as a gateway to understanding the unconscious mind. Though interpretations vary widely, what seems certain is that dreams allow us to consolidate experiences and information and help us to deal with unresolved tensions.

Clinical tests have proved that without REM sleep we get moody and anxious, as well as becoming more prone to infection. Dream research has also shown that dreams may last for no more than a fraction of a second, and that they can be deliberately used to solve problems in the dreamer's life.

Keeping a dream diary

Studying your dreams can give you a unique insight into your inner life. Try keeping a notebook and pen by your bed so that you can jot them down the moment you wake up. With practice, you can do this while you are still half-conscious. Note the settings of your dreams, the people involved, the activities, colors, emotions, and words used. If you want to dream about a particular subject, try meditating on it before you go to sleep.

Coping with insomnia

A good sleep regenerates the body, repairs damaged tissues and cells, and strengthens the immune system, as well as helping you to feel mentally relaxed. Difficulties in sleeping affect about 1 in 5 of us at some stage of our lives – and most people suffer from disturbed sleep from time to time. There's no need to worry if you sleep badly for a short period.

If you suffer from recurrent insomnia, look first at possible causes, such as particular stress factors in your life, and deal with these (pp.60-3). Try simple self-help measures (below) for a few weeks. If none of these work for you, add a natural remedy (p.133). Whatever you do, try to avoid taking sleeping tablets, except for a brief respite at times of intense shock or grief. All sleeping tablets have side-effects, and mar normal sleep, affecting how much and how well you dream. And some tablets are addictive.

Dietary aids

Avoid stimulating drinks, such as tea or coffee, cocoa, or cola drinks, before bedtime, replacing them with a soothing herb tea, such as lemon verbena or chamomile, or a protein snack, such as yoghurt or milk. You can also try taking a protein supplement that contains the amino acid tryptophan. Take it 20 minutes before retiring, together with some vitamin B6 and calcium. These will relax you and give the body the raw materials from which to make serotonin, a natural sleep-inducing substance.

Relaxation techniques

Use a method of relaxation (p.63) or meditation at least once a day. And take some active exercise at mid-day or in the early evening, especially if your occupation involves a lot of mental work and you find it hard to "switch off". If you tend to wake up early, try practicing relaxation or meditation then – or start the day early. You can introduce a mid-day nap to make up for it, without detracting from the next night's sleep.

Sleeping routines

Look at your sleep and pre-sleep rituals and see if there have been any changes. Could the cause be too much or too little activity, perhaps, or the wrong mattress or bedclothes? If old patterns gave you better sleep, try to recreate them. If sleep is slow in coming, try to visualize a single object, or keep repeating a sound or word, while you practice a relaxing breathing exercise (p.59). Most people find this very effective.

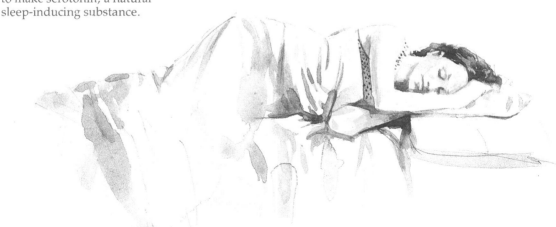

CHAPTER THREE

The cycle of life

According to surveys, most of us feel we have little control over our health. We think of disease as something to be put up with, preferably without grumbling, and regard the stresses our lives may impose as unavoidable hazards. But we can take action in advance.

In this chapter we look at the times of greatest change in life, from conception to the later years, examining the health issues associated with each particular stage, to enable you to anticipate and, where possible, avoid potential problems. Thus you will find advice on ensuring that children grow up with a good posture, for example, or with healthy feet. We also focus on the considerations you may confront in changing to a more natural, health-promoting lifestyle – such as knowing the safe limit of alcohol consumption, or choosing a different form of contraception. We have concentrated on the target areas of preventive health throughout life, bringing in both emotional and physical factors, for emotional contentment naturally results in fewer physical problems. And at all stages we have shown in what way the natural therapies can help.

Planning a healthy future

When you are young it's difficult to believe that the way you live now is going to affect your health later in life. From the perspective of youth, middle and old age seem like afflictions that happen to other people. But there is no doubt that your lifestyle in early adulthood does have a bearing on your fitness later on. Your diet and occupation, your home and working environment, your family and social life are all factors you need to consider deeply in taking more responsibility for your own health. For with a little awareness, you can plan for a happier and healthier future.

A constructive approach to future health strategy would be to look at the health of your parents and grandparents and see what you can do by way of prevention. Diseases and health problems do run in families, partly because we pick up our parents' bad habits, partly because we tend to grow up in the same environment as our parents, and partly because of genetics. So if one of your parents suffers from heart trouble, for example, you would do well to take steps to alter your lifestyle, to prevent this tendency dominating your life later on.

Your responsibility as parents

If you have a family, of course, you have a dual obligation, not only to take care of your own health but to protect the next generation's too. Children learn by example, and are quick to copy their parents' habits, both good and bad. Diet is of prime importance, for the way you feed young children sets the pattern for life. A taste for sweet, salty or refined foods is laid down in childhood and can be extremely difficult to reverse later on, especially in adult life. And too much junk food gives inadequate protection against infection, exposing children to minor illnesses that, with a wholesome diet, they should be able to resist.

Seeing that children get plenty of exercise and fresh air is also important. Far too many spend their lives sitting in front of a television for hours every day and regard walking or other forms of exercise as some sort of punishment. As parents it's a good idea to teach children that exercise is fun – ideally, you should try to find a recreational pursuit you can all enjoy together, such as swimming or yoga or walking.

Finally, don't make the mistake of neglecting your own well-being in your eagerness to give as much as possible to your family. By taking care of your own health and making time for your relationship, you will be able to give far more to your children.

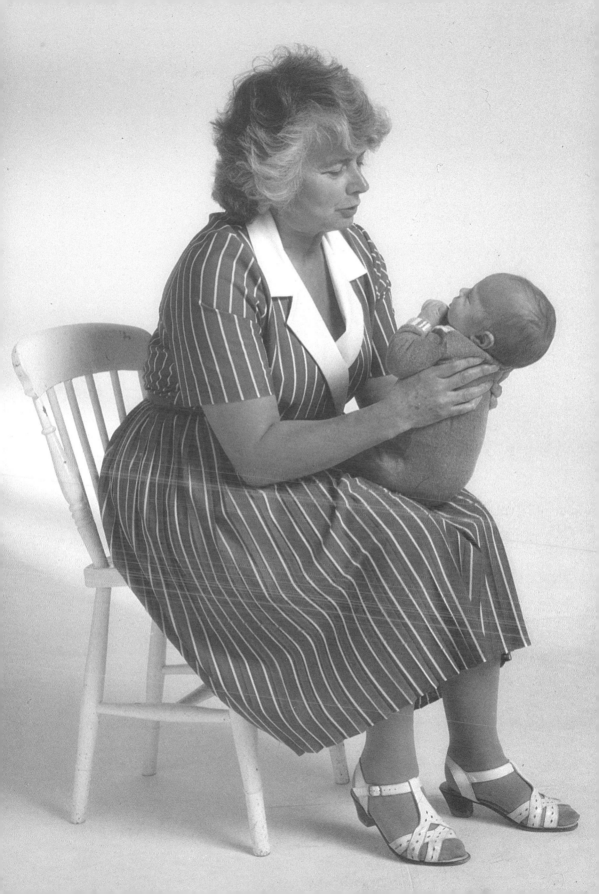

Foundations for life

In the past, it was always thought that starting to care for a baby began with birth. But in recent years it has become clear that the future health of a child can be influenced by preconceptual and ante-natal care. To some extent the health of the fetus depends on the quality of sperm and egg – and this in turn is governed by the health of the parents who produce them.

Today, preconceptual care is a field of expanding interest and research and any prospective parents are advised to consider the guidelines outlined below well before conception. It makes sense for both partners to stop taking medication, alcohol, and tobacco some months ahead of conception. Sperm, for example, take three months to form in a man, so noxious substances may adversely affect sperm a long time before conception.

Longest cycle | 1 2 3 4 5 6 7 8 9 10 11 12 13 14 15 16 17 18 19 20 21 22 23 24 25 26 27 28 29 30 31 | subtract 11 days

Shortest cycle | 1 2 3 4 5 6 7 8 9 10 11 12 13 14 15 16 17 18 19 20 21 22 23 24 25 26 | subtract 18 days

Possible fertility | 1 2 3 4 5 6 7 8 9 10 11 12 13 14 15 16 17 18 19 20 21 22 23 24 25 26 27 28 29 30 31 | fertile period

Record of menstruation

Preconceptual health precautions

Three to six months before you plan to try for a baby, take the following precautions:

Men and women:
● Stop all medication (after discussion with your doctor)

● Stop smoking and drinking

● Take extra care to eat a nutritious, wholesome diet (p.47) – one that is rich in vitamins and minerals and low in refined foods.
Nutritional supplements should not be necessary, but it is advisable to be aware of the specific vitamins and minerals recommended for fertility (p.46)

● Take regular exercise to ensure fitness and suppleness (pp.53-5)

● Go for a general health check-up to test for any possible allergies or diseases that may be potentially hazardous to the fetus

● If possible, get your drinking water analysed for levels of lead, copper, cadmium and aluminium, or drink bottled water only.

Women:
● Stop taking the contraceptive pill and use another, preferably barrier, method (p.101)

● Have a blood test to check that you are immune to rubella (German measles)

● Have a gynecological examination to check for pelvic or vaginal diseases.

Conception time

Keeping a record of menstruation helps to identify a woman's fertile days (and it is useful, if you do conceive, for estimating the date when the baby is due). To get an accurate picture of your average fertile period in each month, you should keep a record of the monthly cycle for at least 8 consecutive months. Count the onset of bleeding as day one; and the day before bleeding as the last day of the last cycle.

For the first day of possible fertility subtract 18 from the number of days in the shortest cycle; for the last fertile day subtract 11 from the days in the longest cycle, as shown above. These 2 days are the boundaries of your average fertile period and if you are trying to get pregnant, this is when to make love most often.

Pregnancy

It's vitally important to attend an ante-natal clinic regularly, and it helps if both partners attend classes to prepare for birth and parenthood, especially if this is your first child.

In pregnancy women have a dual responsibility to stay healthy because anything taken in to the mother's body will affect the baby too. This means taking special care with diet and avoiding any unprescribed medication and environmental toxins and hazards. Several natural therapies offer safe remedies for problems like morning sickness (p.138); others, such as massage, shiatsu, or reflexology, are useful for relaxing the body and helping to ease any aches or pains. Raspberry leaf tea is beneficial in the last few months before birth (p.225).

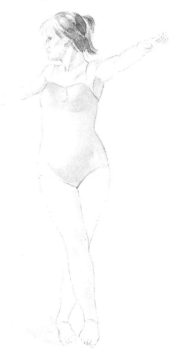

Standing spinal twist

Health in pregnancy checklist
● Have a dental check-up in the early months

● Stay away from tobacco and alcohol – both are demonstrably harmful to the developing fetus; avoid smoky places too

● Avoid X-rays, and environmental pollutants (p.72)

● Avoid unprescribed medication. Use natural remedies where possible

● Keep a balance between activity and rest – both regular exercise and relaxation are important during this time, as well as plenty of sound sleep.

Healthy eating
The needs of most mothers-to-be will be met by a well-balanced diet, but you should pay special attention to getting the nutrients that are needed in greater quantity than normal (p.46). Babies from allergic families can become sensitized while in the womb, so don't binge on any one food during pregnancy. And try to avoid putting on too much unnecessary weight.

Resting
For a comfortable position for sleeping or relaxing, try raising one knee while lying on your front, and place a pillow under the abdomen, as shown below.

Exercise and posture
A good posture is vital in pregnancy. Take special care of your back (p.234) as backstrain is common. You can generally carry on with any sport as long as it feels comfortable. Yoga exercises help to strengthen and stretch the body in preparation for birth, but some poses may need to be modified. The spinal twist (p.289), for example, can be practiced in a standing position, as shown above. Cross your legs, right in front of left, stretch your arms, and twist to the left. Repeat, reversing these directions.

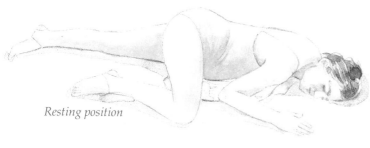

Resting position

Birth

Until very recently most births were controlled by the medical profession and normally took place in hospital. Over the last two decades or so things have changed, however – many alternative ways of giving birth are now available.

In order to get the kind of birth you would most like, you need to ask and prepare for it as soon as you know you are pregnant. Among the options you will need to consider are: whether or not you want some form of pain relief and, if so, what form (see below); in what position you would prefer to give birth; whether you would like your partner to be with you; and whether you would like to have the baby at home or in hospital and, if in hospital, which one suits your requirements best in terms of facilities and policy.

Homeopathic remedies for labor pains
Homeopathic medicines can be taken, without risk to the baby, during the birth as well as in pregnancy and after the delivery. The remedies can help to reduce pain and encourage a safe, straight-forward delivery (p.156).

Easing labor
Giving birth can hurt, and most women want help in handling the powerful sensations they experience. Until recently pain relief in the form of drugs was taken very much for granted, but drugs carry some risk of side-effects for the woman, and they can affect the baby.

Today, other methods of pain relief are available, and women should exercise the right to choose whether they want to rely entirely or partly on medical sedation, or whether they prefer a drug-free alternative, such as: relaxation and breathing exercises, widely taught in classes; acupuncture; hypnosis (generally self-hypnosis); massage; or shiatsu. Perhaps the most natural pain-relieving method is to give birth in an upright position (p.93).

Natural birth techniques have the advantage of

Massage provides reassurance and relaxation in labor.

enabling you to relax, while at the same time retaining the control you need in order to use your body efficiently. Exercising this control may well improve the whole experience of giving birth.

Massage in labor
Massage can provide valuable support in labor. It should either be given by a professional, or by a very well-practiced amateur, and the mother-to-be should be quite accustomed to the process. She can lie on her side, as shown above, while the masseur or masseuse works on the lower back and buttocks to relax the muscles – or sit up with her legs apart, so that pressure in the belly or tension in the thighs can be released.

Active birth

The main purpose of active birth is to help the woman in labor to control the process. During labor she can move about freely and take whatever position she finds most comfortable. If she is standing, sitting, squatting or kneeling, the force of gravity helps the pressure of the baby's head to stretch the cervix, and makes the womb's contractions more effective. The effort required to push the baby out is considerably reduced. The baby benefits from a better supply of oxygen, and labor tends to be shorter. Practicing squatting in the months before the birth will help to open out the pelvic area. Unfortunately, hospital facilities for active birth and staff trained in this approach are still relatively scarce.

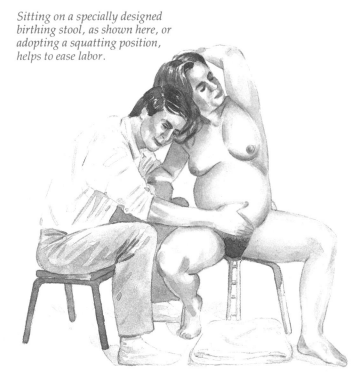

Sitting on a specially designed birthing stool, as shown here, or adopting a squatting position, helps to ease labor.

Bonding

Putting the newborn baby to the breast starts the production of hormones that contract the uterus and expel the placenta. It also gets the mother's milk production going, giving the baby a valuable substance called colostrum, rich in antibodies to protect against disease.

No baby should be taken from its mother straight after birth unless it is too ill to remain outside an incubator. The first contact is when bonding starts and research has found that babies who are handled and caressed right from the start grow and thrive better in every way.

A gentle environment

This is one of the prime considerations of natural birthing (apart from, of course, the well-being of the baby). The French obstetrician Frédéric Leboyer pioneered gentle birth methods, which include the use of a semi-darkened, peaceful room and soft voices, with a view to minimizing what he believed to be the traumatic experience of being born. Modifications of this method include Michel Odent's famous birthing pool, where women give birth in warm water. Sympathetic caring staff and a partner or other trusted friends to be with the laboring woman can also transform the experience.

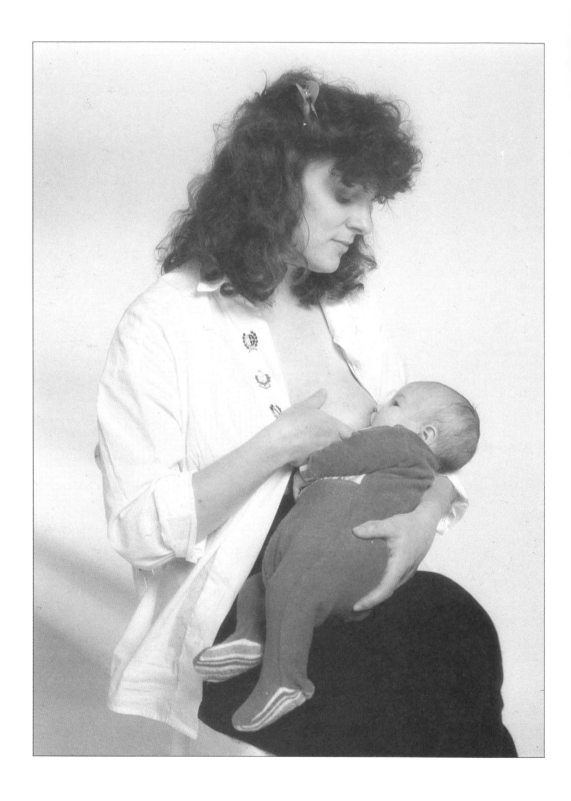

New life

However much you have wanted and planned for a baby, its birth is the starting point of a whole new lifestyle. Your relationship with your partner is transformed by parenthood and the new responsibility for the care and development of another human being. The trend today is for couples to share the physical and emotional demands of parenthood far more than they did a generation ago.

Of the natural therapies, homeopathy is particularly useful for babies and children, providing safe, effective remedies for common problems such as colic, teething troubles and nappy rash (pp.158-9). Always consult a professional if your baby's symptoms are unusual, alarming, or persistently distressing (pp.115-16).

Breast-feeding

The best possible way of nourishing a baby is to breast-feed it. It doesn't simply supply him or her with milk – it is also the child's surest way of feeling close to the mother. Breast milk provides a baby with a host of benefits nutritionally, and by passing on the mother's immunity, it gives a far greater resistance to infection than artificial feeding and minimizes the likelihood of allergies (see Allergies in babies, p.175). You should continue with breast milk as the sole source of feeding for at least 4-6 months before introducing other foods into the diet. While breast-feeding, women need to take particular care with their diet (p.46, p.139, p.175). Homeopathy offers a range of remedies for problems with breast-feeding (p.157).

Bottle-feeding

For the small number of women who cannot breast-feed and for those who choose not to, there are several alternatives. Bottle-feeding with cows' milk formula is the obvious choice, but for those whose babies are allergic to cows' milk, goats' milk or a good quality soya milk are recommended. Though none are as good as breast milk nutritionally, bottle-fed babies can still be comforted and cuddled while feeding in the same way as those who are breast-fed. Bottle-feeding also enables fathers to play a greater part in nourishing the newborn.

Touch and massage

For a baby, touch is essential – both as a source of pleasure and comfort and as a means of bonding and communication. It is by touch that babies discover themselves as well as the world around them. They need toys of different textures and shapes to stimulate their curiosity. Babies should be held, stroked, rocked and cradled, to support and encourage all aspects of their development, physical and psychological.

Massaging your baby, as shown above, is also highly beneficial. It is a familiar part of child-rearing in many countries. Parents find that it improves sleep and feeding and relieves colic.

A natural childhood

It is up to you as parents to teach your children the elements of a healthy life and to instil good habits for the future, through caring and example.

Diet is of crucial importance. Babies can be weaned straight on to adult food from about 4 to 6 months, but it's best to keep them off all sugary, salty, refined foods, and additives (pp.44-5). Watch out for any possible reaction to gluten (pp.338-41), and go very gently with foods which may cause allergies (p.175). Avoid at all costs making food an area of conflict. Let children eat what and how much they like, provided it is healthy food. And establish regular mealtimes and bedtimes right from the start.

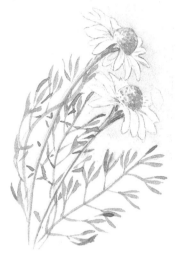

Chamomile, an excellent herb for childhood ailments

Emotional development

Love, care, security and continuity are every bit as important as satisfying your children's physical needs.

A vital part of bringing up young children is to ensure that they will be able to be independent members of the community when they grow up. Clinical experience shows that children who are made to feel secure in the unconditional love of their parents during their earliest years are much more able to stand on their own feet when they go to school, and indeed later on in life. There is no danger of spoiling a child at this time. Children also need your understanding and encouragement in learning to do things for themselves, to fulfil their growing need for independence. Look out for some toys and games that are fun but have an educational value as well. Children learn best through play.

Telling a child about sex should come naturally. There's almost never any need to talk to young children formally on the subject. Just deal with the questions as they come up, and answer as simply and honestly as you can.

Natural therapies in childhood

Children can safely be given natural remedies for common ailments like colds, coughs and headaches, and there are also a number of specific remedies for childhood diseases, such as chickenpox or mumps (pp.158-9). Homeopathy or herbalism are perhaps the most popular complementary therapies for home use; naturopathy (pp.188-207) also provides a great range of preventive and remedial treatments; and the Bach flower remedies (pp.182-7) are excellent for emotional problems and times of change.

The great hazard to be aware of is that sick children, especially very young ones, can go downhill very quickly. Whatever your views about natural medicines, it makes sense to get medical help if your child doesn't get better quickly on the treatment you are trying.

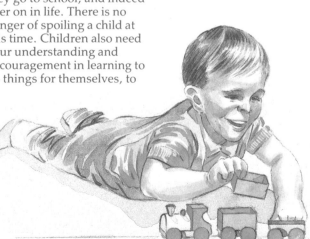

Making strong teeth

Proper food, daily brushing (p.67), and regular dental visits will ensure your children stand the best possible chance of keeping their teeth for life. Give them plenty of calcium-rich foods (p.41) and food that encourages chewing, such as fruit or raw vegetables, to help make strong teeth and gums. To prevent tooth decay, avoid buying food and drinks with sugar in them and keep sweets down to the minimum – make sweets an occasional treat after a meal, getting your children in the habit of brushing their teeth afterwards. Help to brush your children's teeth until school age, and check that they do it properly, at least once a day, when they learn to brush their own teeth.

Growing healthy feet

In adult life, three out of four people suffer from some form of foot problem – and much of it could be prevented by proper foot care in childhood and in the teenage years. The bones of the foot are pliable during the early years and they grow fast. Prevent bunions and other physical distortions from developing by ensuring that socks aren't tight and shoes are wide enough and at least half an inch (1.3 cm) longer than the big toe. If you keep shoes to pass around the family, check the fit carefully. Whenever possible, let your child go barefoot, to strengthen the foot muscles.

Posture

Children who get in the habit of moving and holding themselves badly will develop physical deformities later, such as round shoulders or knock knees. Encourage your child to stand and sit up straight and to walk with straight, forward-pointing feet. Chairs should be low enough for the child's feet to reach the floor and should support the base of the spine; beds should be firm (p.71).

If you do notice any physical defects, seek specialist help from a

Rolfing

Before treatment, the young girl pictured on the right suffered from "swayback" and a forward-tilted pelvis, imbalances which frequently cause chronic backache in later life. After ten sessions of Rolfing this problem was corrected, as shown far right. Two years later the child showed the same much improved posture.

Health checks and precautions

● Keep up to date with vaccinations and routine medical check-ups, especially in the first 5 years

● Take children to the dentist every 6 months from the age of 3 onwards

● Make sure that they get the right nutrients (pp.46-7)

manipulative therapist, such as an osteopath, an Alexander teacher, or a Rolfer. A course of Rolfing sessions often produces a dramatic and lasting improvement in posture, as shown below. Yoga is excellent too, encouraging natural flexibility and a sense of balance.

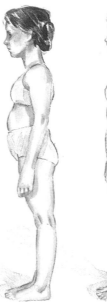

Before Rolfing treatment   *After ten sessions*

● See that your children get sufficient exercise

● Pay close attention to safety factors: protect your children from household hazards (pp.76-7); teach them to beware of strangers, and to tell you if anyone tries to touch them on any part of the body.

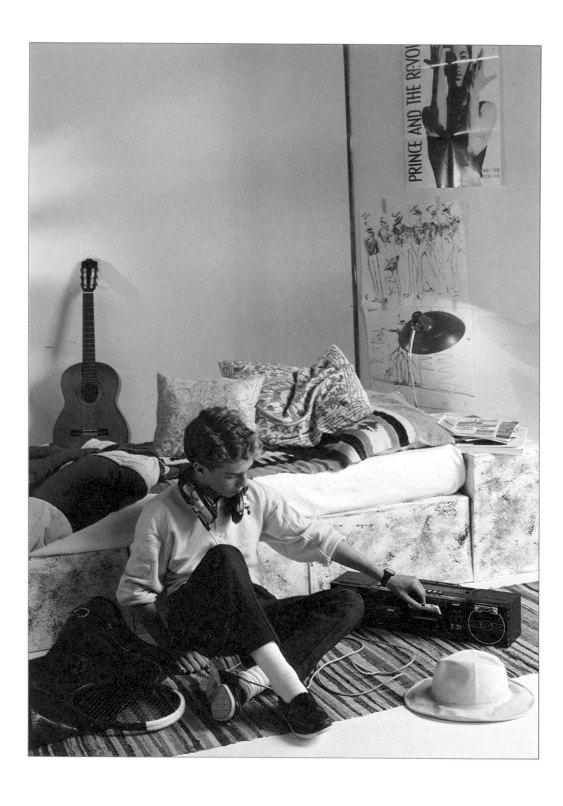

Puberty and teenage years

From the ages of approximately 9 to 18 a young person develops sexually into an adult. This is a time of profound changes, in body shape and hormone production as well as sexual development. In early puberty (from around 9 to 14) physical changes are dominant, while later the focus shifts to the teenager's need to establish his or her own identity and increasingly to take on the role of an adult. Parents can give valuable help at this time, by freely, and with humor, sharing their knowledge of relationship and health issues and of contraception (pp.100-101).

Rebellion is common during adolescence, but frequent battles should be avoided, since the average teenager is all too vulnerable to insecurity and self-doubt. Parental understanding and approval are important, but clear and fair household rules to ensure that all members of the household enjoy some privacy and adequate protection from disruption are also necessary.

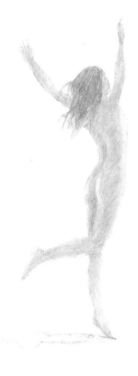

Preventive health care

Teenagers rarely think much about preventive health care, but proper exercise and a well-balanced diet will not only promote health but also help to prevent many common ailments, such as puppy fat, skin disorders, and menstrual problems; various therapies provide remedies (pp.122-40).

The teenage years may be a time of strong peer group pressure, to start smoking, drinking, taking drugs or to indulge irresponsibly in sex. All of these activities are provably damaging to the health, physically and emotionally, and may have long-term consequences. Parents can help by encouraging trust and open communication on all subjects, without reserve.

Growing pains

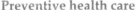

From a parent's point of view it may be difficult to separate teenage moodiness from early signs of health problems, such as anorexia or drug abuse, but a sensitive parent should be able to recognize real trouble when it is brewing, and to know when professional help is necessary. Be alert to any marked change in usual health, behavior or mood patterns and, in particular, to any of the warning signs described below:

• Serious loss in weight or obsessional slimming (anorexia nervosa)

• Vomiting and excessive use of laxatives (bulimia)

• Frequently smelling of alcohol or being out of control – teenage alcoholism is an increasing problem

• Sleeping tablets, sedatives and tranquillizers disappearing – keep them locked up

• Unexplained disappearance of things from the house – money, or belongings which may be being sold to support a drug habit; unexplained bruises, scratches or needle marks; strange smells on clothes (from drug abuse or glue sniffing).

Contraception

The first experience of sexual intercourse is a great milestone in life. A large number of contraceptive devices are available, but unfortunately no method is both 100 percent effective and completely free from long- and short-term health risks. The choice will depend on many factors, such as interest in natural health, sexual habits, and how undesirable an unwanted pregnancy would be. The best-known natural method is the careful identification of "unsafe", fertile days by the female partner. (Withdrawal by the male partner is both unsafe and unsatisfactory and so is not included here.)

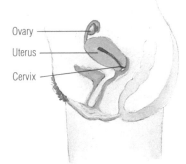

Ovary
Uterus
Cervix

Female reproductive organs

NATURAL CONTRACEPTION		
Method	**Advantages (+)** **Disadvantages (−)**	**Effectiveness**
Calendar A record of the menstrual cycle (p.90) is used to calculate the "unsafe" days in every month when there is a possibility of conception.	+ Costs nothing. No medical side-effects. − Unreliable. Demands constant attention. Bars intercourse for many days in each month.	Must be combined with other natural methods to ensure success.
Temperature This method requires that the woman keeps a record of her temperature (if possible with a basal body thermometer) every morning before rising. Her temperature drops slightly 24 hours before ovulation, then rises to a ½ degree higher than normal and remains high for up to 3 days. Intercourse should be avoided for at least 4 days, from the initial drop in temperature.	+ As above. − Indicates only when ovulation has begun. Demands a strict daily routine. Unreliability is increased by temperature variation during illness.	Must be used with other natural methods. Together with the cervical mucus method its effectiveness is rated high.
Cervical mucus The woman tests her cervical mucus daily, before rising. After menstruation, the vagina is dry, then mucus increases, becoming thick and cloudy at first. When ovulation is about to occur, it becomes slippery, thin and clear. Intercourse must be avoided at this time and for 3 full days afterwards.	+ As above. − As above.	Must be used with other natural methods, eg, temperature, see above.
State of the cervix The woman may be able to assess whether her cervix is open ("unsafe") or closed ("safe") by gently feeling for it internally. When it is receptive to sperm, it is softer and higher up in the abdomen, and its aperture is open.	+ As above. − Unreliable. Requires some experience and skill.	Must be combined with other natural methods.

BARRIER AND MEDICAL CONTRACEPTION		
Method	Advantages (+) Disadvantages (−)	Effectiveness
Sheath/condom A latex rubber sheath (with spermicide) applied to the erect penis acts as a barrier. After intercourse, when the sheath is removed, care must be taken not to spill the semen.	+ Simple to use. No side-effects. Method protects both partners from sexually transmitted diseases. − Interrupts sexual spontaneity. Lessens sensation.	97%
Diaphragm/cap Before intercourse, a dome-shaped rubber device is fitted by the woman over her cervix as a barrier against sperm. Spermicide is applied for added protection.	+ Easy to use. Causes no hormonal changes in the body. − Must first be supplied and fitted by a trained person. Not effective unless correctly inserted. Calls for at least some forethought.	97%
Spermicide Foams, jellies, cream or film are inserted in the vagina before intercourse to kill the sperm. It should only be used together with a sheath or diaphragm.	+ Provides extra lubrication. − May produce allergic reaction, although this is rare.	Only use with another device.
Vaginal sponge A specially designed sponge impregnated with spermicide is placed in the vagina before intercourse.	+ Easy to use. − Expensive.	75-85%
Intra-uterine device (IUD) A plastic or copper device is inserted, by a doctor or other health care professional, into the uterus (womb) to make it hostile to the fertilized egg.	+ Once in place can be ignored, apart from an occasional medical check-up that it remains in place. − Can cause infections, heavy menstruation, and spotting. Not recommended for women suffering from anemia, rheumatism, heart or kidney disease, or fibroids.	96-98%
Combined pill The Pill suppresses ovulation, making the body believe it is pregnant. It is taken 21-22 days running; then stopped for an interval to allow withdrawal bleeding to occur so that the woman appears to be menstruating.	+ Completely reliable if taken regularly. Not intrusive. Makes the timing of menstruation predictable. − Interferes with the hormones estrogen and progesterone. Experts usually advise against using it for longer than 5 years, or after the age of 40. Can damage nutritional balance (p.46).	Almost 100%
Mini-pill This contains no estrogen and is taken daily throughout the month. Suitable for over-35s.	+ As above. − Similar to the Combined pill.	98%

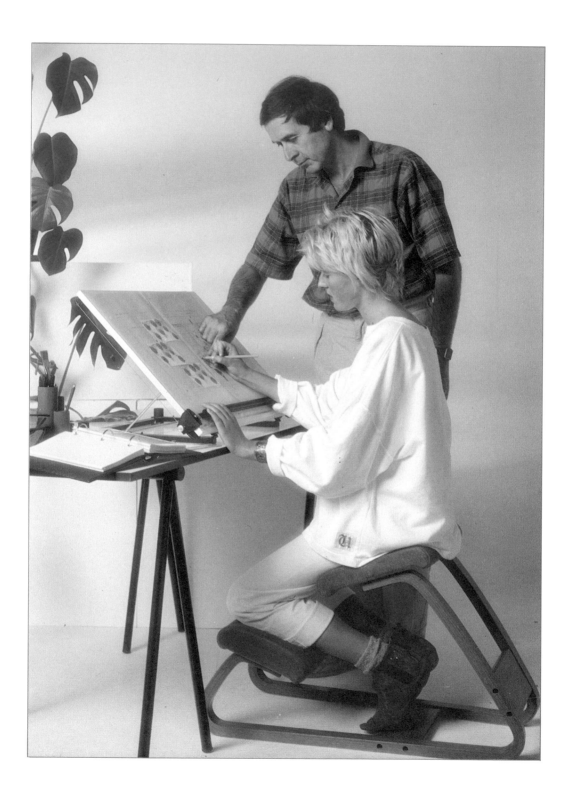

Adult life

Early adulthood is the best time to start a serious life-plan for future fitness and personal development, but you can still make many adjustments in middle years that will enhance and prolong your life. As well as making sure your basic diet is wholesome (pp.46-7), be aware of the dangers of alcoholism (p.105), smoking (p.57), and lack of exercise (p.49), and be sure to keep up with regular preventive health checks, summarized below.

Taking responsibility for your health means being in charge of other aspects of your life too – your relationships, work, and other resources. Think seriously about your whole lifestyle, weighing up alternative choices carefully.

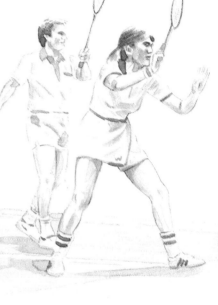

Health checks and precautions

Men and women:
- Keep near your ideal weight

- Have a dental check up every 6 months

- Get your blood pressure checked when you see your doctor, or at least once a year

- Have an electro-cardiogram done every 5 years after the age of 40

- Have your sight tested regularly, if you have poor sight

- Get your hearing tested every 5 years until age 65.

Women:
- Check your breasts once a month (p.104)

- Have a cervical cancer smear every 2 years

- Have a pelvic examination every 3 years.

Staying fit and relaxed

Fitness is important in young adulthood as well as in later years. Regular exercise maintains and builds a strong, supple frame with a sound cardio-respiratory system, and it helps to combat any tendency to put on weight. The form of exercise should be adapted to your lifestyle (p.48), and it should be balanced with relaxation – this becomes even more important as you enter the middle years.

Around the mid-40s the natural ageing process begins to show itself more obviously, especially if you are unfit, overtense, or overweight. This is a time when many people are at their best, emotionally and psychologically, but health risks are increasing. For example, about one in ten people in the West will have a peptic ulcer at some time – usually during middle age. The risk of heart disease, another stress-related problem, also increases at this time of life. Good diet, proper relaxation (p.63), and physical exercise will help to keep you young in mind and body. If you are taking up exercise for the first time in your middle years, look for an enjoyable sport that doesn't put excessive strain on your joints – swimming or walking, for example, rather than more strenuous activities.

Cancer – reducing the risks

Although many types of cancer are ill-understood, certain factors that make its incidence more likely have been clearly identified. It has been estimated that about 20% of all deaths are caused by cancer (in statistics from 10 European countries). In the UK, one in four people develops cancer at some point in their lives.

Physical factors It is well worth reducing the following known and suspected risk factors:

● Don't smoke – a third of all cancers result from tobacco smoke

● Go easy on alcohol – it contributes to cancers of the mouth, throat and larynx

● Watch your weight – obesity is associated with an increased risk, especially of breast cancer

● Take care in strong sunlight and make frequent use of a good sun barrier cream. Excessive exposure can cause skin cancer

● Avoid unnecessary exposure to X-rays and other ionizing radiations

● Make sure you take the necessary precautions if your work involves carcinogenic chemicals

● Eat plenty of green and yellow vegetables – these may reduce the likelihood of cancer

● Avoid too much saturated fat, which is linked with breast and colon cancers

● Include plenty of fiber in your diet – too little is associated with cancer of the colon. And avoid foods that are moldy

● Avoid promiscuous sex under the age of 20, if you are a woman – it appears to be linked with a higher incidence of cancer of the cervix.

Personality factors In addition to physical hazards, many specialists believe there is a link between cancer and personality traits or emotional factors, such as an inability to express anger, lack of self-esteem, and bereavement, since stress appears to weaken the immune system. On the positive side, cancer patients' chances of survival may be substantially increased if they respond to the disease with a fighting spirit rather than with despair or stoic acceptance.

Breast tests

Breast cancer is the commonest cancer in women. If it is detected early and treated promptly the success rate is high. All adult women should examine their breasts once a month after menstruation, to recognize any changes, by way of size, shape, lumps, or skin puckering.

   Start by looking at your breasts in a mirror. Check also with your arms up in the air. Now lie down on a flat surface, with a folded towel or small pillow under one

Breast testing

shoulder. Feel the breast on that side, using the flat of your fingers. Work systematically around the breast in a decreasing spiral, as shown above, and end by squeezing the nipple to see if there is any discharge. Now do the other breast. Finally, feel under your armpits. If you do find anything unusual, see your doctor at once. It may be just a cyst.

The "mid-life crisis"

While in men there is no exact parallel to the menopause, many men undergo a form of "mid-life crisis". In a culture that puts a great emphasis on youth and sex, middle-aged working men often begin to feel that life is passing them by. With regard to sexual activity it is all too easy to over-react to an individual failure. If you think you have a problem, check with your doctor or therapist that you have no physical illness or disability. Try stopping intercourse altogether for some weeks, and return to "courtship" behavior with your partner. Find time for gentle, invigorating exercise, such as yoga or swimming, and plenty of relaxation (pp.62-3).

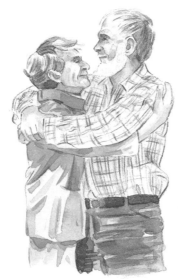

Don't be tempted to use alcohol to overcome fear of failure or sexual boredom. Some therapies offer remedies for loss of sex drive (p.134).

The menopause – treating it naturally

By the age of 48 half of all women will have stopped ovulating, though the exact age is influenced by several factors, such as genetics, smoking, stress, and nutrition. This is a period of transition, which most women go through with no ill effects. Some experience mild symptoms, such as hot flushes, sweating, dizziness, insomnia or headaches, which may be exacerbated by low vitality or a stressful lifestyle. A very small minority suffers more major problems. Unfortunately, the established medical solution, hormone replacement therapy (HRT), has been linked with major health risks and side-effects in some women.

Natural remedies For homeopathic or herbal remedies you must consult a professional. Aromatherapy offers a remedial massage with cypress oil (p.181), and you can also use shiatsu manipulation (p.283). Vitamin E is effective against hot flushes and insomnia, and appears to be especially successful when taken in conjunction with ginseng or vitamin B. Calcium supplements can reduce tension, backache, and hot flushes and, combined with vitamin D, keep the bones strong. The need for regular exercise is greater than ever during the menopause, and a technique such as yoga which balances the body systems can be extremely beneficial.

One standard drink =

a glass of wine

a small glass of sherry

a half pint of ordinary beer or lager

a measure of spirits

a measure of vermouth or aperitif

Alcohol – knowing your limits

What begins as moderate social drinking can easily escalate into a dangerous, self-destructive habit. In the West it is estimated that one in every twelve people, teenagers as well as adults, has a drinking problem. But where is the border line, the safe limit, and how much is too much? If you use one "standard" drink as a measure (see above), you can easily get a clear idea of how drinks compare and add up.

A safe limit for men is 5 or 6 standard drinks, 2 or 3 times a week. For women it is 2 or 3 standard drinks 2 or 3 times a week.

A man who drinks more than 8 standard drinks a day, or a woman who drinks more than 5 a day, is likely to suffer damage to health (p.45).

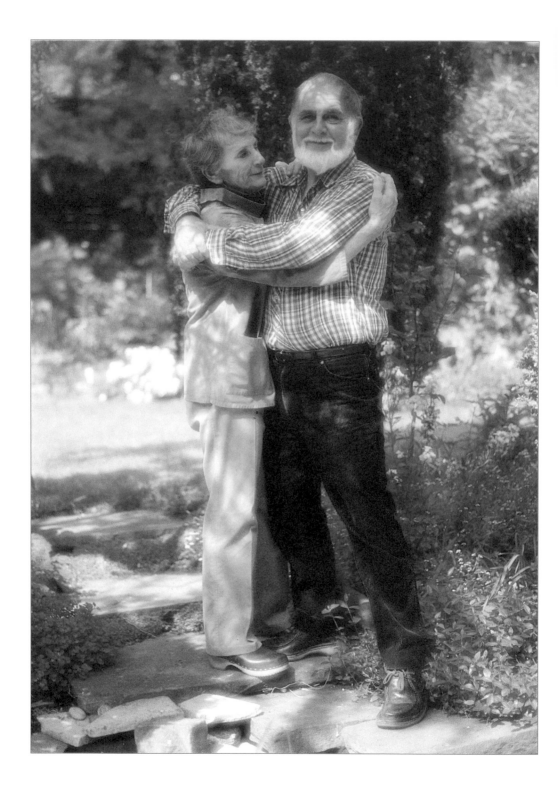

The later years

Old age can be a most fulfilling time of life, with leisure to devote to your physical and spiritual self. It is important to keep yourself active, with new interests, hobbies, and social activities. Practicing meditation as a daily routine, and taking regular, gentle exercise, such as yoga, can work wonders in helping to refresh and strengthen mind and body.

In the West, one recently identified cause of ill health in the elderly is the formidable "cocktail" effect of taking several drugs at once. Try to avoid such multiple prescriptions, and make the most of safe, natural remedies. Several body-mind therapies, such as massage, can solve health problems while giving a new sense of bodily ease and completeness.

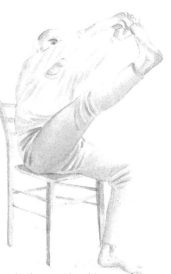

The forward bend is one of many yoga exercises that can be modified according to your level of fitness.

Health checks and precautions

Over the age of 65 you should have the following checks done regularly:

Men and women:
- Blood pressure, every year

- A rectal examination, every 2 years

- A hearing test, every 2 years

- A sight test, every 2 years

- An electro-cardiogram, every 5 years.

Women:
- A pelvic examination, every year

- A cervical cancer smear, every 2 years

- Examine your breasts once a month (p.104).

Optimum health and long life

Enjoying the later years is not just a matter of avoiding things that are bad for you. Anthropological studies of centenarians in the Soviet Caucasus, in Hunza, West Pakistan, and in Vilcambaba in Ecuador have isolated 6 factors shared by the different communities, that seem to promote a long and healthy life. They are:
1 Genetic influences
2 A low-calorie diet (around 1,700-1,900 K.cal.), low in animal foods, but rich in vegetables, fruit and grains
3 A diet low in cholesterol and saturated fats
4 A high degree of physical activity, from regular walking, farming, climbing and so on, guarding against cardiovascular disease
5 A high degree of sexual activity well into old age
6 Continued, active participation in family and community affairs.

Keeping fit in later life

Proper exercise has many health benefits (p.49). It gives you more energy, prevents joints stiffening, makes bones and muscles stronger, and protects you from heart disease. Walking, swimming, and yoga are all excellent forms of exercise, readily adapted to different levels of fitness. Yoga's forward bend (p.288), for example, is still beneficial when practiced in an easy sitting position in a chair, as shown above. If you suffer from stiffness and muscle tension, try osteopathy exercises (pp.232-5), or simply home massage (pp.245-7).

Variety is one of the keys to healthy eating. Make sure that you eat fresh fruit and vegetables, and sufficient protein. Avoid too much sugar or fat. Check that you are getting enough vitamin B, C, D, and iron (p. 46).

Death and bereavement

We tend to think of death as something which happens only at the end of our lives – as the final event of the life cycle. But in fact, it is more accurate to regard dying as a constant accompaniment to living. All through life parts of us die or wear out, parts of the body, objects we own, as well as people we love and share our lives with. The distress we feel reflects the value of what is lost, how much we depend on it to be ourselves, and whether we can replace it in our lives. We grieve most for what we feel we can never replace – an adored pet, a home we love but can never return to, a job we are forced to give up. And naturally, all of us find it hardest to adapt to the loss of our closest relatives and friends.

For most of us, bereavement plays a larger and larger part in life as we grow older. But if, throughout life, we can accept the part played in it by death, recognizing that our understanding of living can only be complete with our own dying, then we can approach both with openness and equanimity.

Therapies for grief

Healing and the Bach flower remedies can be of particular value in helping you to deal with grief. Homeopathy provides several remedies, including Ignatia which is suitable in many situations (p.155 and p.329). Generally it is better for the bereaved to be in touch with their emotions rather than to suppress them with tranquillizers.

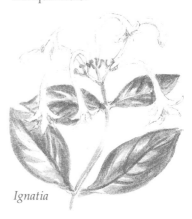

Ignatia

Grief and mourning

In order to come to terms with loss more easily when it happens we need to allow ourselves to grieve freely and openly, accepting and exercising our right to feel sadness, anger and fear, while avoiding the dangers of permanent, hidden resentment.

There are three main stages to the process of mourning, each of which need to be completed in order to move on to the next. In the first, you feel shocked and may try to protect yourself from what has happened by denying it. The second stage is marked by the realization that the loss has really occurred. This is the most painful phase, since you need to accept that the separation from the loved one is permanent. It is common to feel guilty at this time, especially about things that you feel you could, or should, have done. To complete this stage may take months or even years, depending on how important the person was to you and on whether you have help to allow you to talk through your feelings.

The final stage is a period of slow recovery, in which you can begin to function normally again. You may begin this phase in a matter of months if you can accept the process of mourning.

Helping the bereaved

The best way to help someone who is grieving is by offering your love and support. At first the bereaved person may want practical day-to-day help with keeping the household going, arranging the funeral, and so on. But more than anything he or she will need companionship, to be able to talk and express feelings and to feel less alone. Try not to burden the bereaved with your own feelings of loss (unless you too are personally affected by the death). At this time they will not have emotional room for the problems of others.

Death with dignity

Until recently there was little choice for the terminally ill – they either died in hospital, which to many seems impersonal, or at home, among family and friends often ill-equipped to cope with prolonged nursing care. Now the re-established hospice movement, based on a concept designed by Dr Cicely Saunders, offers a welcome alternative. Though normally run along similar lines to hospitals, hospices offer a far more friendly, relaxed and informal environment where visiting is encouraged at all times and patients are free to choose how their days are spent, even drinking or smoking if they wish. One of the inspirations for the hospice movement has been Dr Elizabeth Kubler-Ross, whose work with the terminally ill led her to realize that it is emotional help that dying patients need most. By allowing the dying to work through any "unfinished business" and to make the most of such time as they have left, she helps them to die peacefully and with dignity.

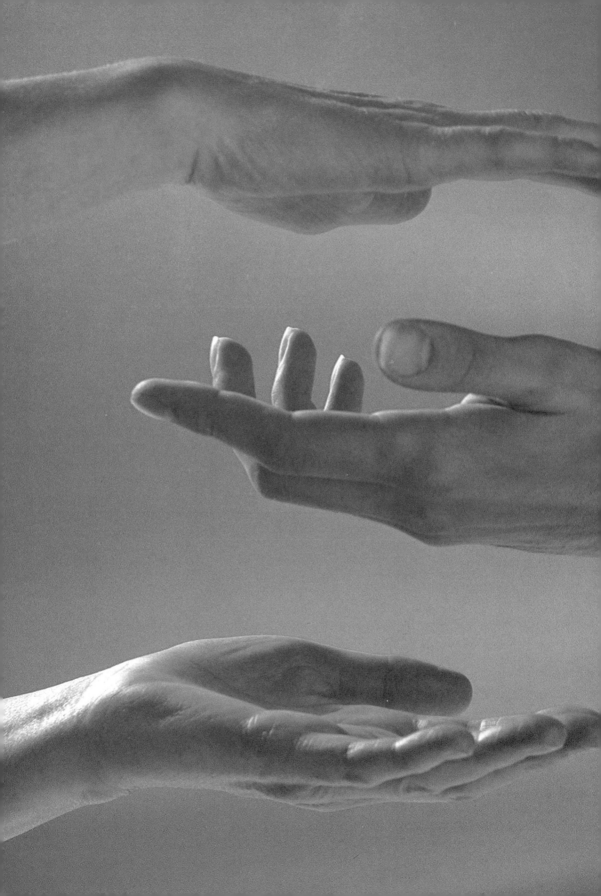

Part Two: HEALING

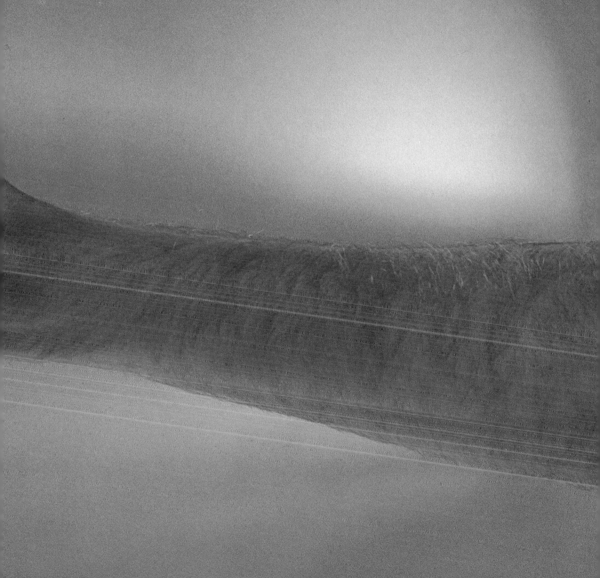

CHAPTER FOUR
Caring for the sick

Almost all ill health starts in the context of the home, and it is the close members of the family or household who first make decisions on how to respond. Overall, very few ailments are ever taken to a doctor or natural therapist, mainly because most ailments are minor and self-limiting. The standard response is to treat them with household remedies or over-the-counter medication.

Safe home remedies and nursing techniques used to be common knowledge. In the extended family, a network of female relatives often took on much of the responsibility for communal health, pooling their knowledge of treatments. But today family units are smaller, and more single people live apart from their families. Responsibility for health often lies with individuals – many of whom are unaware of basic home nursing skills.

In this situation it is essential that every adult learn the rudiments of home care: how to distinguish, as clearly as possible, between minor symptoms and those that require prompt professional care; and how to give safe, effective treatments which relieve temporary pain and discomfort, and speed recovery. The essential home nursing skills are described in the following pages, and these are supported by natural remedies indexed in the Chart of ailments (pp.122-40).

The value of home care
Good home care involves a skilful combination of love, reassurance, nursing and medicinal treatment. Any illness can and should be tackled from several angles. Ensuring that an ill person rests, and taking time to talk through any problems, are as important as administering the right medicine. Above all, don't underestimate the importance of showing your love and concern – many people, especially children, say that they feel better just for being cuddled or comforted for a while. Perhaps the carer

is actually "healing" the patient – certainly the process involved is similar to the healer's laying-on-of-hands, or to therapeutic touch (pp.304-5). All these gestures say: "I care for you and want you well" – and this in itself undoubtedly affects an individual's power to combat illness, be it physical, mental or emotional. The next approach should be some form of home remedy – a pill or a nourishing drink, for example. Given lovingly, such treatment has an enormous placebo effect, in addition to any provable medicinal benefits.

Natural medicines or not?
Drug-oriented medical treatment has until recently enjoyed a near monopoly in health care in the West but, today there are encouraging signs that more people are adopting non-drug approaches to health. However, natural medicine provides not only answers but dilemmas too. Should you tell your doctor that you have tried a herbal tea, a homeopathic remedy or therapeutic massage, for example? Should you go to your doctor at all, or to a natural therapist? And what kind of natural therapy should you choose (p.120)?

Every individual will have to decide for him or herself on the balance to be made between orthodox and complementary treatments. As a general rule, it makes sense to use natural home remedies for minor or long-standing conditions – a child's asthma, for example, or an elderly person's arthritis. A recurrent ear infection will probably improve with a special diet coupled with herbal or homeopathic care. On the other hand, if you have pneumonia, which is potentially fatal, there is little doubt that an antibiotic can save your life. Whichever route you choose, it is essential that you seek a sound professional diagnosis for any ailment that is new for the individual concerned or any persistent symptoms.

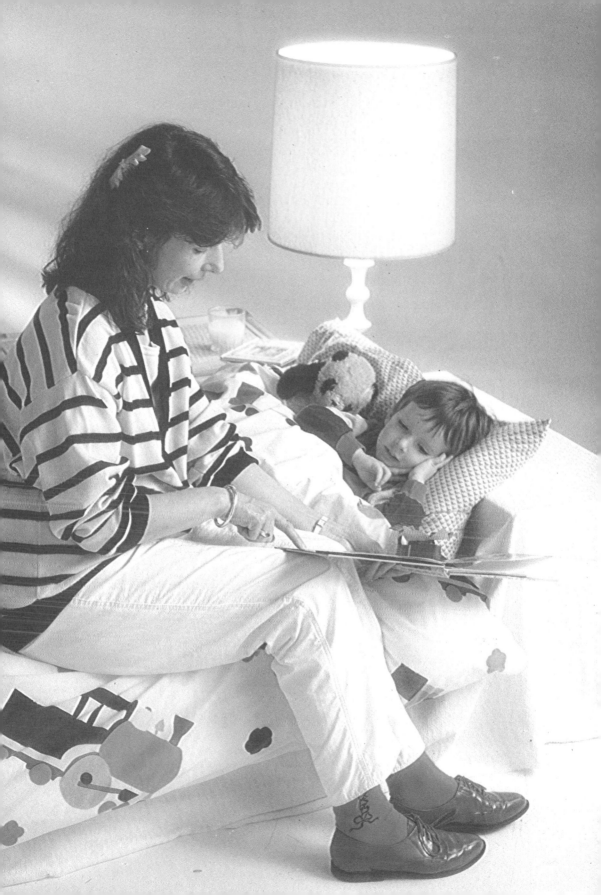

Recognizing illness

Knowing when someone is ill isn't always as clear cut as it may seem. Obviously a raging fever or severe pain demands immediate attention, but the commonest complaints are usually less dramatic. It is important to be aware of signs of stress. They include poor sleep, loss of appetite, reduced sex drive, increased smoking and drinking, bad temper, sighing, and so on. Any of these signs calls for extra love and support, and you should try to find out possible causes. Above all, be alert to changes in behavior – such as a teenager missing meals and being obsessed with his or her weight (see also Growing pains, p.99). The best care involves detecting "dis-ease", as well as recognizing the common signs of illness.

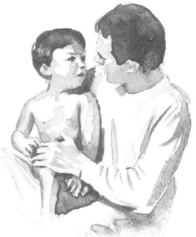

Illness in children

What are the types of things you should look for if a child is simply unwell? Experienced parents can tell at a glance whether or not their child is ill, or even slightly off-color. They are in by far the best position to distinguish between physical ailments and signs of emotional or psychological problems. The child with a tummy ache, for example, may have nothing wrong with his or her abdomen, but may be trying unconsciously to find a way of avoiding school, and seeking care and attention. As you become attuned to a child's individual personality, you will become better and better at interpreting what is going on.

These are the signs to look out for:

● **Activity** Is the child quieter or more active than you would expect?

● **Sleep** Is the sleep pattern disturbed?

● **Eating** Is the child not eating well or being picky?

● **Vomiting and diarrhea** These are always signs that something is wrong, even if only having eaten the wrong thing.

● **Urine** Is the urine very concentrated? If so, be sure to administer fluids liberally.

● **Temperature** A high fever is a sign of infection. A low temperature can occur with some viral illnesses. Be sure you know what is normal, and be careful not to let a fever rage too high (see Medical emergencies, opposite, and Nursing skills, pp.118-19).

● **Skin** Gather the abdominal skin together using all your fingers. If it doesn't spring back immediately when you release it, the child may be dehydrated. Rashes require a doctor's attention – there are many possible causes, and they may signal a childhood illness, such as measles.

● **Breathing** Shallow, rapid breathing is always a sign of trouble, as is fighting for breath or any blueness of skin color. (A newborn baby may have a breathing rate of 50 per minute, but a 6 year old breathes only 30 times a minute and a 10 year old, 25 times a minute.)

● **Eyes** Are they glazed, red, or sunken-looking? Are there dark rings underneath them?

Illness in adults

Adult patients are often more difficult to treat than children. For one thing, sick adults have their own views on what should or should not be done. Many adults ignore their ailments and struggle on, and as a result, their recovery is slow. Bed rest is invariably best for any acute, viral illness, such as flu or a bad cold.

Look out for the following signs:

● **Temperature** See Medical emergencies below.

● **Headaches** Repeated headaches that occur from no apparent cause.

● **Swallowing** Any persistent difficulty in swallowing (the cause can be physical or emotional).

● **Weight** An unintentional loss of more than about 10 lb (4.5 kg) over a 10-week period is cause for concern.

● **Glands** Are any glands swollen or tender? Check especially the lymph glands in the neck and under the armpits.

● **Hoarseness** Hoarseness or difficulty in talking for longer than one week should always be taken seriously.

● **Color** Is there a bluish color round the lips, the insides of the eyelids, or the beds of the fingernails?

● **Bleeding** Any bleeding from the rectum could be a sign of trouble.

● **Urine** Is the urine cloudy, smoky, or red in color? (If it is concentrated, then administer fluids liberally.)

● **Bowel movement** Don't neglect any changes in bowel movements, such as sudden attacks of diarrhea or constipation. Do feces look unusually black?

● **Sight** Is vision sometimes blurry or can haloes be seen surrounding light sources?

● **Moles** A mole, or other skin blemish, that starts to change color or shape, or starts to bleed, especially in middle-aged people, must be seen by a doctor.

● **Coughing** Any persistent cough, especially if you are a smoker, needs investigating.

● **Signs specific to women:** Look out for any lumps in the breasts or any changes in breast shape (p.104). Also, any bleeding or discharge (except milk during lactation) from a nipple. Any unusual vaginal discharge, pain on passing urine, and spots of blood between periods or after the menopause are also causes for concern.

● **Signs specific to men:** Any difficulty in passing urine or any discharge from the penis.

Medical emergencies

Be on the lookout for the signs below and call a doctor at once if any member of the family exhibits one of them. Babies and children, especially, can deteriorate quite rapidly in medical terms, and 24 hours can be a long time in a child's illness. It is vital to have your doctor's telephone number where everybody knows where to find it – perhaps by the telephone itself. In case of emergencies, it is important to know the rudiments of first aid (pp.331-7).

Any one of the following may signal an emergency:

● Fainting

● Fits and convulsions

● Temperatures of more than 103° F (39.4° C)

● Choking that can't be cleared instantly

● Suddenly turning blue for more than a few moments

● Heavy bleeding from a wound for more than a few minutes

● The soft spot on a baby's head bulging or sinking in

● Sleepiness or disorientation a few hours after a shock, a blow to the head, or a fall.

Organizing a sickroom

The main thing that you can do for someone who is sick is to administer tender loving care – and then wait for the person's own body to heal itself. The illness, may indeed, be unconsciously aimed at receiving the love and attention the person feels is lacking. It can be a time of growth, a special opportunity to show love and affection.

The first step is to ensure that the sufferer rests, and is left in peace. He or she should know that the carer has taken charge. If a sick person is confined to bed, it is essential that you make the bedroom comfortable and organized to cater to his or her needs. If the illness is highly infectious, an isolation area may be necessary. If you are nursing very young babies, the chronically ill, or the elderly, you should make sure you have the benefit of regular medical advice and support.

Bedside table
Position a bedside table so that it is accessible, yet not so close to the bed that it will hinder any movement. On the table, stand a reading lamp, a container of water, fruit juice, and a clean glass. A buzzer or bell on the table will allow the person to attract your attention whenever necessary. There should also be space for a radio, book, sketch pad, etc.

Food trays and backrests
If meals are taken in bed, a free-standing tray is useful – one that is placed over the lap and has supports resting on either side of the bed. A firm backrest, specially shaped to give support, makes sitting up in bed more comfortable. Alternatively, use 2 or 3 well-filled pillows as a backrest.

Bedding
Ideally the bed should be positioned to allow you access to the person from either side. Light, warm, bedclothes are best.

Change sheets frequently, and keep pillows plumped up – clean, tidy bedding is a comfort to the ill person.

Room temperature

Keep the sickroom at a normally comfortable temperature, about 70° F (21° C). Old people are particularly susceptible to chills, so take care to maintain the temperature. Unless it is extremely cold outside, keep a window slightly open to keep the air fresh. In hot weather, cool drinks and a fan to circulate air will help to prevent overheating.

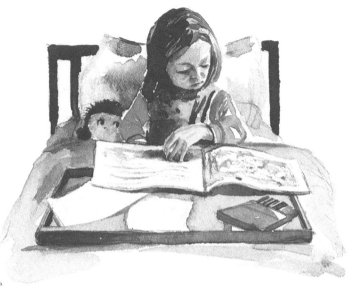

Humidity

Centrally heated and air-conditioned rooms tend to be dry, and this may cause discomfort, particularly if the person has a respiratory complaint. To overcome this, stand a bowl of water in a corner of the room or use a humidifier. Essential oils or aromatic herbs steeped in hot water may be soothing.

Clothing

Pajamas or night dresses should be loose, comfortable, and warm. A bedjacket is a good idea when sitting up in bed, reading or eating, etc.

Giving medicine to children

It is usually a parent's responsibility to ensure that proper doses of medicine are taken by the sick child. Give a glass of something the child likes to wash away any unpleasant taste afterwards. Tablets can be crushed and mixed with something like jam to disguise the taste. Capsules, once wetted can be easier for a child to swallow. Herbal medicines can be sweetened with honey.

Entertaining a sick child

Anybody who has nursed sick children at home will know that, unless a child is extremely ill, their needs are different from those of sick adults. Adults usually want peace and quiet and like to be left alone for much of the time, whereas children, more often than not, need company and some form of entertainment if they are not to become unbearably bored. Television, radio, videos, and records can be a great help, but don't neglect books, drawing pads, jigsaw puzzles, coloring-in books and construction kits (depending on the age of the child). If you provide construction kits or coloring-in books, give the child a large tray on which to work, and a few extra pillows to act as a backrest.

Bed baths

A complete bed bath is generally not necessary, unless the individual is chronically sick. But most people, even if they are only in bed for a few days, will appreciate the chance to freshen up twice a day. If the person feels too ill to get to the bathroom, provide a towel, a bowl of warm water and a sponge, and wash the face, hands and armpits. If there is a fever it may be necessary to sponge more of the body (see Fever, p.119)

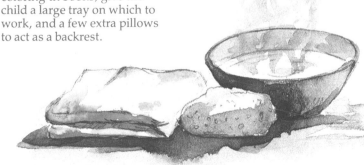

Nursing skills

Learning the basic skills of nursing is an essential part
of holistic health care – of taking more responsibility
for your own and your family's well-being. Try to
anticipate the needs of the child or adult who is
unwell, whether that means giving frequent drinks or
providing occupation. Check the person's
temperature regularly and be on the alert for any
deterioration or alarm signs that call for professional
help. Make sure that the diet is appropriate to the
person's condition and don't forget to look after
yourself too, so you don't get too strained, impatient,
or tired.

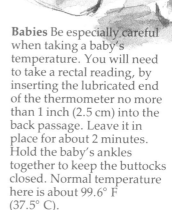

Using an indicator strip

Taking a temperature

A thermometer gives the
most accurate temperature
reading. Always ensure that
it is hygienically clean (wash
well with soap and warm
water, and rinse). When it is
not in use, keep it in the case
in which it is supplied. Before
use, remove it from the case
and shake it sharply (holding
the non-bulb end), so that the
level of mercury is below the
98.6° F (37° C) mark of normal
body temperature.

Normal method Place the
bulb end of the thermometer
under the tongue, close the
mouth, and wait for 3-5
minutes. Don't hold the
thermometer by the bulb end
when checking the reading,
since this will cause the
mercury to rise.

Under 7s With small children
you should place the
thermometer in the armpit,
making sure that it is firmly
held (but not crushed)
between arm and body. Wait
for 3 minutes. A normal
reading with this method is
about 97.6° F (36.5° C).

Indicator strips A less
accurate but much easier
method of taking a
temperature is to use an
indicator strip, available in
some pharmacies. Press the
strip against the forehead for
about 1 minute. The body's
heat causes chemicals within
the strip to change color,
indicating the approximate
temperature – this is accurate
enough for most home
nursing purposes.

Babies Be especially careful
when taking a baby's
temperature. You will need
to take a rectal reading, by
inserting the lubricated end
of the thermometer no more
than 1 inch (2.5 cm) into the
back passage. Leave it in
place for about 2 minutes.
Hold the baby's ankles
together to keep the buttocks
closed. Normal temperature
here is about 99.6° F
(37.5° C).

Apart from a raised
temperature, you must be
alert to other symptoms, such
as persistent vomiting,
rashes, diarrhea, or red or
dull eyes. Call a doctor if you
are at all worried.

Taking a child's temperature

Special diets

A sick person's diet should be appropriate both to the age and to the illness. Most doctors and natural therapists will give advice on an individual's needs. Naturopaths advise a range of healing diets that are suitable for many conditions (pp.192-3), but you will also need to consult the relevant ailment (pp.196-207).

Drinks Liquids often form a large part of an ill person's diet and may be the best means of giving nutrition. Fizzy, glucose drinks should be given in moderate quantities only. Lemon barley water is more nutritious (p.226), and diluted natural fruit drinks. Savory tastes can be satisfied by beef or vegetable extract drinks, and vegetable or chicken broths. Herbal teas, which have their own medicinal properties, may be welcome too (pp.163-75).

Meals Unless the person is fasting, small quantities of nourishing, well-balanced food should be served at regular intervals. Protein should be present – a little meat, fish, eggs, or cheese – and if the patient is vegetarian, vegetable proteins (grains, legumes, dairy products) should be correctly combined (p.43). Meals must have fiber too, in the form of unrefined cereals, for example. Fresh fruit will provide vitamins, fiber, and fructose (p.38). Grapes (and honey) are a natural source of energy-boosting glucose.

Invalid fare should also look appetizing and be easy to eat. Light smooth food (purées, for example) will slip down most easily, especially if the person is weak or has a sore throat.

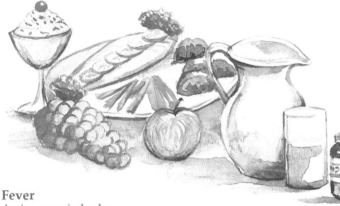

Fever

An increase in body temperature is extremely common, and it is not necessarily dangerous unless it climbs higher than 103° F (39.4° C). With temperatures lower than this, give plenty of liquids in order to prevent dehydration. If a child's raised temperature sticks at about 102° F (40° C), you can reduce it by sponging the arms, neck, forehead, and legs with tepid water. Do not dry the skin afterwards, since the natural evaporation of water has a cooling effect.

If this does not reduce the temperature, you should call a doctor.

Vomiting and diarrhea

When someone vomits, it may help to support the head and to apply gentle yet firm pressure to the stomach. When the attack is over give some water to freshen the mouth, and clean the face with a wash cloth. Do not offer solid food for several hours after the vomiting, but try to give nourishment in liquid form, to strengthen the body and prevent dehydration. If a child vomits over a period of hours it's wise to call a doctor.

If vomiting is accompanied by diarrhea, do your best to give plenty of liquids. If you succeed, proceed to give substantial nourishment, such as a little porridge, or a vegetable broth. When a sick person cannot take even plain or boiled water, try rice water (the strained water from cooked rice). Or give hot milk and nutmeg (p.198).

If the condition persists get professional help. Loss of nutrients and body fluids is a serious matter.

CHAPTER FIVE

The natural therapies

In this chapter we deal with twenty-five of the most popular natural therapies currently practiced today, ranging from complete health care systems, such as homeopathy, to complementary therapies, such as biofeedback, that can be readily used in conjunction with other treatment methods. The therapies have been chosen both on the grounds of their importance and popularity and on the basis of their suitability for home use, but precedence has been given to those therapies with a strong self-help application. Thus you will find that naturopathy, for example, has much more space devoted to it than, say, acupuncture, despite the importance of the latter.

The therapies are grouped into two large sections – "medicinal" and "body-mind". Medicinal therapies are those in which, by and large, you take something by mouth or apply it to your skin, as in herbalism or aromatherapy. Body-mind therapies include both manipulative or physical treatment methods, such as osteopathy and Rolfing, and therapies which make use of the power of the mind to affect the health of the body, such as autogenics and meditation.

How the therapies are presented
The section on each therapy has been prepared in collaboration with a highly experienced practitioner in the field. An introductory part defines what the therapy is and for which ailments it is especially effective, and outlines some of the clinical trials that have proven its value. It also describes in detail what to expect if you consult a practitioner. The majority of therapies then have a substantial self-help section, with ailments listed according to a common order, from respiratory, digestive and skin disorders to musculoskeletal, urinogenital, gynecological and miscellaneous conditions. Some therapies also have special entries for children's and babies' ailments.

Selecting a remedy
The main problem you face when looking at which natural therapy to turn to in a domestic setting is the wealth of choice. Many of the therapies – especially those, such as homeopathy or herbalism, that are whole systems of medicine in themselves – have answers for most of the common ailments. Also, contrary to popular belief, both medicinal and body-mind therapies have effective remedies for a wide spectrum of ailments, whether they seem primarily physical or psychological in origin or not. Thus either homeopathy or shiatsu, for example, could be used to treat indigestion or insomnia. In practice, however, medicinal therapies are likely to appeal to people who prefer to take a pill or a potion when they are ill, while body-mind therapies tend to suit those who believe more in the curative power of touch or exercise or in the healing powers of the mind. The Chart of ailments (pp.122-40) lists the remedies for all the commonest ailments.

The remedies or treatment methods selected for home use have been chosen by the therapists, both for their safety and their effectiveness, bearing in mind the risks inherent in advising treatment without a proper diagnosis having been made first. But you should be sure to follow directions on dosages, applications, methods, and so on, and to take heed of any cautionary notes. If you wish, you can use remedies from different therapies in combination. So, for example, if you had a stiff neck, you could take a homeopathic remedy, practice osteopathic exercises and use meditation to reduce stress. It is also safe to try a natural remedy as an additional measure to an orthodox medicine – although, as in the case of homeopathy, the orthodox drug may act as an "antidote" to the natural remedy. If a health problem is slow to respond to home treatment, of course, you must consult a professional.

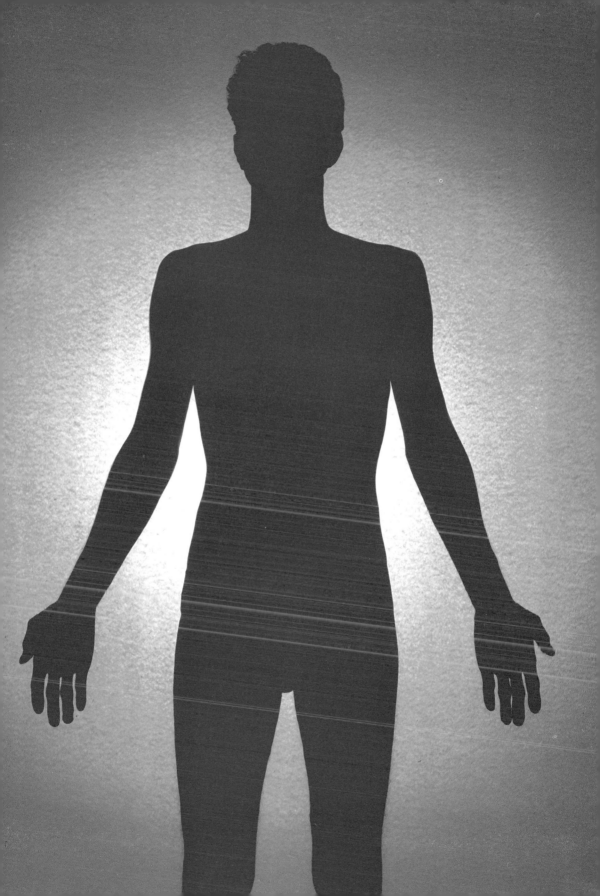

Chart of ailments

This chart acts as a guide and index to the great range of self-help remedies and treatments described in the Natural therapies chapter. It also includes first aid remedies which are covered in Chapter 6. The therapies beside each ailment are given in a common order: medicinal; then manipulative and spiritual. The ailments are ordered largely by body system.

The list of self-help remedies is intended both to help you choose between the many alternatives given in this chapter, and as a reminder of where to find the remedies. It is essential, however, that you read the introduction and the self-help section of the selected therapy, to be sure that a treatment is suitable, and to follow the instructions on dosage, application, etc. NB Just because a therapy is not included here, it does not mean that it has no effective remedy for that ailment, only that it is necessary to consult a practitioner to pursue it (eg, acupuncture for migraine).

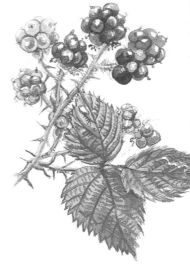

Blackberries, a folk remedy for diarrhea

Ailments	Therapies	Remedies
General respiratory ailments Strengthen resistance with exercise and a good diet (p.47); keep away from sources of infection when you can.	**Yoga** p.290 **Reflexology** pp.261-2	Basic asanas, breathing exercises, nasal wash, corpse pose Head and sinus reflexes; lung and chest reflexes
Sore throats There are numerous causes for this ailment. Avoid airborne pollutants (p.72), which aggravate soreness, as will breathing cold and dry air. Rest your voice and keep warm.	**Homeopathy** p.149 **Herbalism** p.166 **Aromatherapy** p.179 **Naturopathy** p.196 **Traditional medicine** p.219 **Shiatsu** p.282	(*With bright red tonsils*) Belladonna; (*with hot and cold feeling*) Mercurius solubilis; (*throat feels scratched*) Hepar sulphuris, or Baryta muriatica Red sage and vinegar gargle; tincture of myrrh gargle Geranium gargle, or lemon gargle, or pine inhalation (*General*) basic health diet, (*local*) throat compress, red sage gargle, (*supplementary*) vitamin B, bioflavonoids, garlic tablets Lemon juice; garlic; cider vinegar; malt vinegar or sodium bicarbonate gargle Pressure points between ribs, and on hands

Lemon

Ailment	Therapies	Remedy
Voice loss See Sore throats, p.122.	**Naturopathy** p.197	(*General*) basic health diet, friction rub, relaxation, (*local*) throat compress, red sage gargle, (*supplementary*) vitamin B, bioflavonoids, compound mineral supplement
Tonsillitis See Sore throats, p122.	**Aromatherapy**	See Sore throats, above
	Naturopathy p.197	(*General*) fasting, raw diet, (*local*) throat compress, red sage gargle, abdominal pack, (*supplementary*) vitamin B, bioflavonoids, garlic
Colds A cold with a fever requires bed rest. For preventive care, follow the advice given under General respiratory ailments, above.	**Homeopathy** pp.148-9	Allium cepa, or Euphrasia, or Arsenicum album, or Natrum muriaticum, or Nux vomica, or Kali iodatum; (*early stages*) Aconite, or Wyethia; (*thick catarrh*) Pulsatilla, or Calcarea sulphurica, or Hepar sulphuris; (*sinusitis*) Kali bichromicum, or Silica
	Herbalism p.166	Composition essence; elderflower; (*feverish flu*) yarrow
	Aromatherapy p.179	(*Colds or sinusitis*) eucalyptus inhalation, or lemon gargle, or pine inhalation, or hyssop inhalation
	Naturopathy p.196	(*General*) Epsom salts bath, fasting, raw diet, trunk pack, (*catarrh*) raw or light diet, friction rub, (*local*) inhalation, hot and cold spraying, (*supplementary*) bioflavonoids, garlic tablets, compound mineral supplement, red sage gargle
	Hydrotherapy p.214	Strong hot blackcurrant tea, cold water pack to trunk
	Traditional medicine p.219	Mustard bath; citrus fruit; cold water to nose; garlic
	Massage p.248	General invigorating massage; gliding, kneading and percussion
	Shiatsu p.282	Points between ribs, on arms, legs, and between vertebrae
Flu Bed rest is essential. If you or your family are susceptible to flu, consider vaccination (flu can be a killer in later life).	**Homeopathy** p.149	(*Typical flu*) Gelsemium; (*with extreme aching*) Eupatorium perfoliatum; (*with extreme restlessness*) Rhus toxicodendron
	Herbalism	See Colds, above
	Aromatherapy p.179	Cinnamon bath, massage, or inhalation
	Naturopathy	See Colds, above

Pulsatilla

Ailments	Therapies	Remedies
Coughs Cold, dry air triggers coughs, so keep warm and try to ensure a humid atmosphere (p.72). Don't suppress a productive cough. For croup and whooping cough, see p.139.	**Homeopathy** p.147	Hepar sulphuris, or Rumex, or Pulsatilla; (*hard cough*) Bryonia, or Causticum, or Phosphorus; (*with spasmodic wheezing*) Ipecacuanha; (*with gagging*) Nux vomica; (*dry, violent cough*) Spongia
	Herbalism p.167	(*Coughs or catarrh*) coltsfoot, or wild lettuce, or white horehound, or Irish moss; (*especially bronchitis and hard, non-productive coughs*) mullein; (*children's coughs*) wild cherry bark; (*cough with fever*) yarrow
	Aromatherapy p.179	Hyssop inhalation
	Naturopathy p.196	(*General*) raw diet, basic health diet, breathing, friction rub, (*local*) hot-and-cold compress, inhalation, (*supplementary*) bioflavonoids, garlic tablets, red sage gargle
	Traditional medicine p.220	Licorice root; lemon juice and olive oil; hot mustard bath; hot mustard chest compress
Hyssop inhalation	**Massage**	See Asthma, p.125
Sinusitis Avoid mucus-forming foods (see Catarrh, below). Amongst several other natural therapies, acupuncture helps (p.269), and reflexology on head and sinus reflexes (p.261).	**Homeopathy**	See Colds, p.123
	Aromatherapy	See Colds, p.123
	Naturopathy	See Catarrh, below
	Hydrotherapy	See Catarrh, below
	Shiatsu p.282	Pressure points on hands, between vertebrae, and on nose
Catarrh Atmospheric humidity helps (p.72). Avoid mucus-forming foods, notably dairy products, sugar, and refined carbohydrates.	**Homeopathy**	See Colds, p.123
	Herbalism	See Coughs
	Naturopathy p.196	(*Catarrh or hayfever – general*) fasting, raw diet, friction rub, (*local*) hot-and-cold sponging, inhalation, (*supplementary*) vitamin B, bioflavonoids, garlic tablets, red sage gargle
	Hydrotherapy p.214	(*Catarrh or sinusitis*) hot-and-cold compress and foot bath, cold sitz bath
	Traditional medicine p.220	Juniper tea, or olbas oil, or cranberries
Juniper tea		

Ailments	Therapies	Remedies
Asthma Avoid cold air, airborne pollutants (p.72) and pollens. Try to reduce house dust. Watch out for allergic reactions to foods and drugs. Avoid excess weight gain. Practice deep, relaxed breathing (p.59). 　Useful body-mind therapies include the Alexander technique (pp.294-7), radionics, hypnotherapy (pp.306-13), and biofeedback (pp.320-1).	**Herbalism** p.166 and p.172	Elecampane, or mullein, or hyssop, or passion flower
	Naturopathy p.197	(*General*) breathing, relaxation, raw diet, (*local*) hot compress, inhalation, massage, (*supplementary*) vitamins A, B, bioflavonoids, compound mineral supplement
	Hydrotherapy p.214	Swimming (especially breast-stroke)
	Traditional medicine p.220	Cranberries and warm water
	Massage p.248	(*Asthma or coughs*) back massage, cupping and kneading chest
	Yoga p.291	(*Asthma or bronchitis*) back rolls, pelvic lift, cobra, kapalabhati, abdominal contraction, deep relaxation
Bronchitis Strengthen your resistance with exercise (p.53), correct breathing (pp.58-9), and a healthy diet (p.47). Avoid polluted atmospheres if possible. If you smoke you should try to cut down or give up (p.57). Cut out mucus-forming foods (see Catarrh).	**Herbalism**	See Coughs, above
	Aromatherapy p.179	Clove or hyssop massage; eucalyptus inhalation; pine bath
	Naturopathy p.197	(*General*) basic health diet, (*local*) hot-and-cold compress, inhalation, postural drainage, (*supplementary*) vitamin B, bioflavonoids, garlic tablets
	Hydrotherapy p.214	Cold water pack; (*with coughing*) hot pack
	Yoga	See Asthma, above
General digestive ailments A healthy diet (p.47) is essential. Many body mind therapies also improve digestive ailments since the digestive system is affected by your emotional state.	**Herbalism** p.168	(*Colitis, constipation, diarrhea, indigestion, ulcers, etc*) slippery elm; licorice; meadowsweet; dandelion; fennel; peppermint; rosemary; matricaria; wild thyme; feverfew
	Yoga p.291	(*Colitis, ulcers, hemorrhoids, constipation, etc*) dietary changes, bending asanas, kapalabhati, abdominal contraction; (*obesity, thinness*) regular meals, rest, corpse pose, basic asanas, leg raises, abdominal contraction
Gallstones Eat fewer refined foods, less animal fat, and more dietary fiber.	**Traditional medicine** p.222	Olive oil and lemon juice; cod liver oil and apple juice

Ailments	Therapies	Remedies
Diarrhea This is commonly caused by an infection. It is important to replace fluid loss. *Agrimony*	**Homeopathy** p.150	Sulphur; (*profuse*) Podophyllum; (*with vomiting*) Arsenicum album, or Veratrum album; (*with flatulence*) Carbo vegetabilis; (*from worry*) Argentum nitricum
	Herbalism p.168	Cranesbill, or marsh mallow tea; (*especially for children*) agrimony, or meadowsweet
	Naturopathy p.198	(*General*) fasting, light diet, hot-and-cold compress, (*emergency*) hot milk and nutmeg, (*supplementary*) vitamin B, compound mineral supplement, slippery elm gruel
	Traditional medicine p.220	Cider vinegar, or arrowroot, or blackberries
	Shiatsu p.282	Pressure points on hips, thighs, shins, and soles of feet
Constipation Too low an intake of dietary fiber and too little fluid cause constipation. Increase your intake of fiber by eating more whole foods, eg, fresh fruit and vegetables, wholemeal flour products and legumes.	**Naturopathy** p.198	(*General*) basic health diet, fasting, raw diet, abdominal tone exercise, hot-and-cold compress, sitz bath, (*supplementary*) garlic tablets, herbal laxatives
	Traditional medicine p.221	Stewed prunes, or molasses, or bran
	Osteopathy p.235	(*Pelvic congestion*) dietary adjustment, and diaphragm and abdominal toning exercise
	Shiatsu p.282	High-fiber diet and exercise, pressure points on abdomen, legs, elbows, between vertebrae
Indigestion, stomach ache, flatulence Avoid smoking, strong tea or coffee, and spicy, sugary, or fatty foods. Try to avoid unnecessary stress. If stomach aches persist, consult a doctor. For colic, see p.139. *Angelica*	**Homeopathy** p.150	(*Indigestion – too much food and alcohol*) Nux vomica, or Pulsatilla; (*with burning pain*) Arsenicum album; (*with much gas*) Carbo vegetabilis, or Lycopodium; (*constant nausea*) Ipecacuanha
	Aromatherapy p.180	(*Indigestion or flatulence*) garlic oil massage
	Naturopathy p.199	(*Indigestion, stomach ache, flatulence, or colic – general*) fasting, light diet, (*local*) hot-and-cold compress, (*supplementary – indigestion or stomach ache*) vitamin B, pawpaw extract, slippery elm gruel; (*flatulence or colic*) pawpaw extract
	Traditional medicine p.221	(*Indigestion*) lemon juice or cider vinegar; herbal teas; bran and oatmeal; juniper berries; angelica root; (*stomach ache*) cinnamon and milk or water; (*flatulence*) angelica root; mustard seeds
	Shiatsu p.282	(*Indigestion*) pressure points on shinbones

Ailments	Therapies	Remedies
Vomiting, nausea Vomiting may be a sign of a more serious disorder, so be alert to warning signs (p.115). Replacing lost body fluids is important (p.119).	**Homeopathy** p.150	(*Too much food and alcohol*) Nux vomica; (*constant nausea*) Ipecacuanha (See also Indigestion, p.126)
	Naturopathy p.199	(*Nausea – general*) fasting, puréed apple and yoghurt, light diet, (*local*) hot-and-cold compress, (*supplementary*) lecithin, compound mineral supplement
Hemorrhoids A very common western complaint, said to affect 50 percent of the population over the age of 50. It is usually associated with constipation. Prevention is easy: eat more dietary fiber, drink more water, and open bowels regularly.	**Homeopathy** p.150	Nux vomica, or Hamamelis; (*with back pain*) Aesculus
	Naturopathy p.198	(*General*) basic health diet, abdominal toning, (*local*) cold water spraying, sitz bath, (*supplementary*) vitamins B, E
	Traditional medicine p.221	Pilewort, Canadian pine or golden seal
	Osteopathy	See Constipation, p.126
	Shiatsu p.283	Dietary adjustment, pressure points on abdomen, head, and between vertebrae
Worms Prompt treatment and close attention to personal hygiene are essential.	**Traditional medicine** p.222	Pumpkin seeds, or wormwood infusion
Mouth ulcers, bleeding gums, toothache, bad breath Brush teeth and gums thoroughly (p.67), take vitamin C, and avoid foods with preservatives. Brushing the tongue helps cure bad breath.	**Homeopathy** p.151	Plantago, or Kreosotum; (*local*) Plantago Mother Tincture
	Herbalism p.169	Tincture of myrrh mouthwash, or red sage mouthwash
	Aromatherapy p.180 and p.181	(*Bleeding gums*) sage gargle; (*gingivitis*) lemon gargle; (*toothache*) oil of cinnamon; (*bad breath*) peppermint oil
	Naturopathy p.199	(*Bleeding gums – general*) basic health diet, raw diet, (*with digestive disorders*) light diet, (*local*) herbal toothpaste, red sage gargle, (*supplementary*) vitamin B, bioflavonoids, garlic tablets, compound mineral supplement
	Traditional medicine p.221	(*Toothache*) oil of cloves, or dried clove

Plantago

Ailments	Therapies	Remedies
Local skin disorders, urticaria, psoriasis Avoid harsh soaps, detergents, etc (p.66). Exercise and a good diet will improve skin. Urticaria is an allergic complaint (see also p.136, Allergies). Psoriasis is linked with certain drugs and medications, heredity and stress.	**Homeopathy** p.152 **Herbalism** p.169 and p.170 **Aromatherapy** p.180 **Hydrotherapy** p.214 **Traditional medicine** p.222	(*Urticaria*) Apis mellifica, or Urtica urens (*Infections or minor wounds*) witch hazel, or marigold, or chickweed compress; (*warts*) greater celandine, or petty spurge, or thuja (*Warts*) garlic oil (*Psoriasis*) tepid salt or coal tar bath (*Skin irritations*) calamine lotion
Boils, sores, abscesses Keep them covered with sterile dressings, replaced frequently. Pay attention to diet. Take plenty of vitamin C. *Oil of thyme*	**Homeopathy** p.151 **Herbalism** **Aromatherapy** p.180 **Naturopathy** p.200 **Traditional medicine** p.222	(*Boils or abscesses*) Belladonna, or Hepar sulphuris, or Silica See Acne, below (*Boils or sores*) oil of thyme (*General*) fasting, raw diet, basic health diet, friction rub, (*local – boils*) poultice, (*local – abscesses*) Epsom salts bath, compress, (*supplementary – boils*) vitamins A, B, bioflavonoids, compound mineral supplement, (*supplementary – abscesses*) vitamin A, bioflavonoids, garlic tablets Fig, bread, or potato poultice
Acne, spots Avoid refined foods, especially sweets and chocolates, caffeine-containing drinks (p.45), and stressful situations. Take vitamins A and E.	**Herbalism** p.170 **Naturopathy** p.200 **Aromatherapy** p.180	Dietary adjustment, and carrot, beetroot, or cabbage juice (*General*) fasting, raw diet, friction rub, trunk pack, (*local*) salt water or calendula, (*supplementary*) vitamin B, bioflavonoids, garlic tablets, compound mineral supplement Juniper or lavender oil
Earache Stay out of cold winds, and try to reduce mucus by adjusting your diet (see Catarrh, p.124).	**Homeopathy** p.151 **Naturopathy** p.201 **Traditional medicine** p.223	Aconite, or Belladonna, or Hepar sulphuris, or Chamomilla, or Pulsatilla; (*early stages*) Ferrum phosphoricum (*General*) fasting, raw diet, (*local*) ear drops, hot salt compress, (*supplementary*) yeast-free vitamin B, bioflavonoids, garlic tablets Hot salt bag; olive or castor oil ear drops

Ailments	Therapies	Remedies
Dandruff and hair loss Dandruff may be related to a poor diet (p.170).	**Traditional medicine** p.223	(*Dandruff*) rosemary, or witch hazel and eau de Cologne rub; (*hair loss*) bay rum and jaborandi lotion; castor oil
Eye problems Avoid bad lighting (p.73). Try eye exercises (p.67). Make sure you eat well (p.47), and rest enough. Have your eyes professionally tested if in doubt.	**Homeopathy** p.152 **Herbalism** p.170 **Naturopathy** p.201 **Hydrotherapy** p.214 **Traditional medicine** p.223	(*Conjunctivitis*) Pulsatilla, or Euphrasia, or Argentum nitricum (*Eyestrain*) eyebright; (*styes*) witch hazel (*Styes – general*) raw diet, fasting, (*local*) seasalt or eyebright, (*supplementary*) vitamins A, B, bioflavonoids, compound mineral supplement (*Conjunctivitis*) salt water eyebath, cold compress (*Eyestrain*) salt water or honey eyebath, or eyebright
Chapping, chilblains, corns, ingrowing toenails, athlete's foot, sweaty feet A good diet and good circulation help prevent chapping and chilblains. Corns and ingrowing toenails usually result from tight footwear. In cases of athlete's foot, always dry feet well, and air them often.	**Homeopathy** pp.151-2 **Aromatherapy** p.180 **Naturopathy** p.200 **Hydrotherapy** p.214 **Traditional medicine** p.222	(*Chilblains*) Pulsatilla, or Agaricus, or Apis mellifica, or Tamus ointment; (*ingrowing toenails*) Magnetis polus Australis (*Corns*) garlic oil applied locally; (*sweaty feet*) cypress (*Local – chilblains*) foot bath, (*local – chapping*) calendula ointment, (*supplementary – chapping or chilblains*) bioflavonoids, vitamin E, kelp, compound mineral supplement (*Chapping or chilblains*) hot-and-cold bathing, compress (*Chapping or chilblains*) myrrh; balsam; (*corns*) turpentine; lemon; (*ingrowing toenails*) lemon; (*athlete's foot*) cypress
Herpes, impetigo, eczema, shingles In cases of herpes, shingles, or impetigo, avoid skin contact with others and pay close attention to personal hygiene. For detailed advice on herpes, see p.69. Eczema sufferers should avoid scratching, and wearing wool or nylon next to the skin.	**Homeopathy** p.151 **Herbalism** p.169 **Aromatherapy** p.180 **Naturopathy** p.201 **Traditional medicine** p.222	(*Herpes*) Natrum muriaticum, or Rhus toxicodendron; (*shingles*) Rhus toxicodendron (*Eczema*) marigold compress, or chickweed compress (*Weeping eczema*) juniper, or lavender; (*dry eczema*) geranium, or hyssop (*Eczema or impetigo*) raw diet, fasting, (*local – eczema*) sodium bicarbonate, (*supplementary – eczema*), vitamins A, B, compound mineral supplement, (*supplementary – impetigo*) plus bioflavonoids (*Herpes*) potatoes

Ailments	Therapies	Remedies
Backache, sciatica, lumbago Pay attention to posture (p.232 and p.296). Avoid poorly designed furniture (p.71) and adjust your car seat if necessary (p.240). Try to minimize strain (p.234). Manipulative therapies such as osteopathy (pp.228-35) and chiropractic (pp.236-41) are very successful. Applied kinesiology, reflexology, Rolfing (pp.250-67) and Alexander technique (pp.294-7) are also helpful.	**Homeopathy** **Naturopathy** p.202 **Hydrotherapy** p.215 **Traditional medicine** p.223 **Osteopathy** pp.232-3 **Chiropractic** pp.240-41 **Massage** p.249 **Shiatsu** p.283 **Yoga** p.292	See Rheumatism, p.131 (*General – backache*) rest; (*lumbago*) stretching; (*local*) compress, Epsom salts and sitz baths, (*supplementary – backache or lumbago*) bioflavonoids, compound mineral supplement, (*sciatica*) plus vitamin B and dolomite (*General*) pool exercise, swimming, hot-and-cold foot bath, (*sciatica*) plus hot water pack on lower back (*Sciatica*) warm olive oil massage General exercises, lower back and posture exercises, morning stiffness routine, hot-and-cold water pack Correct posture, rest, cold compress, remedial exercises Gliding, kneading, friction and percussion on back (*Backache*) hot towel on lower back, points between vertebrae, on sacrum, ankles and hip bones; (*sciatica*) points between vertebrae, on legs and hips Basic asanas, corpse pose, shoulder rotation, back rolls
Arthritis Prevention means eating well (p.47), with plenty of calcium and zinc, and keeping active – yoga is excellent (pp.284-93). Other beneficial therapies are listed under Backache, above. *Copper bracelet*	**Herbalism** p.171 **Naturopathy** p.203 **Hydrotherapy** p.215 **Traditional Medicine** p.223 **Massage** p.249 **Yoga** p.292	Kelp or devil's claw; celery seed; bogbean; wild thyme (*General*) basic health diet, raw diet, relaxation, (*local – rheumatoid arthritis*) cold compress, hot-and-cold compress, (*local – osteoarthritis*) hot-and-cold compress, Epsom salts bath, (*supplementary*) bioflavonoids, compound mineral supplement, dolomite Hot packs, cold packs, or ice packs; (*later*) hot baths, pool exercises, hot-and-cold hand or foot baths Sulphur compress; cod liver oil, orange juice; olive oil, camphor, cayenne massage; honey and cider vinegar; dandelion; copper bracelet (*Arthritis, rheumatism, stiff shoulders, fibrositis, etc*) general body massage Basic asanas, shoulder, hand, and foot rotations

Ailments	Therapies	Remedies
Rheumatism, fibrositis, gout Rheumatism, like arthritis, responds to a good diet and gentle exercise (see above). Relaxation and correct posture combat the inflammation of fibrositis. In cases of gout adjust your diet (p.47) and avoid rich foods in particular (p.170).	**Homeopathy** p.152	(*Rheumatism or backache*) Arnica, or Rhus toxicodendron, or Bryonia, or Nux vomica
	Herbalism p.170	(*Fibrositis or gout*) thyme; feverfew. (For rheumatism, see Arthritis, p.130)
	Aromatherapy p.180	(*Rheumatism or gout*) chamomile or cypress, or eucalyptus, or rosemary
	Naturopathy p.202	(*Rheumatism or fibrositis – general*) raw diet, relaxation, (*local*) compress, Epsom salts bath, (*supplementary – rheumatism*) vitamin B, bioflavonoids, garlic tablets, kelp, compound mineral supplement
	Hydrotherapy p.215	(*Rheumatism or fibrositis*) hot packs, hot baths, hot-and-cold compress, breathing, relaxation
	Traditional medicine p.223, p.224	(*Gout*) potato juice; turpentine compress, (*rheumatism*) hot salt or salt and cayenne pepper compress; asparagus tea;
	Massage	See Arthritis, p.130
Stiff or frozen shoulder, stiff neck Keep yourself supple with regular stretching exercises. Avoid poorly designed beds, car seats, furniture, etc.	**Homeopathy** p.153	(*Stiff neck*) Rhus toxicodendron, or Nux vomica, or Actea racemosa
	Herbalism	See Fibrositis, above
	Naturopathy p.203	(*Stiff neck*) neck rolls, relaxation, hot-and-cold compress, massage
	Hydrotherapy p.215	(*Shoulder*) cold packs, exercises; (*recovery*) hot packs
	Shiatsu p.283	(*Shoulder*) points between vertebrae, on neck, shoulders
	Massage	See Arthritis, above
Muscular cramps Possible causes, include fatigue, mineral deficiency, stress, and alcoholism. *Evening primrose*	**Homeopathy** p.152	Cuprum metallicum
	Herbalism p.171	Kelp, cramp bark or evening primrose oil
	Hydrotherapy p.214	Hot-and-cold baths, cold frictions
	Massage p.249	Gliding, kneading, and chopping strokes over affected area
	Shiatsu p.283	(*Stomach cramps*) clockwise massage on belly, pressure points on abdomen, legs, and between vertebrae

Ailments	Therapies	Remedies
Nervous disorders Many body-mind therapies offer simple but highly effective self-help methods including: massage; touch for health (pp.242-55); yoga; Alexander technique (pp.284-97); hypnotherapy (pp.310-13); biofeedback (pp.320-21).	**Aromatherapy** pp.180-1	(*Nervous disorders*) basil, chamomile, or orange blossom bath; (*irritability*) oil of cypress, or chamomile bath
	Bach flower remedies p.187	Rescue Remedy; Examination Mix (see also Negative emotional states, p.40)
	Naturopathy p.204	(*Nervous stress – general*) relaxation, basic health diet, increased protein, (*supplementary*) vitamins B, E, bioflavonoids, compound mineral supplement, dolomite
Stress, anxiety, depression Stress and anxiety are often part and parcel of modern living. Bottling up your emotions can be damaging. Try to be more open (pp.80-1). Eat well (p.47), take regular exercise (p.53), and practice relaxation (p.63). See also Negative emotions, p.140.	**Homeopathy** p.154	(*Stress*) Nux vomica, or Ignatia, or Sepia; (*anxiety*) Gelsemium, or Argentum nitricum, or Aconite
	Herbalism p.172	(*Anxiety or insomnia*) chamomile, or lime flowers, or valerian, or hops, or rosemary; (*with neuralgia, headaches*) betony; (*with spasmodic asthma, neuralgia*) passion flower
	Naturopathy	See Nervous disorders, above
	Hydrotherapy p.214	(*Anxiety or insomnia*) tepid bath, hot-and-cold compress, cold friction, deep breathing
	Traditional medicine	See Tiredness, p.134
	Yoga p.293	(*Anxiety or tiredness*) corpse pose; (*depression*) more active asanas, eg, kapalabhati, salute to the sun, and relaxed breathing
Neuralgia Neuralgia is often the result of nerve inflammation. It usually clears quickly. Several natural therapies are helpful, including acupuncture (pp.268-73) and manipulative disciplines such as chiropractic (pp.236-41).	**Homeopathy** p.153	(*From cold, dry weather*) Aconite; (*right-sided pain*) Magnesia phosphorica; (*left-sided pain*) Colocynthis; (*stinging pains involving eye*) Spigelia
	Herbalism	See Stress, anxiety, above
	Aromatherapy p.180	Chamomile oil massage
	Naturopathy p.204	(*General*) relaxation, (*local*) hot-and-cold compress, (*supplementary*) vitamin B

Hops

Ailments	Therapies	Remedies
Headaches, migraines Anxiety and stress should be avoided if at all possible. The causes of migraine are numerous, and include food sensitivity, stress, too much or too little sleep, certain smells, lights, or a stormy atmosphere. Many body-mind therapies can give relief, including Touch for Health (pp.253-5), reflexology (pp.256-63), acupuncture (pp.268-73), healing (pp.298-303), meditation (pp.314-17), hypnotherapy (pp.310-11) and biofeedback (pp.320-1).	**Homeopathy** p.153	(*Worse for movement*) Bryonia; (*like a band around head*) Gelsemium; (*hangover-type*) Nux vomica; (*violent, bursting*) Belladonna; (*blinding, hammering*) Natrum muriaticum
	Herbalism p.173	Feverfew, infusion of fresh leaves
	Naturopathy p.203	(*General*) basic health diet, extra protein, (*local – headache*) cold, or hot-and-cold compress, (*emergency – migraine*) relaxation routine, rest in dark, and cold compress
	Hydrotherapy p.214	Hot-and-cold compress to forehead and base of skull
	Traditional medicine p.224	Herbal teas; vinegar and brown paper or vinegar inhalation; onion poultice; aromatic massage, lemon peel
	Massage p.248	Massaging neck and shoulders, and face
	Shiatsu p.283	Points beside vertebrae, and on neck, shoulders, hands, legs, face
	Yoga p.292	Upper back, shoulder and neck exercises, eg, shoulderstand, fish, cobra, (*migraine*) dietary adjustment
Insomnia There are many ways to help a good night's sleep (pp.86-7). Try food supplements, eg, tryptophan. Practice deep breathing, and relaxation (p.63). *Shiatsu treatment for insomnia*	**Homeopathy** p.154	(*From over active mind*) Coffea; (*apprehension*) Arsenicum album; (*emotional stress*) Ignatia
	Herbalism	See Stress, p.132
	Aromatherapy p.180	Chamomile or orange blossom bath
	Naturopathy p.204	(*General*) cold spraying of lower legs, and feet, or cold footbath, walks in fresh air, relaxation routine
	Hydrotherapy	See Stress, p.132
	Traditional medicine p.224	Honey, or skullcap, or hops, or garlic
	Shiatsu p.283	General and light stretching exercise, foot massage, points on face, head, feet, between vertebrae
	Yoga p.292	Basic asanas, back rolls, corpse pose

Ailments	Therapies	Remedies
Tiredness, fatigue Avoid overwork, lack of exercise, lack of sleep, and boredom. Make sure you get enough magnesium, potassium, vitamin C, and folic acid (pp.40-1). *Garlic*	**Homeopathy** p.154	(*From over-exertion*) Arnica; (*effort and worry*) Kali phosphoricum; (*with anxiety*) Arsenicum album; (*with depression*) Sepia; (*in workaholics*) Nux vomica
	Aromatherapy p.181	Clove bath; cypress or garlic oil massage; lemon, lavender, peppermint, sage or thyme bath
	Naturopathy p.200	(*General*) relaxation, basic health diet, protein snacks, (*supplementary*) vitamins B, E, bioflavonoids, compound mineral supplement, kelp
	Hydrotherapy p.214	Stimulating cold water friction
	Traditional medicine p.225	(*Fatigue or depression*) ginseng
	Yoga	See Stress, anxiety, p.132
Loss of sex drive Apart from the various psychological reasons, the condition can be caused by diseases of the nervous system, hormone deficiencies, alcohol, drugs and smoking.	**Aromatherapy** p.181	Sacral massage with oil of rosemary
	Hydrotherapy p.214	Cold baths, showers, or sitz baths, and cold frictions
	Traditional medicine p.225	Ginseng or cold water baths
	Yoga p.293	Half shoulderstand, forward bend, kapalabhati, pelvic lift
Bladder disorders, cystitis, kidney stones Anxiety or depression can cause cystitis. Other causes include poor hygiene, low consumption of plain water, dietary fiber, and intolerance of tea, coffee, and alcohol. Avoid wearing tight clothes. Wear cotton next to the skin. In case of kidney stones, eat a diet rich in fiber, drink plenty of water, take vitamin B6, and magnesium supplements, and cut down on salt.	**Homeopathy** p.157	(*Cystitis – with burning pains*) Cantharis; (*with painful urging and little result*) Nux vomica; (*sudden onset*) Aconite; (*from cold wet weather*) Dulcamara
	Herbalism p.173	(*Cystitis or kidney stones*) corn silk, or buchu, or marsh mallow, or couch grass, or eryngo
	Aromatherapy p.181	(*Bladder problems*) juniper bath, or juniper massage; (*fluid retention*) caraway, cypress or rosemary bath
	Naturopathy p.205	(*Cystitis – general*) fasting, raw diet, hot-and-cold spraying and sitz baths
	Hydrotherapy p.214	(*Cystitis*) daily hot-and-cold sitz baths

Ailments	Therapies	Remedies
High blood pressure High blood pressure is more common in older people and fat people. As preventive care, avoid too much stress, take regular exercise, cut down on salt, sugar, saturated fats, alcohol, and caffeine. Several therapies are effective, including meditation, autogenics, and biofeedback (pp.314-21).	**Herbalism** p.174 **Naturopathy** p.204 **Yoga** p.293	Lime flowers, or vervain; valerian (*General*) basic health diet, fasting, raw diet, foot bath, relaxation routine, gentle exercise, (*supplementary*) vitamin E, lecithin, garlic tablets Corpse pose, and meditation (pp.316-17)
Low blood pressure This may cause dizziness or even fainting. If it persists it may be a symptom of a more serious disorder.	**Naturopathy** p.205 **Yoga** p.293	(*General*) basic health diet, rest, exercise, (*supplementary*) vitamin E, compound mineral supplement Basic asanas, breathing exercise
Palpitation Palpitation can develop after rheumatic fever or as a result of a heart disorder. It also occurs normally in stress.	**Aromatherapy** p.181	Basil massage, or orange blossom bath
Anemia Anemia sufferers benefit from extra iron and vitamin C.	**Herbalism** p.174	Nettle infusion, or watercress, or kelp tablets
Varicose veins Varicose veins can be prevented, at least in part, by increasing the intake of dietary fiber, drinking more fluids, avoiding long periods of sitting or standing, taking regular exercise, and avoiding very hot baths.	**Homeopathy** p.156 **Aromatherapy** p.181 **Naturopathy** p.205 **Traditional medicine** p.225 **Yoga** p.293	Hamamelis, or Pulsatilla; (*acute phlebitis*) Vipera Lemon oil bath, lemon and almond oil applied locally (*General*) brisk walks, (*local*) cold spraying, rest,(*supplementary*) bioflavonoids, vitamin E, compound mineral supplement Witch hazel compress; calendula compress; hay-flower compress; cider vinegar Basic asanas, especially inverted postures

Ailments	Therapies	Remedies
Addiction Acupuncture (pp.268-73) and hypnotherapy (pp.310-13) are successful. Self-help groups, eg, Alcoholics Anonymous, play a major role.	**Naturopathy** p.207 **Bach flower remedies** p.187	(*General*) basic health diet, fasting, relaxation, friction rub, exercise, (*supplementary*) vitamin B, bioflavonoids, compound mineral supplement Drug Detoxification Mix
Allergies and food allergies Try to identify and avoid the offending food, or other harmful substances. Stop smoking (p.57), since this reduces the body's ability to cope, and come off the Pill. See also Allergies in babies, p.139.	**Herbalism** p.175 **Naturopathy** p.206, p.207	Eyebright; nettle; marsh mallow; wild thyme; hyssop (See also Children's and babies' ailments, p.139) (*General*) basic health diet, fasting, raw diet, (*food allergies*) regular meals, protein snacks, (*local*) for skin troubles, see Acne and Eczema, p.128; for catarrhal symptoms, see Catarrh, p.124, (*supplementary – food allergies*) bioflavonoids, compound mineral supplement, and (*allergies*) vitamin A
Hay fever Several natural therapies claim to relieve hay fever, including reflexology (pp.256-63) and radionics (pp.306-9). *Honeycomb*	**Homeopathy** **Herbalism** p.175 **Naturopathy** p.206 **Hydrotherapy** p.214 **Traditional medicine** p.226	See Colds, p.123 Hyssop (See also Allergies, above) (*General*) fasting, raw diet, basic health diet, breathing exercise, (*local*) hot-and-cold face bathing, (*acute*) cold bathing, nasal wash, (*supplementary*) vitamin A, bioflavonoids, garlic tablets Cold water face-plunge, cold friction, cold sitz bath Honeycomb, or onion, or brewers' yeast, or comfrey tablets
Feeling faint, fainting, emotional shock Fainting may be a symptom of a more serious disorder, such as anemia, or bleeding. It is usually caused by missing a meal, or being in a stuffy atmosphere.	**Homeopathy** p.329 **Bach flower remedies** p.184, p.329 **Naturopathy** p.206	(*Feeling faint – from emotional upset*) Ignatia; (*with fright and trembling*) Gelsemium; (*with shock and fear*) Aconite; (*slight pain*) Hepar sulphuris; (*hot room*) Pulsatilla; (*shock, needs air*) Carbo vegetabilis Rescue Remedy (*Feeling faint – general*) basic health diet, regular meals, light protein snacks

Ailments	Therapies	Remedies
Fever Check the sufferer's temperature frequently (p.118), and look out for warning signs of serious illness (p.115).	**Homeopathy** p.155	(*First sign*) Aconite; (*sudden onset*) Belladonna; (*dry heat*) Bryonia; (*very chilly*) Nux vomica; (*restless*) Arsenicum album; (*hot and cold*) Sulphur; (*weak and trembly*) Gelsemium; (*worse at night*) Mercurius solubilis; (*with flushing and paleness*) Ferrum phosphoricum; (*in children*) Pulsatilla
	Herbalism	See Coughs, p.122
	Naturopathy p.207	(*General*) fruit and vegetable juices, vegetable broth, fresh fruit, yoghurt, (*in younger children*) cool or tepid sponging, cold compresses, (*in adults*) trunk pack
	Hydrotherapy	See Colds, p.121
	Traditional medicine p.226	Barley water, or chicken soup
Vaginal infections Try the same prevention as for cystitis (p.134), plus a diet low in yeasts and refined carbohydrates.	**Homeopathy** p.157	Mercurius iodatus flavus
	Herbalism p.173	Acidophilus tablets; tea tree oil or cream; vinegar bath
	Aromatherapy p.181	Sage bath or bidet
	Naturopathy p.205	(*General*) fasting, yeast-free diet, (*local*) goats' milk yoghurt, acidic gel, (*supplementary*) vitamin B, bioflavonoids, garlic tablets
Menstrual problems Exercises to stretch and relax muscles, and to tone the pelvic region, can be helpful. Dietary adjustment may also help some women with pre-menstrual tension, see Special needs, p.46.	**Homeopathy** p.157	Magnesia phosphorica, or Colocynthis, or Chamomilla
	Herbalism p.174	Ginger, or black haw bark decoction, or caraway infusion
	Aromatherapy p.181	(*Scanty periods*) oil of basil massage; (*pain*) caraway oil bath
	Hydrotherapy p.214	Contrast sitz bath daily
	Traditional medicine p.225	(*Pain*) raspberry leaf tea; (*delayed period*) syrup of beetroot, or hot mustard bath
	Shiatsu p.283	(*Pain*) general exercise, and pressure points on the legs, abdomen, feet, and beside the lumbar vertebrae
	Yoga p.293	Corpse pose, half shoulderstand, forward bend, pelvic lift, kapalabhati

Raspberry leaf tea

Ailments	Therapies	Remedies
Aches and pains in pregnancy Several natural therapies, notably massage (pp.242-9) and yoga (pp.284-93) helpful.	Shiatsu p.283	(*Backache*) pressure points on hip bones, between lumbar vertebrae, on feet; (*headaches*) points on neck, between vertebrae, on ankles, forehead, between eyes; (*constipation*) points between vertebrae, on head and shinbones; (*hemorrhoids*) points between vertebrae, on sacrum
Morning sickness If vomiting is frequent, replacement of lost body fluid is important.	Homeopathy p.156	(*With heavy and full feeling*) Pulsatilla; (*with persistent nausea*) Ipecacuanha; (*worse for thought of food*) Nux vomica; (*with empty feeling*) Phosphorus
	Shiatsu p.283	Pressure points beside the vertebrae, and on the neck
Labor pains Changing the birthing position may ease the pain (p.95). Most ante-natal classes teach helpful breathing techniques.	Homeopathy p.156	(*To encourage a straightforward delivery*) Caulophyllum; (*to encourage rapid delivery*) Arnica; (*"false", weak labor pains*) Gelsemium, or Caulophyllum; (*"can't bear the pain"*) Chamomilla; (*weepy, discouraged*) Pulsatilla; (*exhausted, feels chilly*) Carbo vegetabilis; (*tired out, feels achy*) Arnica
	Traditional medicine p.225	Raspberry leaf tea
Breast-feeding problems Mothers should pay close attention to their diet (see also p.139).	Homeopathy p.157	(*Poor milk flow*) Pulsatilla; (*blocked ducts (engorgement)*) Silica, or Phytolacca; (*early mastitis*) Bryonia; (*mastitis*) Belladonna; (*cracked nipples*) Castor equi
Menopausal problems Supplements of vitamin C, D, E, and calcium have been found to reduce problems such as hot flushes and depression. Good all-round nutrition is important.	**Aromatherapy** p.181	Oil of cypress massage
	Bach flower remedies p.186	(*Major changes in life*) Walnut
	Traditional medicine p.225	Ginseng
	Shiatsu p.283	Points on legs and between lumbar and thoracic vertebrae
Feverish disorders Check the temperature frequently (p.118), and be on the lookout for signs of deterioration (p.115).	Naturopathy p.207	(*Measles, chickenpox, flu, etc*) fasting, packs and compresses; (*rashes*) sodium bicarbonate or bran baths (See also Fever, p.137)

Ailments	Therapies	Remedies
Children's and babies' ailments Infants and young children require the gentlest of medicines, and natural therapies are oriented toward safe mild treatments. Herbal remedies help to soothe allergic problems, but the cause must be dealt with too (see Orthodox treatment).	**Homeopathy** pp.158-9	(*Teething*) Chamomilla, or Pulsatilla, or Calcarea phosphorica; (*nappy rash*) Calendula cream; Chamomile cream; (*croup*) Aconite, or Spongia, or Hepar sulphurica; (*colic*) Magnesia phosphorica; Colocynthis; Dioscorea, or Ipecacuanha; (*nappy rash*) Calendula or Chamomile cream
	Herbalism p.165, p.168, p.175	(*Croup*) wild cherry bark; (*allergies in babies*) matricaria (German chamomile), or dill, or fennel; (*diarrhea*) agrimony, or meadowsweet
	Naturopathy	For colic, see Indigestion, p.126
	Traditional medicine p.223	(*Nappy rash*) cornstarch dusted on affected area; (*bed-wetting*) honey, or cinnamon
Chamomile	**Orthodox treatment**	(*Allergies or colic*) It is most important to identify and eliminate offending foods (p.170). Cows' milk may provoke allergic reactions. If breast-feeding, try cutting out cows' milk and dairy products for a couple of weeks. Problem foods which may cause colic include onions, garlic, Chinese foods, cabbage, beans, green leafy vegetables and alcohol. (*Nappy rash*) The baby's bottom must be washed well, dried thoroughly, and a gentle barrier cream should be applied.
INFECTIOUS DISEASES	**Vaccination**	Vaccines have been developed for several childhood diseases. Parents should discuss having their children vaccinated, and the implications of vaccination, with their doctor. Vaccines against particular infectious diseases, such as cholera, may be required by law if you are travelling to certain countries.
Whooping cough	**Homeopathy** p.159	Cuprum metallicum, or Carbo vegetabilis, or Drosera, or Kali carbonicum, or Coccus cacti
	Herbalism p.167	Wild cherry bark
Scarlet fever	**Homeopathy** p.158	Belladonna
Mumps	**Homeopathy** p.158	Aconite, or Belladonna, or Bryonia, or Pulsatilla, or Mercurius, or Pilocarpus
Chickenpox	**Homeopathy** p.158	Antimonium, or Rhus toxicodendron, or Pulsatilla, or Mercurius, or Pilocarpus
Measles	**Homeopathy** p.158	Aconite, or Belladonna, or Bryonia, or Pulsatilla, or (*with sensitive eyes*) Euphrasia

Ailments	Therapies	Remedies
First aid For commonsense first aid measures consult Chapter 6, First Aid and Emergencies, pp.324-37.	**Homeopathy** pp.324-8	(*Burns*) Urtica urens or Cantharis; (*cuts*) Hypericum, or Ledum, or Hypercal; (*sunburn*) Belladonna, or Ferrum phosphoricum, or Kali carbonicum, or Cantharis; (*sprains*) Ledum, or Arnica, or Rhus toxicodendron, or Ruta graveolens, or Bryonia; (*bruises*) Arnica, or Ledum, or Ruta graveolens, or Bellis perennis; (*frostbite*) Agaricus muscarius; (*splinters*) Ledum, or Hypericum; (*nosebleeds*) Ferrum phosphoricum, or Vipera; (*bites and stings*) Ledum, or Apis mellifica, or Urtica urens; (*motion sickness*) Cocculus, or Tabacum
	Herbalism pp.324-7	(*Burns*) witch hazel, or chickweed, or marigold; (*cuts*) witch hazel; (*sunburn*) marigold; (*sprains*) comfrey; (*bruises*) comfrey, or witch hazel, or marigold; (*splinters*) slippery elm poultice; (*nosebleeds*) witch hazel
	Aromatherapy pp.324-8	(*Burns*) lavender oil; (*cuts*) clove, or lavender, or eucalyptus; (*wasp stings*) cinnamon
	Traditional medicine pp.324-8	(*Burns*) leek, or potato, or onion, or aloe vera; (*cuts*) witch hazel, or lemon, or sodium bicarbonate; (*sunburn*) sodium bicarbonate, or black tea; (*sprains*) olive oil, or wintergreen, or Tiger Balm; (*frostbite*) cucumber, or potato, or onion; (*splinters*) kaolin poultice; (*nosebleeds*) lemon juice; (*bites and stings*) sodium bicarbonate, or garlic, or lemon, or witch hazel, or vinegar, or cornstarch, or plantain, or onion; (*poison ivy*) cider vinegar, or aloe vera; (*motion sickness*) brewers' yeast, or yeast-free vitamin B, or lemon
Negative emotional states	**Bach flower remedies** pp.185-7	(*Fear*) Mimulus, Cherry Plum, Aspen, Red Chestnut; (*lack of interest in the present*) Clematis, Honeysuckle, Wild Rose, Olive, White Chestnut, Chestnut Bud; (*over-sensitivity to influence and ideas*) Agrimony, Centaury, Holly; (*loneliness*) Water Violet, Heather, Impatiens; (*depression and anguish*) Mustard, Larch, Pine, Elm, Sweet Chestnut, Star of Bethlehem, Willow, Oak, Crab Apple; (*uncertainty*) Cerato, Scleranthus, Gentian, Gorse, Hornbeam, Wild Oak; (*over-concern for the welfare of others*) Chicory, Vervain, Vine, Beech, Rock Water

Arnica

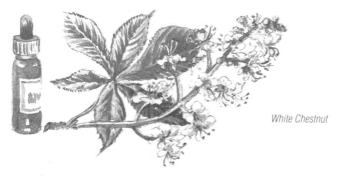

White Chestnut

Medicinal therapies

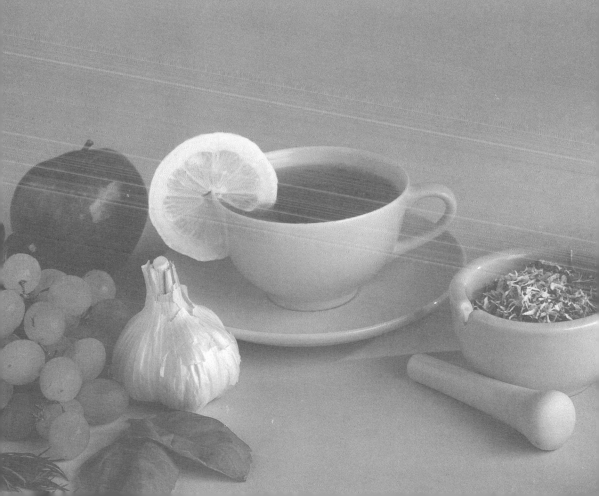

Homeopathy

Homeopathy is a comprehensive medical system practiced both by highly qualified lay persons and by physicians fully trained in orthodox medicine. It is based on the principle of "curing like with like" and relies on a unique system of diagnosis and treatment to arouse the immune system to overcome sickness and restore health, by prescribing remedies that induce symptoms similar to the disease. Unlike allopathic medicine which suppresses symptoms, homeopathy regards the symptoms of disease as part of the body's attempt to defend itself from illness.

In the New World, Europe, India and Pakistan, homeopathy is one of the leading natural medicines and the major alternative to allopathy (orthodox medicine). It has obtained official recognition in many countries of the world, the main exceptions being China, Japan and Africa (apart from South Africa). The official pharmocopoeias of France and the German Federal Republic have separate sections for homeopathic medicines. And in 1938, the US Food, Drug and Cosmetic Act finally recognized the homeopathic pharmacopoeia as the legal equivalent of the allopathic one.

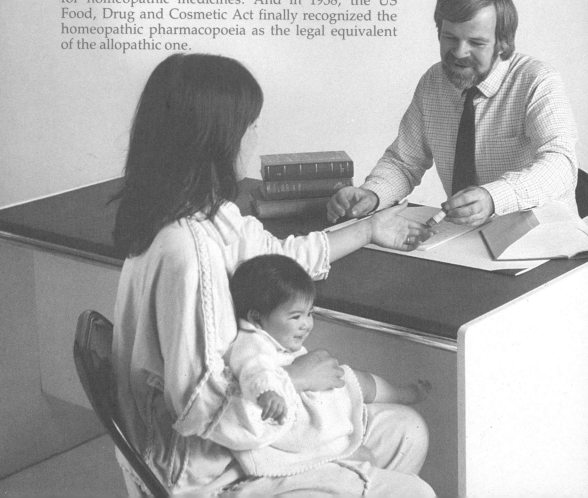

Hahnemann and the law of similars

The "law of similars", which is the guiding principle of homeopathic prescribing, was discovered by Samuel Hahnemann, a Leipzig physician, in the last years of the 18th century – at precisely the time that Edward Jenner was advocating cowpox vaccination for the prevention of smallpox, using the same general principle. In brief the law states that a remedy can cure disease if it produces symptoms very similar to those of the disease in a healthy person. The homeopath's task is to find the remedy whose action on the body is most similar to the patient's condition.

Treatment with "similars" was, of course, well known to medicine before Hahnemann's time – in fact it was mentioned as early as the 4th century BC in the Hippocratic Corpus. Hahnemann, however, gave it a new definition through his discovery that the curative powers of medicinal substances could be found by giving them to healthy people, called in homeopathy the "proving". His work led him to the conclusion that the curative power of a medicine was identical to its power to cause symptoms in the healthy. It followed that symptoms which medicinal substances caused in healthy "provers" were the best guides to using these substances for cure.

Hahnemann spent the rest of his life "proving" a variety of substances from the animal, vegetable and mineral worlds, ascertaining the symptoms produced in healthy people, then giving the corresponding substance to a patient presenting with a similar collection of symptoms. This work has been carried on by his followers, and today homeopathy has provings of about 1,500 medicinal substances.

The infinitesimal dose

Hahnemann made another major discovery in the course of his research – the principle of the minimum or infinitesimal dose, the dilution of medicines 1:1,000, 1:1,000,000, 1:1,000,000,000 parts and beyond. He found that progressively diluting the dose of a remedy and "succussing" or shaking it vigorously at each stage of dilution – a process known as "potentization" – makes the remedy more rather than less powerful. Potentization releases the intrinsic curative energy of a substance. In homeopathy, therefore, dosages are most powerful when given in the lowest concentration or highest dilution.

Research

Of the enormous amount of research done on homeopathy, two topics stand out as being of particular interest – the infinitesimal dose and homeopathic clinical trials.

The infinitesimal dose is an aspect of homeopathy that has provoked amazement and disbelief in unsympathetic observers. Even more scepticism has been aroused by homeopathy's further contention that a medicine can be powerfully operative on the body when diluted to such a degree that, statistically speaking, there is little probability of any molecule of the active medication remaining in the dilution (the so-called "ultramolecular" dose). The most important experiment demonstrating the existence of a medicinal power in the ultramolecular dose was performed by Dr William E. Boyd (see also p.307) in Edinburgh in the late 1940s. Boyd proved that a microdilution of mercuric chloride accelerated the rate of hydrolysis of starch by diastase.

In recent years, several clinical trials of homeopathic medicines have been conducted, and their results reported in the general medical press. In a 1978 trial in Glasgow, Scotland, three groups of rheumatoid arthritis patients were compared – one group was treated with aspirin, another with a placebo, and the third with homeopathic remedies. The homeopathic group was found to be appreciably better than the other two a year after the trial.

Consulting a homeopath

The first time you consult a homeopath, be prepared for a lengthy visit. The initial consultation may take an hour or more, but subsequent visits will normally be shorter. The homeopath's first task is to obtain a comprehensive picture of you and your symptoms, seeking out details, such as your mental or emotional state, which are often ignored in allopathy, but are vitally important for the correct homeopathic prescription. He or she will then choose a homeopathic medicine that most closely matches your symptoms (see Symptoms and characteristics, pp.147-59).

Patients are often surprised to find homeopathy based on symptoms rather than causes of disease. As a vitalist healing system, homeopathy is in fact opposed to discovering the cause of disease inside the body. It maintains that the human body is

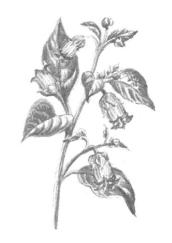

Homeopathic Belladonna
Belladonna is a classic example of Hahnemann's principle that "like cures like". Every part of the plant, a deadly poison, produces symptoms that range from acute fever and delirium to dryness of the mouth and constricton of the throat. In homeopathic preparation it is an important fever and inflammation remedy.

continually reacting to its environment, though in health signs of this reaction generally pass unnoticed. In sickness, however, the signs of reaction stand out and it is these that are called symptoms. Symptoms are seen as positive phenomena, indicating the body's attempt to restore balance. Where allopathy sees symptoms as part of the disease, and seeks to suppress them, homeopathy sees symptoms as part of the *cure*, indicating the body's attempt to restore balance. The homeopath is therefore only interested in symptoms, in how the body is reacting to the cause, and prescribes a remedy to assist the reaction.

"The highest ideal of therapy is to restore health rapidly, gently, permanently; to remove and destroy the whole disease in the shortest, surest, least harmful way, according to clearly comprehensible principles."
Samuel Hahnemann,
Organon of Medicine, 1810

Common and specific symptoms

Every individual has his or her own unique set of symptoms or way of reacting to and restoring equilibrium with the environment. Only the remedy that produces symptoms "most similar" to those of the individual will be curative, so the practitioner must be able to distinguish the "most similar" medicine from all the others. This is done by ranking your symptoms according to importance. Homeopathy divides symptoms into "common" and "specific" or "peculiar" (strange or unusual). Common symptoms are those that are found in most states of disease and manifested by most participants in the "provings" of medicines – examples are headaches, stomach pains, nausea, and neuralgia. "Specific" symptoms are found infrequently, in few patients or provings, and it is these that are most important for prescribing. By obtaining details about the common symptoms, homeopathy endeavors to convert them into specific ones.

If, for example, you glance at Headaches on page 153, you will find a number of different remedies described. Each will act curatively only on a specific type of headache, as defined by the specific symptoms. In choosing the correct remedy to prescribe, the homeopath will ask questions precisely directed to distinguish one remedy from another. For a headache, he or she might ask whether you feel better or worse when lying down or moving around, if both Bryonia and Gelsemium seem appropriate. When several of the specific symptoms found in the proving of a given remedy have been ascertained, the homeopath can be reasonably certain that this is the right remedy for you at this particular time.

Homeopathic medicines

Homeopathic medicines are easy to administer, and completely safe for all, including infants, the pregnant and the elderly. Most of the remedies are taken by mouth and are available in the form of pills, tablets or granules – it does not matter which you use. Some remedies are for external application, in the form of creams, ointments or tinctures. For home treatment the recommended potency for all remedies is 6th centesimal (6x). Select the remedy from those on pages 147-59 which matches your symptoms most closely. Use only one at a time. If your first choice does not help or it's not successful despite a good trial, choose another remedy based on your present symptoms, or consult a homeopath. The remedies listed are a limited selection from the vast pharmacopoeia. (See also First aid, pp.324-30.)

Caution Always seek medical advice for serious or persistent ailments.

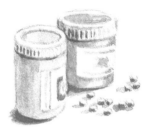

Dosage

Take one pill or tablet or a few granules at a time. It is the frequency of dosage that matters, rather than the quantity. The more ill you are, the more often you need to take a remedy – for a high fever or acute earache, for example, take a dose every 15 minutes; for problems of intermediate urgency, every 1 to 4 hours; for complaints that have been going on for days, weeks or longer, one dose 3 times a day.

Take the remedies when your mouth is clean – that is, free from the odor or taste of anything you may have been eating, drinking, sucking or smoking. Put nothing in your mouth for 15 minutes before or after taking a remedy.

When an ailment shows marked improvement, increase the interval between doses. Discontinue treatment once relief is obtained. If, after taking the medicine, your symptoms get worse, stop taking the remedy. An aggravation of symptoms is usually followed by a pronounced overall improvement. Repeat the remedy only if the original symptoms occur.

Antidotes

During treatment, avoid the following, which can antidote homeopathic remedies:
- anything with a strong odor, especially menthol, eucalyptus, camphor, oil of cloves, and any products containing them, plus extra strong peppermints, strong toothpastes, mouthwashes and essential oils
- coffee (unless decaffeinated)
- any drug treatment – but always consult your doctor before stopping any treatment.

Taking a homeopathic remedy

When taking homeopathic medicine internally, either tip the remedy onto your clean palm or onto a teaspoon to transfer it to your mouth. Chew it up and dissolve it thoroughly before swallowing. Do not wash it down with drinks. For external treatment, apply creams and ointments in the normal manner, but dilute tinctures (known as Mother Tinctures in homeopathy), using a ½ teaspoon of tincture to a cup of water.

Storage of medicines

Store remedies in their original containers, away from anything that smells strong, especially items listed in Antidotes, and soaps, perfumes, mothballs, etc. Keep them away from direct sunlight, heat, X-rays and strong magnetic fields.

Ailments and remedies

If you are new to homeopathy, you may be surprised at the wording and detail of the symptoms that distinguish one remedy from another. Alongside more familiar details of physical symptoms you will find descriptions of an individual's mental state or type, for example, or the time of day, temperature, or climatic condition in which symptoms appear better or worse. By closely observing the sufferer's condition, you can use these symptom pictures to arrive at the remedy that is right for the individual.

Ailments	Symptoms and characteristics	Remedies
Coughs	Dry hard cough – Coughing causes pain and holding of head and chest – Excessive thirst – Worse in warm room and from cold dry weather	Bryonia
	Hard cough – Great difficulty in expectorating – Better for cold drinks – Involuntary urination from coughing – Hoarseness with rawness of the throat	Causticum
	Hard tickling cough – Worse from talking and in cold air – May be hoarse – Tight chest – Headache from coughing	Phosphorus
	Cough induced by every breath of cool air, forcing person to keep mouth covered – Violent tickle in throat	Rumex
	Cough worse in warm air – Worse from lying down – Dry in the evening, loose in the morning	Pulsatilla
	Spasmodic suffocating cough – Loose and rattling cough and respiration, early in illness – Wheezing and sensation of weight on chest – Intense nausea with clean tongue	Ipecacuanha
	Dry, teasing, spasmodic cough with gagging and retching – Feverish, person cannot move or uncover without feeling chilly – Worse for cold dry windy weather	Nux vomica
	Worse for cold dry weather – Coughs when any part of the body is uncovered and from breathing cold air – Better in warm moist atmospheres	Hepar sulphuris
	Very dry violent cough sounding like a saw being driven through a board	Spongia

Bryonia

Ailments	Symptoms and characteristics	Remedies
Colds, catarrh, hay fever and sinusitis	First stages of a cold – Sudden onset – After exposure to cold dry weather	Aconite
	Early stages of a cold with much dryness and itching of the back of the nose and throat	Wyethia
	Streaming eyes and nose – Nose very sore – Tearing sensation in the larynx on coughing – Better in the open air	Allium cepa
	Streaming eyes and nose – Eyes very sore	Euphrasia
	Streaming eyes and nose – Both very sore	Arsenicum album
	Cold starts with sneezing – Nose runs like a tap – Indicated especially if cold sores present – Sinusitis may be present	Natrum muriaticum
	Nose blocked and running – Better in the open air, yet person feels very chilly and must keep warm – Very irritable – After exposure to cold weather	Nux vomica
	Thick yellow-green catarrh – Better in the open air – Often indicated for affectionate people who are prone to weepiness and desire consolation and company	Pulsatilla
	Thick yellow catarrh – Better in the open air – Important in sinusitis (If not effective try Kali bichromicum)	Calcarea sulphurica
	Very stringy discharge – Yellow-green catarrh – Important in sinusitis	Kali bichromicum
	Streaming hot sore nose – Violent sneezing – Sinusitis often present – Better in the open air	Kali iodatum
	Sinusitis pain starting at the back of the head and settling over the eyes – Sinusitis without any discharge	Silica
	Thick yellow catarrh – Feels very chilly and sensitive to draughts – Very irritable – Sinusitis may be present – After exposure to cold dry weather	Hepar sulphuris
	Excessive saliva – Raw nose – Much sweating – Very sensitive to temperature changes – Sinusitis may be present – Worse from radiant heat	Mercurius solubilis

Pulsatilla

Silica

Ailments	Symptoms and characteristics	Remedies
Colds, etc (continued)	Dull, heavy head – Heavy eyes and limbs – Feels shivery, like flu – Lack of thirst despite fever	Gelsemium
	Nose runnier in warm room, stuffed up outside – Streaming eyes and nose – Nose sore – After exposure to cold wet weather	Dulcamara
	Unbearably itchy, raw, tingly nasal passages – Can't leave nose alone – Constant picking and rubbing at nose and lips	Arum triphyllum
	Violent sneezing, worse in open air – Can't tolerate the odor of flowers – Especially in hay fever	Sabadilla
Sore throats *Belladona*	Bright red tonsils and throat, which feel dry and burning – Skin similarly very hot and flushed	Belladonna
	Very coated tongue – Very bad breath – Excessive saliva – Much sweating – Feels alternately hot and cold	Mercurius solubilis
	Feels as if the throat has been scratched or a fishbone is present – Neck and throat very sensitive to touch – Better for warm drinks	Hepar sulphuris
	Rather nondescript sore throat – No strong symptoms	Baryta muriatica
	See also Fever (p.155)	
Flu *Rhus toxicodendron* 	Typical flu symptoms	Gelsemium
	Extreme aching of limbs, including the bones – Constant aching of eyes	Eupatorium perfoliatum
	Extremely restless – Very achy and stiff muscles – Worse at rest and at night – Better for continued motion – Feels very chilly, better for warmth	
	See also Colds, catarrh, hay fever and sinusitis (above) and Fever (especially Bryonia and Arsenicum album) (p.155)	

Ailments	Symptoms and characteristics	Remedies
Diarrhea	Simultaneous diarrhea and vomiting – Considerable weakness, chilliness and restlessness – From food poisoning	Arsenicum album
	Simultaneous diarrhea and vomiting – Very copious and violent diarrhea – Considerable weakness and exhaustion – Extreme chilliness with cold sweat especially on forehead – Indicated if Arsenicum album doesn't help	Veratrum album
	With much gas and flatulent distension – Not much vomiting – Not restless – Feels very cold but desires air, especially fanning	Carbo vegetabilis
	From worry and excitement	Argentum nitricum
	Drives person out of bed in early morning (5.00 am)	Sulphur
	Profuse and offensive diarrhea, in early morning (4.00 am) – Much flatus passed with stool – Feels very weak and faint afterwards	Podophyllum
Indigestion, vomiting	With much distension and gas – Relieved by belching – Feels chilly but desires the open air	Carbo vegetabilis
	With much distension and gas – Relieved by passing flatus	Lycopodium
	From over-indulgence in food and alcohol – Much retching, wants to vomit but can't – Vomiting gives relief	Nux vomica
	Constant nausea – Unrelieved by vomiting	Ipecacuanha
	From too rich food – Better in the fresh air – Taste of food remains a long time	Pulsatilla
	With burning stomach pains – Chilly and restless	Arsenicum album
Hemorrhoids	Painful, itching hemorrhoids	Nux vomica
	Bleeding hemorrhoids	Hamamelis
	With back pain and sensation of small, painful sticks in rectum	Aesculus

Carbo vegetabilis

Nux Vomica

Ailments	Symptoms and characteristics	Remedies
Boils and abscesses	When first forming – Red, hot and painful	Belladonna
	When pus has formed – Very sensitive to touch	Hepar sulphuris
	When slow to clear	Silica
Herpes	First try	Natrum muriaticum
	If Natrum muriaticum not effective	Rhus toxicodendron
Ingrowing toenails		Magnetis polus Australis
Earache	Sudden onset – Hot, frightened and restless – After exposure to cold dry weather	Aconite
	Skin is very hot and flushed bright red – Throbbing pain – Crying out in sleep – May be with delirium	Belladonna
	Frantic, irritable, can't bear the pain – If it's a child, must be carried – One cheek flushed, the other pale – Often happens during toething.	Chamomilla
	If it's a child, weepy, clingy, needing attention and company – Often with thick yellow nasal catarrh – Has no thirst despite having a fover	Pulsatilla
	Early stages of an earache – No distingulshing symptoms	Ferrum phosphoricum
	Ear very sensitive to touch – Patient very chilly, irritable, and sensitive to draughts	Hepar sulphuris
Toothache	If Plantago not effective (For local treatment Plantago Mother Tincture can be dabbed on painful areas)	Kreosotum

Chamomilla

Ailments	Symptoms and characteristics	Remedies
Chilblains	Worse when hot	Pulsatilla
	Worse when cold	Agaricus
	When there is much swelling (worse when hot)	Apis mellifica
	As a local application	Tamus ointment
Urticaria,	With much swelling – Skin tight and shiny	Apis mellifica
	With much itching	Urtica urens
Conjunctivitis	Burning eyes with acrid discharge – Strong sensitivity to light	Euphrasia
	With yellow pus	Argentum nitricum
	If Argentum nitricum doesn't help	Pulsatilla
	For bathing the eyes use Euphrasia Mother Tincture – 2 or 3 drops in an eyebath with a standard eyebath solution	
Rheumatism, backache	From over-exertion – Feels bruised – Considerable sensitivity to touch and pressure	Arnica
	Worst at rest and on beginning to move – Improves with gentle movement ("limbers up") – Worse from cold wet weather – Better for warmth	Rhus toxicodendron
	Worse with any movement – Better at rest	Bryonia
	Turning over in bed causes pain – Needs to sit up in order to turn over in bed – Worse on waking in the morning – Worse for first movements but improves with continued movement – Not worse at rest (compare Rhus toxicodendron)	Nux vomica
Cramp		Cuprum metallicum

Arnica

Ailments	Symptoms and characteristics	Remedies
Shingles		Rhus toxicodendron
Stiff neck	Stiffness and pain at rest and on first movements – Improvement with continued gentle movements and warmth – From cold wet weather and draught	Rhus toxicodendron
	Worse on waking in the morning – Worse on first movements, limbering up with gentle movement, but not worse at rest – From cold dry weather and draughts	Nux vomica
	If Rhus toxicodendron or Nux vomica not clearly indicated	Actea racemosa
Headaches	Worse for the slightest movement, even of the eyes	Bryonia
	Like a band around the head or at the back of the head spreading from the neck up into the forehead – Head feels dull, heavy or bursting – Worse when lying down – From exposure to the sun	Gelsemium
	Hangover-type headache – Splitting headache – Often with nausea and stomach complaints – From over-indulgence in food, alcohol and tobacco – Irritable and over-sensitive	Nux vomica
	Violent, bursting, throbbing headache with red, hot face – Sudden onset – Worse from the slightest jarring, movement, stooping, light or noise – Better for sitting up – From exposure to the sun	Belladonna
	Blinding, hammering headache, often worse between 10.00 am and 3.00 pm – Often with visual disturbance – Desires salt – Dislikes being fussed over when ill	Natrum muriaticum
Neuralgia	Facial neuralgia caused by cold dry weather	Aconite
	Worse for any movement or draught – Better for warmth and firm supporting pressure – Usually right-sided	Magnesia phosphorica
	Symptoms like Magnesia phosphorica but usually left-sided	Colocynthis
	Sharp, stinging pains in the face, especially involving the eye – Usually left-sided – Very sensitive to touch	Spigelia

Ailments	Symptoms and characteristics	Remedies
Insomnia	From over-active mind – Mind crowded with ideas and thoughts	Coffea
	From apprehension, with great restlessness and anxiety	Arsenicum album
	From emotional stress, with lowness of spirits – Person often sighs	Ignatia
Stress	For the person who is irritable, has high expectations of himself or herself and others – Drives self hard – Tends to over-indulge in food, alcohol and tobacco – Feels awful on waking	Nux vomica
	Emotional stress, grief and disappointment	Ignatia
	For the person who can't cope any more – Feels tired out, weepy, irritable and indifferent to loved ones	Sepia
Anxiety	From anticipation of an engagement, eg, an examination or meeting – Feels paralysed and weak (especially at the knees) with trembling	Gelsemium
	In rather impulsive and hurried person – From anticipation of engagements – May get strong compulsions, eg, not to tread on the lines between paving stones – Worse for heat	Argentum nitricum
	Great anxiety with fear and restlessness – Panic attacks – From sudden shocks, eg, road accident or earthquake	Aconite
Tiredness, fatigue, exhaustion	From over-exertion	Arnica
	After mental effort and worry	Kali phosphoricum
	With anxiety and restlessness	Arsenicum album
	With depression, weeping, irritability, indifference to loved ones – Feels unable to cope any more	Sepia
	In workaholics – Feels irritable and intolerant of inefficiency	Nux vomica

Ailments	Symptoms and characteristics	Remedies
Grief	Disbelief, cannot cry, speechlessness, sighing, hysterical reactions, and psychosomatic symptoms, such as trembling, paralysis, etc (Ignatia is best used in higher potencies such as 30 or 200x)	Ignatia
	Complete weakness, debility, apathy, and indifference as a result of shock	Phosphoric acidum
Fever	For first sign of fever – Sudden onset – Intense thirst – Dry heat – With restlessness and fear – Following exposure to cold dry weather	Aconite
	Sudden onset – Flushed, bright red skin – Radiates intense heat – Feels as if "burning up" – Sweat on covered parts – Often with delirium	Belladonna
	Very dry heat – Very dry tongue and mouth – Intense thirst and gulps drinks down – Worse from the least movement – Worse from heat – Irritable and resents any interference	Bryonia
	Feels very chilly – Can't get warm enough – Very irritable and hypersensitive	Nux vomica
	Very restless, anxious and fearful – Feels very chilly and rapidly exhausted – Thirsty for small frequent drinks	Arsenicum album
	Feels alternately hot and cold – Feet feel hot, so uncovers them – Very red lips – Fever with no obvious cause – When no other remedy clearly indicated	Sulphur
	Feels weak and trembly – Eyes and limbs feel heavy – Aches all over – Back-of-head headache, feels dull – Chills up and down the back – Lack of thirst despite fever	Gelsemium
	Feels alternately hot and cold – Profuse sweats – Profuse saliva – Foul breath – Very sensitive to changes of temperature – Worse at night	Mercurius solubilis
	Flushes and pales easily – When no other remedy clearly indicated	Ferrum phosphoricum
	For the weepy child who won't be put down or leave your side – Lacks thirst despite fever – Worse for heat	Pulsatilla

Aconite

Ailments	Symptoms and characteristics	Remedies
Varicose veins		Hamamelis
	In affectionate, gentle and emotional people	Pulsatilla
	Acute phlebitis with or without thrombosis	Vipera
Morning sickness	Feels heavy and full – Worse from fatty and rich foods – Wants fresh air – Feels insecure and desires company and affection – Lack of thirst – Worse in the evening	Pulsatilla
	Persistent nausea unrelieved by vomiting	Ipecacuanha
	Worse from the thought and smell of food – Feels empty – Better for eating – Often has a fondness for vinegar – Tired, weepy and irritable	Sepia
	Much retching and straining, especially in the mornings – Irritable and tense – Desires stimulants	Nux vomica
	Feels empty – Desires cold drinks but soon vomits them back – Nausea on putting hands in warm water – In very sympathetic and open people	Phosphorus
Labor pains	To encourage an easy, straightforward delivery (take a dose daily for the last 3 weeks of pregnancy)	Caulophyllum
	To encourage a rapid delivery and reduce bruising, swelling and pain after delivery (take early in the second stage, then immediately after the baby is born, then half-hourly for 2 or 3 hours, then 3 times a day for 2 or 3 days, or as necessary)	Arnica
	"False" irregular, short and weak labor pains	Caulophyllum
	"False" labor pains with weakness and trembling	Gelsemium
	"Can't bear the pain" – Irritability	Chamomilla
	Feels weepy, easily discouraged and "can't go on" – Needs company and consolation	Pulsatilla
	Feels exhausted and chilly but needs open air, especially fanning	Carbo vegetabilis
	Feels tired out from long exertion – Feels achy and bruised	Arnica

Sepia

Ailments	Symptoms and characteristics	Remedies
Breast-feeding	For poor milk flow, take a dose half an hour before each feed	Pulsatilla
	For blocked ducts (engorgement)	Silica
	For early mastitis (hot, hard and painful) – Feels better for support	Bryonia
	For mastitis – Hot, hard and throbbing pain – Red streaks radiating from nipple – Very tender	Belladonna
	Hard sensitive lumps in breast – Area involved becomes purple in color – Feeding is very painful	Phytolacca
	Cracked nipples	Castor equi
Cystitis	Burning pains, better for cold applications	Cantharis
	Frequent painful urging with little result – Better for warm applications	Nux vomica
	Very sudden onset – From getting chilled in cold dry weather	Aconite
	From getting chilled in cold wet weather	Dulcamara
Vaginal infection		Mercurius iodatus flavus
Menstrual cramps	Cramping pains, better for warmth	Magnesia phosphorica
	Person is doubled up and can't keep still due to the pain – Irritable – Better for firm pressure	Colocynthis
	Feels the pain is unbearable – Irritable and snappy	Chamomilla
Premenstrual tension	Feels tired, irritable, weepy, chilly and unable to cope	Sepia

Phytolacca

Childhood ailments

Homeopathic medicines are completely safe for even the youngest child. Several remedies for common childhood ailments are listed below, but other medicines useful for children suffering from headaches, earaches, and fever, can be found on the preceding pages.

Ailments	Symptoms and characteristics	Remedies
Measles	See Fever (p.155), especially Aconite, Belladonna, Bryonia and Pulsatilla	
	Eyes very sore and sensitive to light	Euphrasia
Mumps	See Fever (p.155), especially Aconite, Belladonna, Bryonia, Pulsatilla, and Mercurius	
	If none of the above match the symptoms	Pilocarpus (Jaborandi)
Chickenpox		Antimonium tartaricum
	Feels very itchy	Rhus toxicodendron
	Child feels weepy and very clingy, needs a lot of attention – Not thirsty and worse for heat	Pulsatilla
Scarlet fever		Belladonna
Teething	Cross, irritable, vexed and restless – Only wants to be carried – Also for illness associated with teething, eg, colds, coughs, and diarrhea	Chamomilla
	Weepy, wants affection and cuddling	Pulsatilla
	Peevish and not helped by either Chamomilla or Pulsatilla	Calcarea phosphorica

Ailments	Symptoms and characteristics	Remedies
Whooping cough *Drosera*	Violent paroxysms of coughing, with cramps of the extremities (especially fists clenched tight) and blueness of the face – Much relief from cold drinks	Cuprum metallicum
	With gagging, vomiting and redness of the face	Carbo vegetabilis
	Worse after midnight – Worse lying down – Coughing hurts tummy, and child wants tummy pressed firmly – With nosebleed	Drosera
	With bag-like swelling between upper eyelids and eyebrows – Worse at 3.00 am	Kali carbonicum
	Vomits mucus that hangs in long strings from the mouth – Coughs at 11.30 pm – Better for cool air and cold drinks	Coccus cacti
Croup	Sudden onset – Considerable anxiety on awakening	Aconite
	Very dry, barking cough, like a saw going through a board	Spongia
	A looser, more rattly cough	Hepar sulphuris
	If uncertain which to give, start with Aconite; if that doesn't work, go on to Spongia; if that doesn't help, try Hepar sulphuris	
Colic *Ipecacuanha*	Doubling up with pain – Relieved by heat	Magnesia phosphorica
	Writhing around in pain – Eased by firm pressure – Very irritable	Colocynthis
	Eased by stretching out or bending backward	Dioscorea
	Cutting pains – Intense nausea with each spasm	Ipecacuanha
Nappy rash	(Consult a homeopath if the problem persists)	Calendula or Chamomile cream

Herbalism

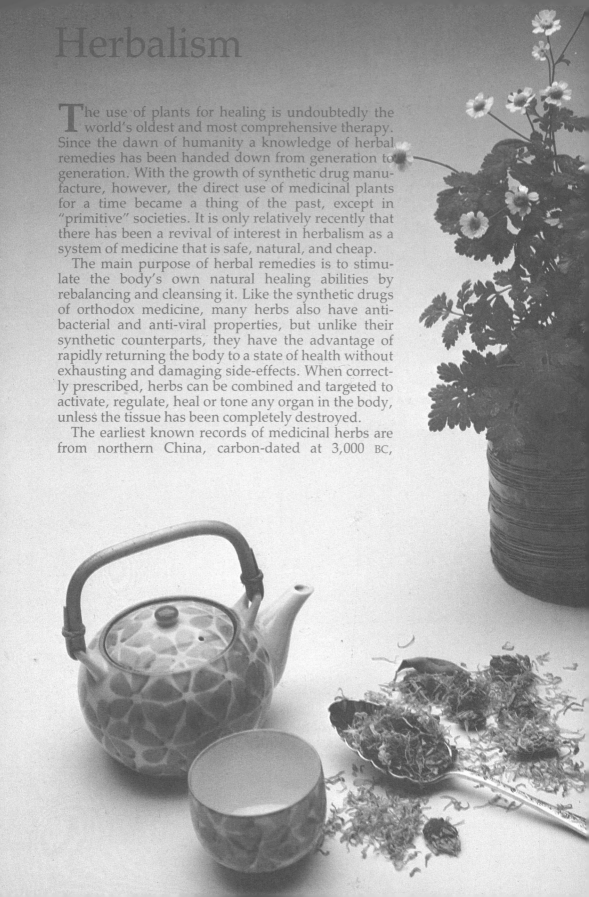

The use of plants for healing is undoubtedly the world's oldest and most comprehensive therapy. Since the dawn of humanity a knowledge of herbal remedies has been handed down from generation to generation. With the growth of synthetic drug manufacture, however, the direct use of medicinal plants for a time became a thing of the past, except in "primitive" societies. It is only relatively recently that there has been a revival of interest in herbalism as a system of medicine that is safe, natural, and cheap.

The main purpose of herbal remedies is to stimulate the body's own natural healing abilities by rebalancing and cleansing it. Like the synthetic drugs of orthodox medicine, many herbs also have anti-bacterial and anti-viral properties, but unlike their synthetic counterparts, they have the advantage of rapidly returning the body to a state of health without exhausting and damaging side-effects. When correctly prescribed, herbs can be combined and targeted to activate, regulate, heal or tone any organ in the body, unless the tissue has been completely destroyed.

The earliest known records of medicinal herbs are from northern China, carbon-dated at 3,000 BC, which is about contemporary with the first Egyptian papyrus that recorded the use of medicinal herbs in the western world. Those that we can identify in these records, such as myrrh and frankincense, are still in use today. Herbal remedies continued to form the major part of medical practice, East and West, for several millennia. The herbals that are perhaps most famous date from the European Renaissance (after the advent of printing). The extraordinary range of publications then – most notably Nicholas Culpeper's *Complete Herbal* (1653) – reflected an insatiable demand for knowledge about medicinal plants. At that time, however, herbalism was often explained in terms of astrology and folklore.

From the 16th century onward, the split between herbalism and allopathic medicine became wider and wider. Swiss alchemists initiated the use of toxic minerals such as mercury and antimony, and surgical intervention became standard practice in many areas. By the 19th century, published knowledge of herbalism had increased considerably through advances in scientific botany, and a number of North American Indian herbal remedies had been added to the pharmacopoeia, the list of medicinal drugs. But herbal cures were increasingly out of fashion.

Over the last decade or so, the World Health Organization (WHO) has been encouraging a revival of traditional herbal medicine in developing countries. In the USA, despite a great resurgence of interest, the professional practice of herbalism is illegal in most states.

The findings of science

About 40 percent of modern, pre-packaged medicines now used in orthodox medical practice are synthetic variants of plant constituents, and several well-known "wonder drugs" such as digitalis and aspirin are in fact extracted from traditional medicinal herbs. Unfortunately, the process of extracting single constituents, and using them singly, usually produces unwanted side-effects, because it destroys the inherent balance of the whole herb.

Universities and other research establishments have confirmed the value of the traditional use of whole herbs, and they have also started substantiating the herbalist's tradition of picking plant remedies at certain times of day. They have found that at

particular times the plants contain a higher proportion of the alkaloids, oils and other chemical compounds from which their healing properties derive.

Consulting a herbalist

The way herbalists work varies enormously, according to training and experience. In the UK, the
National Institute of Medical Herbalists (NIMH) has
established a well-defined discipline, requiring rigorous training. The NIMH-trained medical herbalist
will always give you a careful examination and take a
detailed medical history before diagnosing an ailment
and making a prescription.

Today, the qualified medical herbalist combines a
sophisticated understanding of the human body with
knowledge of a greatly expanded herbal pharmacopoeia. Most important of all, he or she is trained to
search out the root cause of ailments and symptoms.
Diarrhea, for example, may have many possible
causes – among them a viral infection, an unsuitable
diet, nervous stress, an allergy, or a contaminated
water supply. Many herbs will correct the symptoms
temporarily but it takes an experienced practitioner to
identify the cause. For this reason it is wisest to
consult a professional, even if you have read about
the virtues of a remedy and matched it to an ailment.

Herbalism versus orthodox medicine

It is important to understand the difference between
the trained herbalist's approach to an illness or
allergy and the allopathic one. Allopathic medicine
regards, say, tonsillitis as an invasion of the throat by
a specific agent, probably a streptococcus, which will
need to be treated with an antibiotic. The infection
may subside rapidly with this treatment; the root
cause, however, will not have been dealt with.

The herbal approach is based on the assumption
that the infection is secondary to a lifestyle with
which the sufferer's body cannot cope. In children
the most usual cause is a diet that is rich in dairy
products or highly processed foods, while in adults it
is more likely to be a lack of nutrients, an allergic
condition, or some other dietary factor. When the
necessary adjustment has been made and the symptoms have been alleviated with gentle herbal remedies, there is far less likelihood of re-infection, and
thus of drastic procedures such as surgery.

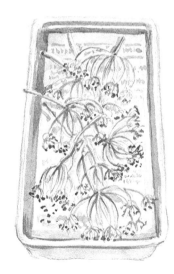

*To dry seeds such as fennel or
caraway, place the seed heads on
a tray in a well-aired room and
leave them until the seeds fall,
ready to be gathered and stored.*

Herbal remedies for home use

Herbal preparations are excellent for home health care. They are gentle, easy to use, and very effective – especially when combined with a balanced diet and a healthy lifestyle.

Gathering and storing herbal remedies

There is nothing to equal the value of a plant freshly picked from a garden or wild area where it is flourishing. But make sure that the area has not been sprayed with chemicals, and that it is legal to pick the plants. Take with you a good, well-illustrated *Flora* so that you can identify the plants with certainty. An amateur can easily confuse plants such as comfrey, elecampane and mullein with a poisonous plant like foxglove. Gather your remedies on a dry morning, once the dew has evaporated, and choose only the healthiest-looking plants. If possible you should pick and dry your plants at least annually, as the longer herbs are kept, the weaker their virtues become.

Drying your herbs
The faster herbs dry the better, so that they retain both color and scent. As soon as possible after gathering your plants, lay them out on a sheet of greaseproof paper in an airy room, preferably with a through draught. Never dry herbs in the sun. When the stems are also used, as with sage, peppermint or meadowsweet, it's best to make small bunches and hang them from the ceiling of a well-aired room or in a dry loft space, if it is warm enough. If any herbs become mouldy, throw them away.

Storing herbs
Home-dried or bought herbs should be stored in a dark closet in airtight glass jars. You can use old lidded jam jars or larger storage jars, but whichever you choose, always label them clearly the moment you fill them, or the contents may be confused later on. Refrigerated herbs deteriorate rapidly after thawing out, so they should be used immediately.

If you have bought your dried herbs you should make a note of the date of purchase and check their condition carefully. You cannot always be certain where or when they were picked. If they have lost scent and color, or smell musty, you should replace them.

Making your own remedies

There are various ways of preserving herbs other than by drying them – alcoholic tinctures and fluid extracts, essential oils, syrups, vinegars, capsules, pills and tablets are all manufactured and on sale. For the layman, however, it is best to use dried herbs in the form of infusions or decoctions, or in pills bought from a reliable supplier. The recipes below are for the standard infusion and decoction. They are most powerful when freshly made, and should be taken as soon as you notice the first symptoms. Any different proportions of herb to water will be specified under the appropriate remedy on pages 166-75.

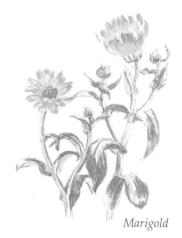

Marigold

Infusions

For an infusion, the herbs are steeped in boiling water, which is probably the easiest and most effective way of taking a herbal remedy. The proportions for a standard infusion are 1 oz (28 g) of the dried herb (or 3 oz (84 g) of the fresh herb) to 1 pint (560 ml) of water. For a small amount use 1–2 teaspoons of dried herb to a cup of water. Put the herbs in a warmed teapot or other china (not metal) container, and pour on boiling water. Leave to steep for 10 minutes, then strain off the herbs and use. Infusions should be freshly made, and they should never be kept for longer than a day.

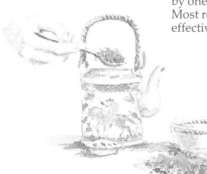

Decoctions

A decoction is the more appropriate method when a herb is tough, woody, or very fluffy, or when the roots are used. For a decoction, the herbs are simmered in water to extract as much goodness as possible. The proportions for a standard decoction are 1 oz (28 g) of the dried herb, torn or cut into small pieces, to 1½ pints (840 ml) of water. For a small amount, use 1 teaspoon of the dried herb to a large cup of water. Put the herbs in an enamel, glass or stainless steel pan (never use aluminium) and add the water. Bring to the boil and simmer for about 10 minutes or until the liquid is reduced by one third, then strain. Most remedies are more effective when still hot.

Dosages

For adults, the dose of most infusions and decoctions is 1 cup (about ¼ pint or 140 ml) 3 times a day. This rarely upsets anybody, but it is wise to take smaller quantities of a remedy at first. If a herb disagrees with you slightly, try a weaker version, using only ½ oz (14 g) to 1 pint (560 ml) of water. To flavour infusions, you can add culinary herbs, such as mint and thyme, or a little honey or apple juice for sweetening (this is especially useful for children). Adding herbs will increase the value of the remedy.

Dosages for children The precise dosages vary according to age and physical development, and the chosen remedy. One teaspoon at a time is often sufficient for small children.
Caution Do not allow any illness, whether it is general aches and pains, diarrhea or catarrh, to continue untreated. Always consult a qualified medical herbalist if an illness persists, as proper diagnosis is essential.

Herbs for the medicine chest

The herbs described here are tried and trusted
remedies. For precise instructions on their use, see
the relevant ailment on pp.166–75. Herbs for first aid
use are given on pp.324–30. You should try out the
remedies before you need them so that if one
disagrees with you, you can look for an alternative
that suits you better, and that will be helpful when
you need it.

Remedy	Ailments	Properties
Elderflower (Sambucus nigra)	**Colds, flu, catarrh, sinusitis**	Helps clear out infection and induces sweating. Available as a ready-made medicine Composition Essence
Coltsfoot (Tussilago farfara)	**Coughs, catarrh**	Soothing and anti-spasmodic, ideal for irritating coughs. Sometimes available in traditional cough sweets and sticks
Red sage (Salvia officinalis)	**Sore throats, mouth ulcers**	Anti-infective and soothes inflamed mucous membranes. Available as a ready-made extract
Wild thyme (Thymus serpyllum)	**Digestive ailments arthritis, allergies**	A powerful anti-bacterial agent, calming and healing, and a digestive tonic
Peppermint Mentha piperita)	**Digestive ailments**	Antiseptic, stimulates the digestive system, relaxes the stomach, and eases tension
Meadowsweet (Filipendula ulmaria)	**Diarrhea, digestive ailments**	Astringent and digestant, very useful in simple diarrhea
Slippery elm (Ulmus fulva)	**Digestive problems**	A soothing and healing bark. Available in tablet or powder form, and as an invalid food (though this rarely contains much bark)
Chamomile (Chamaemelum nobile)	**Insomnia, anxiety**	Excellent gentle sedative, relaxing, a tonic to the digestive system
Rosemary (Rosemarinus officinalis)	**Indigestion, headaches**	This aids digestion, and calms nervous tension
Valerian (Valeriana officinalis)	**Anxiety, insomnia, stress**	Relaxes muscle spasms, helps digestion, reduces tension and produces a healing sleep. Available in pill form
Witch hazel (Hamamelis virginiana)	**Cuts, bruises, sprains**	Excellent antiseptic and astringent used externally. The distilled water is widely available, ready-bottled, from pharmacies or health stores
Marigold (Calendula officinalis)	**Cuts, burns, bruises**	An excellent healing herb for local skin problems

Ailments and remedies

Take care that you match the remedy to the individual's overall condition – herbs that are diuretic will increase fluid secretions, those that are astringent reduce fluid secretions. Always make up your remedies according to the proportions given and in the stated quantities – and seek advice from a medical herbalist if a problem persists.

Caution During pregnancy it is advisable to seek professional advice before taking home remedies.

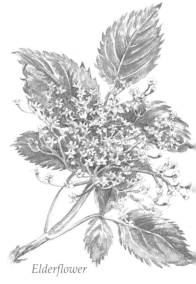

Elderflower

Sore throats
Action is best taken the moment your throat feels sore even if the discomfort is only slight, as this indicates that an infection is starting. At this stage gargling will often be sufficient to soothe the throat and stop the infection developing.

Myrrh (*Commiphora molmol*) Tincture of myrrh makes a simple gargle and is readily available in pharmacies. Use 5–10 drops in half a tumbler of warm water. Myrrh is antiseptic and astringent.

Red sage (*Salvia officinalis*) Simmer 2 oz (56 g) of the dried leaves (or 4 oz of freshly picked leaves) in ⅕ pint (112 ml) of vinegar for 10 minutes in a covered pan. Strain this liquid, then add an equal measure of water, and bottle ready for use. Dilute to taste for gargling. A few drops of myrrh can be added to this mixture.

Colds and flu
In the event of a viral infection, such as a cold or flu, or once a sore throat has taken hold, the best policy is to go to bed, no matter what "has to be done". Not only does this avoid spreading the infection to others, but a few hours' rest and medication will often clear the condition quickly. Demanding physical activities carry the risk of chills, which really give viral infections a chance to fell the sufferer – and may create further complications, such as bronchitis.

Elderflower, peppermint and composition essence This is an excellent cold remedy, that you should purchase from health stores, as it is too complicated to make at home. For dosage, follow the manufacturer's advice (different preparations vary in strength).
Caution Not to be taken by anyone with high blood pressure.

Elderflower (*Sambucus nigra*) This is a diuretic. It helps the body to sweat out any accumulated toxins. Make a standard infusion (p.164), and take 1 cup, hot, 3 times a day. Elderflower combines well with yarrow (p.167) in feverish conditions like flu.

Yarrow See Coughs, p.167.

Asthma
Several cough remedies (see opposite) can be used in cases of asthma, notably elecampane, mullein, and hyssop, for strengthening the lungs. For possible underlying causes or aggravating factors see Allergic reactions, p.175.

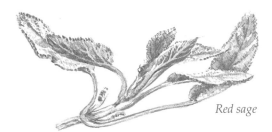

Red sage

Coughs, catarrh

With coughs, as with any catarrhal condition, you should avoid all milk products for some time and eat a light diet, consisting mainly of salad, fresh vegetables and some easily digested protein, such as fish. You can flavor the remedies that follow with honey – few cough remedies would be chosen for their taste.

Yarrow (*Achillea millefolium*) This is a classic remedy for fevers from coughs, colds, or flu. It induces sweating, lowers blood pressure, and it is both a diuretic and an astringent. Take 1 cup of a standard infusion (p.164), 3 times a day.

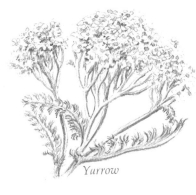

Yarrow

White horehound (*Marrubium vulgare*) A standard infusion of the aerial parts makes a good expectorant and relaxes the bronchial passages. It also inhibits spasm. Take 1 small cup, 3 times a day.

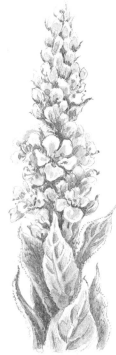

Mullein

Mullein (*Verbascum thapsus*) For bronchitis, and hard, non-productive coughs with chest soreness, mullein has a long tradition of medicinal use. It is also a diuretic. Take a standard infusion of the leaves freely, in combination with coltsfoot or white horehound if desired.

Wild cherry bark (*Prunus serotina*) Mainly used for children, this remedy is especially beneficial for whooping cough, and good for coughs that are persistent and irritating. It is mildly sedative and astringent. Take 1 small cup of a standard decoction, 3 times a day.

Wild lettuce (*Lactuca virosa*) This acts as a mild sedative and is particularly useful for irritable coughs. Take 1 small cup of a standard infusion, 3 times a day.

Irish moss (*Chondrus crispus*) This is very beneficial in chest conditions and helps bring up phlegm. Take 1 small cup of a standard infusion, 3 times a day.

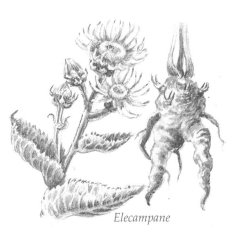

Elecampane

Elecampane (*Inula helenium*) A standard decoction (p.164) of the root is especially indicated for bronchial catarrh. It brings up phlegm, induces sweating and kills bacteria, and it also combines well with coltsfoot or white horehound. Take 1 small cup, 3 times a day.

Coltsfoot (*Tussilago farfara*) This soothes inflamed tissues and acts as a diuretic. For most people, a half-strength standard infusion is strong enough – ½ oz (14 g) of leaves to 1 pint (560 ml) of freshly boiled water. Take 1 small cup, 3 times a day.

Elderflower See Colds, opposite.

Hyssop See Anxiety, p.172.

Diarrhea

In most cases diarrhea is the body's reaction to a poison in the system and, as such, you should simply allow it to run its course, with only gentle medication. Childhood diarrhea needs prompt treatment, however, since the body may lose excessive amounts of liquid (see also Allergies in babies, p.175).

Agrimony *(Agrimonia eupatoria)* An excellent remedy for mild childhood diarrhea. Agrimony is both an astringent (reduces fluid secretions) and a digestive tonic. Take 1 cup of a standard infusion (p.164), hot, 3 times a day.

Meadowsweet *(Filipendula ulmaria)* This is an excellent digestive medicine, particularly useful for children, but it should not be taken indefinitely. Take 1 cup of a standard infusion, 3 times a day.

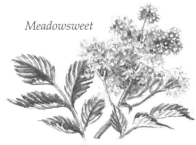

Meadowsweet

Cranesbill *(Geranium maculatum)* A strong astringent, take 1 cup of a standard decoction (p.164) of the rhizome, 3 times a day.

Marsh mallow *(Althaea officinalis)* This "tea" is very soothing. Take 1 cup of a standard infusion of the leaves, 3 times a day.

Digestive problems

Though nervous tension is generally blamed for a large variety of ailments, in fact many of them, including colitis, constipation, flatulence, diarrhea, indigestion, ulcers, depression, migraines, headaches, and fatigue, are due mainly to a diet that is unsuitable for the individual – especially one consisting chiefly of processed, pre-packaged foods and too much tea and coffee. The most acute reactions are usually caused by the nitrates which are added to most processed proteins, and which occur naturally in yeast extracts. If any of the conditions listed above are chronic problems, consult a medical herbalist. If the symptoms are transient, the following herbs will be helpful.

Feverfew *(Chrysanthemum parthenium)* This pungent herb is one of the best-known herbal remedies for migraine. Take 1 small cup of a standard infusion, 3 times a day, or add a leaf to a salad or sandwich, if preferred. Tablets are also now available from health food stores.

Rosemary *(Rosemarinus officinalis)* Take 1 cup of a standard infusion, 3 times a day, to aid digestion and calm nervous tension.

Peppermint *(Mentha piperita)* Take 1 small cup of the standard infusion as necessary.

Wild thyme See Arthritis (p.171).

Licorice *(Glycyrrhiza glabra)* Take 1 cup of a standard decoction of the root (p.164), 3 times a day, or chew small sticks of licorice.
Caution Licorice has an anti-diuretic property, so it should not to be taken by anyone with kidney problems, hypertension, or high blood pressure.

Slippery elm *(Ulmus fulva)* This soothing and healing bark is available in tablet or powder form. You may make hot or cold infusions from the powder, using ¼ oz (7 g) of powder to 1 pint (560 ml) water.

Meadowsweet *(Filipendula ulmaria)* See Diarrhea.

Dandelion root *(Taraxacum officinale)* This is a good liver tonic. Take 1 cup of a decoction, 3 times a day.

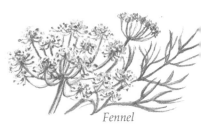

Fennel

Fennel *(Foeniculum vulgare)* An excellent digestive tonic. Take 1 small cup of a standard decoction of the seeds, 3 times a day.

Matricaria *(Matricaria chamomilla)* 1 small cup of a standard infusion, taken after meals, strengthens the digestive system, combats inflammation and helps reduce pain. Matricaria is also know as German chamomile.

Mouth ulcers

A common cause of mouth ulcers, and bleeding gums, is a reaction to substances found in toothpastes, particularly to a detergent, sodium lauryl sulphate. Varying types of treatment will be required, so advice from a medical herbalist is essential.

Myrrh (*Commiphora molmol*) Tincture of myrrh makes an excellent mouthwash for several mouth disorders, including toothache. For instructions on dilution, see Sore throats (p.166). Take the remedy 3 or 4 times a day.

Red sage (*Salvia officinalis*) Use a standard infusion of the leaves (p.164) as a mouthwash.

Local skin problems

There are many herbal remedies which are excellent for healing skin conditions and minor external wounds (see also First aid and emergencies, p.324 onward). They ward off infection, relieve pain and can reduce scarring. Use either compresses, made by soaking gauze in an infusion of the herbal remedy and binding it to the damaged area, or an ointment, if available. It is wise to try out ointments on undamaged skin before you have an emergency to cope with, so that you can be sure you will not suffer any reaction to the ointment base used in manufacturing.

Marigold (*Calendula officinalis*) A compress made from a standard infusion (p.164) of the flowers or petals of marigold is one of the best remedies for local skin problems, such as eczema, minor burns and bruises. It combats infection and helps to reduce swelling.

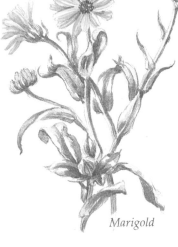

Marigold

Chickweed (*Stellaria media*) A compress of a standard infusion, or an ointment, is excellent for healing skin problems. It also softens the skin. The remedy is suitable for abrasions, eczema, itchy skin eruptions, abscesses and indolent ulcers. The fresh herb is particularly useful.

Witch hazel

Witch hazel (*Hamamelis virginiana*) For healing cuts, bruises and sprains, there is nothing to beat witch hazel, a remedy learned from the North American Indians. Besides being strongly antiseptic, it also reduces swelling and scarring. You can apply it neat to a wound, or diluted if the skin is broken (it may sting at first but this will soon stop). Distilled witch hazel is widely available in pharmacies and drug stores.

Eczema

Both marigold and chickweed (above) relieve itching and combat infection. For possible causes and contributing factors see Allergic reactions, p.175.

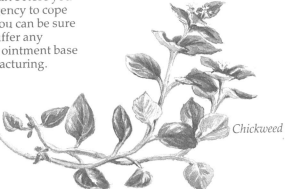

Chickweed

Acné, spots

Acne, spots, boils, dandruff, styes, and chapped hands, are often closely related to food allergies, and generally indicate an unbalanced diet. Cut down on carbohydrates and cut out all dairy produce, sugar, fats, oils and preserved foods. Eat fresh salads, vegetables, fresh meat or fish (p.47). For acne especially, fresh vegetable juices are recommended.

Carrot juice An excellent liver cleanser. Take half a glass once or twice a day.

Beetroot juice Another invaluable vegetable juice, take half a glass once or twice a day.

Cabbage juice This is another cleanser, widely used in French folk medicine. You can add small quantities of the extracted juice to other vegetable juices or soups, but it may cause indigestion.

Styes

If styes are severe and recur frequently you must consult a qualified medical herbalist.

Witch hazel (*Hamamelis virginiana*) Use 1 part distilled witch hazel to 4 parts boiled, cooled water for an excellent stye remedy. Bathe the eyelid every 2-4 hours.

Eyestrain

Eyestrain is often caused by poor light, glaring light, or by wearing glasses or lenses with the wrong prescription. It is important to correct the cause of the problem.

Eyebright (*Euphrasia officinalis*) A cooled standard infusion (p.164) of eyebright is useful. Lie down for up to 20 minutes with pads or small compresses soaked in the cool infusion placed over the eyelids.

Warts

Most warts are harmless and painless, and disappear naturally in time. They may sometimes serve as a useful warning, since they tend to flourish in children who eat a lot of sweets or unsuitable foods. In this case they indicate a clear need to improve dietary habits (p.47).

Greater celandine (*Chelidonium majus*) A drop of the yellow latex from a leaf stalk of the plant, carefully applied to the wart (not to the surrounding skin), is a very efficient cure. If it does not work after a few applications, do not persist with it.

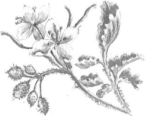

Greater celandine

Petty spurge (*Euphorbia peplus*) This is an efficient alternative to greater celandine.

Thuja (*Thuja occidentalis*) Paint the wart carefully with a few drops of tincture of thuja, morning and night. This will reduce and weaken the wart, and often clear it altogether.

Fibrositis, gout

These ailments have a number of different causes, from chronic or acute inflammation in an internal organ, to dietary imbalance and reactions to foods, or vitamin and mineral deficiencies. Gout responds particularly well to a change in dietary balance, away from rich foods. Yeast-based flavorings often aggravate the pain, as do alcohol and certain high-purine foods, such as liver and salmon.

Wild thyme See Arthritis (below).

Feverfew (*Chrysanthemum parthenium*) Take 1 cup of a standard infusion (p.164), 3 times a day. This is particularly useful if the cause of the reaction in the joint is an allergy to food additives or dietary imbalance. The taste is fairly unpleasant, however, and many people prefer to eat the leaves (1 leaf each day) in a sandwich, disguising the taste with a strong savory spread

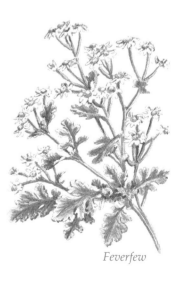

Feverfew

Arthritis, rheumatism

Arthritis is a complex condition which may be largely allergic in origin. There are many possible causes of the joint pains and spasms and muscular aches it gives rise to, including viral and bacterial infections, reactions to drugs, fungicides, or pesticides; or to any of the host of chemicals contained in food, toothpastes and cosmetics. Yeast in food and drinks, such as alcohol, chocolate and sweets also commonly triggers arthritis. It is essential to see a qualified medical herbalist as soon as possible, because if treated in time, the problem is seldom serious. The same herbal remedies work for rheumatism.

Kelp or devil's claw
(*Harpagophytum procumbens*) As mineral supplements, tablets of either of these are excellent. They are usually available in health stores. *Caution* Some people experience indigestion with herbal tablets.

Celery seed (*Apium graveolens*) These seeds are anti-rheumatic and diuretic. You can use them either as a decoction or an infusion. For celery seed tea, make a decoction using 1 oz (28 g) of seeds in 2 pints (1.1 litres) of water, simmered for 20 minutes, and take 1 small cup 3 times a day. A cup of standard celery seed infusion (p.164) can be added to home-made vegetable soups or to vegetable or meat stews (though it is best for arthritis sufferers to avoid too much meat). Fresh celery stalks are also useful.

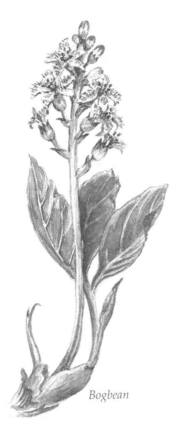
Bogbean

Bogbean (buckbean)
(*Menyanthes trifoliata*) Another useful arthritis remedy, bogbean is also a diuretic. Make a standard infusion of the leaves, and take 1 small cup, 3 times a day.

Wild thyme (*Thymus serpyllum*) This plant has powerful anti-bacterial properties as well as helping digestion, aiding healing, and inducing a calmer state of mind. Take 1 small cup of a standard infusion, 3 times a day.

Cramps

Many herbal remedies will help with the unpleasant symptoms of cramp, but choosing the right one obviously depends on the problem's cause. This may be a mineral deficiency, such as lack of zinc, calcium, or magnesium. But cramp is also sometimes an indication of a circulatory or arthritic problem. Correct diagnosis is important.

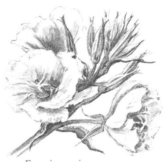
Evening primrose

Evening primrose (*Oenothera bienis*) The oil of this herb is available in capsule form. If cramp is accompanied by headaches or nausea, make sure that the evening primrose capsules are combined with a marine oil supplement – this generally eliminates the problem.

Kelp Kelp tablets will help only if mineral deficiency is the cause.
Caution Some people experience indigestion with these tablets.

Cramp bark (*Viburnum opulus*) Take 1 small cup of a standard decoction (p.164), 3 times a day. This herb is a sedative and an astringent.

Anxiety and insomnia

We all suffer from anxiety and insomnia at some time. Both can be due to an infinite number of factors including noise, emotional problems, overwork, excitement, exhaustion, or indigestion. If the condition persists, advice from a qualified medical herbalist is essential. For a temporary condition, you will benefit from infusions of any of the following plants, which have a long tradition of medicinal use.

Chamomile (*Chamaemelum nobile*) This is an excellent, gentle sedative, and you can take a standard infusion (p.164) of the flowers freely. Don't confuse it with German chamomile (*Matricaria*), which has different virtues.

Lime flowers (*Tilia*) Use the flowers to make a standard infusion, which you can drink freely. It will tone the nervous system, increase urine flow and sweating, and act as a mild astringent.

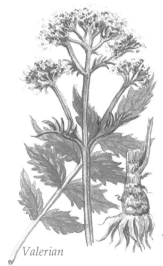
Valerian

Valerian (*Valeriana officinalis*) This is probably the best-known herbal sedative, available in powder and pill form. It also relaxes muscle spasm and helps digestion. The rhizome and root are usually used in powder form, or cut into small pieces. Take 1 small cup of a standard infusion when needed.

Rosemary See digestive problems (p.168).

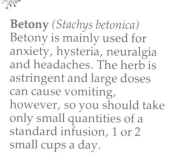
Lime flowers

Betony (*Stachys betonica*) Betony is mainly used for anxiety, hysteria, neuralgia and headaches. The herb is astringent and large doses can cause vomiting, however, so you should take only small quantities of a standard infusion, 1 or 2 small cups a day.

Hops (*Humulus lupulus*) This is a well-known nerve relaxant, but you should not use it for depression. Take 1 small cup of a standard infusion of the flowers, 3 times a day.

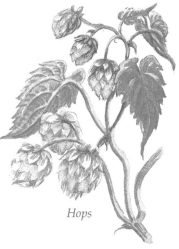
Hops

Passion flower (*Passiflora incarnata*) For nervous conditions, such as spasmodic asthma, neuralgia, and insomnia, take 1 small cup of a standard infusion of the leaves. Passion flower is also available in tablet form (follow the manufacturer's instructions on dosage).

Hyssop (*Hyssopus officinalis*) For centuries people have used hyssop to soothe anxiety, and for chronic nasal catarrh, asthma, colds and coughs. It helps bring up phlegm, induces sweating and also tones the digestive system. Take 1 small cup of a standard infusion, 3 times a day. Use only the dried aerial parts of the shrub.
Caution Not to be taken during pregnancy.

Cystitis, kidney stones

These ailments are commonplace, yet one of their causes is very simple to remedy. Many people of all ages drink insufficient plain water. Fruit juices, squashes, cola drinks, coffee and other beverages are no substitute and can cause reactions such as cramp or pain and stiffness in the kidney area. Another frequent cause of cystitis is an allergy to yeasts, especially in wines and other alcohols, stock cubes and yeast extracts. To remedy these conditions you need herbs that are diuretic. It is best to consult a medical herbalist.

Corn silk *(Zea mays)* A standard infusion (p.164) of corn silk soothes the symptoms of cystitis and kidney stones. This is an excellent healing medicine, soothing inflamed tissues, and acting as a diuretic. You may drink it freely.

Buchu *(Barosma betulina)* This herb has antiseptic and diuretic qualities. Make a standard infusion, and drink it freely.

Couch (cough grass) *(Agropyron repens)* This is especially useful for clearing kidney gravel and stones. It soothes inflamed tissues and encourages urine flow. Make a standard infusion, and drink it freely.

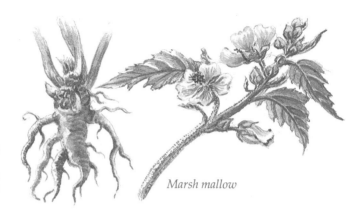

Marsh mallow

Marsh mallow *(Althaea officinalis)* Either the roots or leaves of this herb make a soothing, healing and mildly diuretic medicine. If you are using root chips, make a decoction of 1 oz (28 g) to 2 pints (1.1 litres) of water, simmer for 10 minutes, and strain; take 1 small cup, 3 times a day. With the leaves, make a standard infusion.

Eryngo *(Eryngium maritimum)* Also known as sea holly, this herb is useful for a whole range of urinary conditions. Take 1 small cup of a standard decoction (p.164) of the dried roots, 3 times a day.

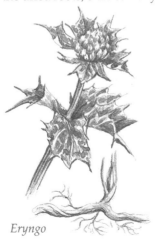

Eryngo

Vaginal infection

Amongst many causes of infection, two of the most common are antibiotics and the contraceptive pill. If you are infected, drink water, avoid yeast-containing substances and cut out dairy products. Wine, fruit juices, tea and coffee may aggravate the condition. Seek advice from a medical herbalist if attacks are frequent or prolonged.

Acidophilus Taken over a long period, these tablets are helpful.

Tea tree oil *(Melaleuca alternifolia)* This is very effective applied locally. Use a little of the pure oil, or dilute a few drops in a little water, and bathe the genital area. You can also use a tea tree cream.

Vinegar Some people obtain temporary relief by adding vinegar to their bath water.

Headaches

Migraines and headaches are often related to an unsuitable diet. See Digestive problems (p.168).

Anemia

The causes of this condition are various but most people respond well to herbal remedies. It may be due to a lack of absorption or utilization of iron, and possibly of a number of other nutrients, or to heavy blood loss from an accident, or hemorrhage from heavy periods or hemorrhoids, for example. Whatever the cause, anemia requires careful investigation by a trained medical herbalist.

Kelp Kelp tablets are rich in all minerals, and contain alginates.
Caution Some people experience indigestion with these tablets.

Watercress An excellent salad ingredient, fresh watercress is rich in the nutrients which are short in anemia.

Nettle (*Urtica dioica*) Nettles are rich in iron and other minerals and trace elements. Make a standard infusion (p.164), and drink it freely.

Menstrual problems

Help from a qualified medical herbalist is essential for these problems, as the causes are very varied and require careful professional assessment. The following herbs may ease the pain.

Ginger (*Zingiber officinale*) Use powdered ginger, or the fresh root finely chopped, to make a standard decoction (p.164). Take 1 small cup when necessary.

Black haw bark (*Viburnum prunifolium*) This relieves cramping pains. Make a standard decoction of the powdered bark. Take 1 small cup, 3 times a day.

Caraway (*Carum carvi*) A standard infusion (p.164) of the seeds helps to relieve menstrual pain, and soothes digestive disorders. It is astringent and anti-spasmodic. Take 1 small cup, 3 times a day.

High blood pressure

Many herbal remedies will help this condition, but it is essential to consult a qualified medical herbalist who will prescribe remedies according to individual requirements.

Lime flowers (*Tilia*) A standard infusion (p.164), taken when needed, is calming and relaxes nervous tension.

Vervain (*Verbena officinalis*) This is a mild sedative, useful in depression and debility. Take 1 small cup of the standard infusion, 3 times a day.

Valerian (*Valeriana officinalis*) Take 1 small cup of the infusion when needed.

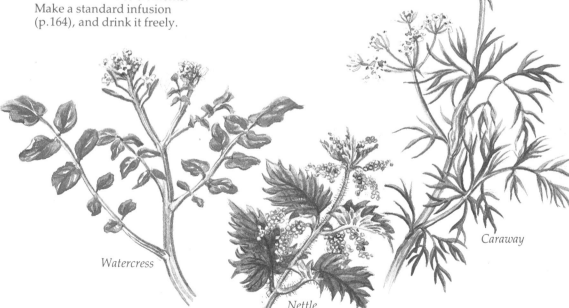

Watercress

Nettle

Caraway

Allergic reactions

An allergy to specific foods or chemical substances underlies or aggravates diverse conditions, including asthma, hay fever, eczema, catarrh, sinusitis, coughs, tonsillitis, and sore throats.

Among common allergens which may damage and inflame the digestive tract are cows', goats' or sheep's milk products, food colorings, flavorings and preservatives, and food containing chemical residues, such as pesticides, fungicides and herbicides, or the antibiotics and steroid hormone residues in meat. Other common causes are the contraceptive pill and a variety of man-made chemicals, from gases and sprays to soap powders and toothpastes. Alcohol in any quantity, especially red wine, may aggravate allergic conditions.

The majority of allergic reactions respond well to herbal remedies, especially when combined with a diet rich in salads and lightly cooked organically grown vegetables (see pp.46–7), but the mainstay of treatment must be to eliminate the cause.

Eyebright (*Euphrasia officinalis*) This herb may help some cases of hay fever and catarrh. Prepare a standard infusion (p.164) and take 1 small cup, 3 times a day.

Nettle (*Urtica dioica*) The common nettle helps soothe some allergic reactions. Make a standard infusion of the leaves and take as required.

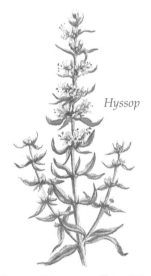

Hyssop

Hyssop (*Hyssopus officinalis*) This is especially useful for hay fever. Take 1 small cup of a standard infusion, 3 times a day.
Caution Not to be taken during pregnancy.

Marsh mallow See Cystitis, p.173.

Wild cherry bark (*Prunus serotina*) Take 1 cup of a standard decoction, 3 times a day.

Wild thyme (*Thymus serpyllum*) This helps some cases. Take 1 small cup of a standard infusion, 3 times a day.

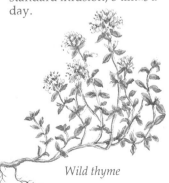

Wild thyme

Allergies in babies

Allergic syndromes sometimes originate during pregnancy. The result may be a difficult, yelling baby with problems ranging from eczema to colic and diarrhea. If breast-feeding, the mother can discover the cause by eliminating all suspect foods from her diet and then re-introducing them one at a time. A varied, balanced diet with few dairy products is advisable. Problems also arise with bottle-fed babies. They are often allergic to the cows' milk which constitutes the basic part of "baby formula" milk. Soya milk, which is obtainable especially formulated for babies, is usually a successful substitute in these cases. The contraceptive pill is not advisable during breast-feeding.

Matricaria (*Matricaria chamomilla*) Give 1 small spoon of a standard infusion (p.164) after meals.

Dill (*Anethum graveolens*) Give 1 small spoon of a standard infusion after meals. This stimulates the digestive system.

Fennel (*Foeniculum vulgare*) 1 small spoon of a standard infusion after meals aids digestion.

Aromatherapy

Aromatherapy uses essential oils extracted from plants, leaves, bark, roots, seeds, resins, and flowers to treat a range of common ailments, as well as for their effects on the mind and emotions. For the greatest therapeutic effect the oils are massaged into the skin, inhaled, or used in the bath. Occasionally they are taken internally, but only with great caution, and on the advice of a qualified therapist.

Many of the oils are expensive to buy initially, because an enormous quantity of plants is needed to obtain even a small amount of essential oil. As a self-help therapy, however, it need not be costly, since the oils are very powerful and a little goes a very long way. The quickest and most remarkable results have been achieved with essential oils in healing wounds and promoting the formation of scar tissue, and in the treatment of acne and other skin problems, rheumatism, premenstrual tension, and poor circulation as well as of many nervous disorders, such as headaches, migraines, stress, and insomnia.

Aromatherapy is one of the most ancient healing arts. Hieroglyphics from as far back as 4,500 BC confirm that the ancient Egyptians used aromatic

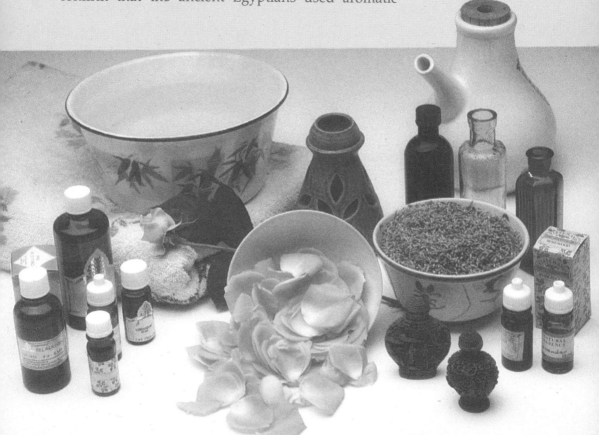

substances in medicine. The antiseptic powers of essential oils were also used to stop the putrefaction of corpses in the mummification process. The Greeks, too, used plant essences – for aromatic baths and scented massages, as well as for healing wounds.

Modern advances

It was not until early this century that the term "aromatherapy" was coined by a French cosmetic chemist, Professor Gattefossé, who was the first to appreciate fully the tremendous healing properties of essential oils. He related how, after accidentally burning his hand, he plunged it by chance into lavender oil and was amazed at how quickly the pain ceased and the skin healed, without blistering. More recently, Dr Jean Valnet and Marguerite Maury have both made considerable contributions to the therapy and to its acceptance as a healing art.

"But of the greatest interest is the effect of the fragrance on the psychic and mental state of the individual. Powers of perception become clearer and more acute, and there is a feeling of having seen more objectively and therefore in truer perspective."
Marguerite Maury

Modern research has confirmed the therapeutic properties of essential oils. At Milan University, for example, depression and anxiety have been successfully treated by Dr Paolo Rovesti, using aerosol-sprayed oils, and in the USSR a type of eucalyptus oil has been found beneficial in the treatment of a strain of influenza – an important finding, since very few natural anti-viral agents have been identified.

Like vitamins and minerals, many essential oils are taken up selectively by different organs of the body. You can test this for yourself by rubbing the soles of your feet with a cut garlic clove, then smelling your breath a few hours later.

Consulting a professional

The first time you visit an aromatherapist, he or she will want to find out about your diet, lifestyle, and present symptoms, as well as taking note of your past illnesses and treatments, in order to establish a basis for diagnosis. Some therapists use a pendulum to find the right oil. Once your particular remedy is chosen, a few drops of the oil are either massaged into the skin, inhaled, or added to a hot bath.

Generally, a local application of oil in massages or baths is given for skin problems, muscular pain, urinogenital and nervous disorders, while inhalation is preferred for respiratory disorders and some nervous problems. A course of weekly treatments may be indicated, and oils prescribed for home use.

Using aromatherapy oils

Aromatherapy is easy to practice at home. The oils can be purchased through a professional aromatherapist, and at some pharmacies and health stores. The therapeutic properties of the oils are dependent on the purest possible means of extraction, however, so it is important to buy from a reliable source. If relaxation is your first priority then choose according to the aroma that you find most attractive. Otherwise, follow the advice given in Ailments and remedies, pages 179-81 (and in First aid, pp.324-30).

Once purchased you should keep your oils in tightly sealed dark glass bottles. Store them in a place that's cool but not freezing, as low temperatures destroy the odoriferous molecules. Oils for self-help are inhaled, used in the bath, or massaged into the skin, either diluted or neat.

Caution If you suffer from any allergic condition such as asthma, you should consult an aromatherapist before using essential oils.

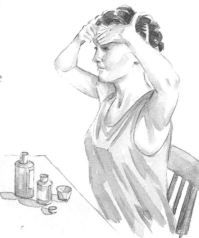

Massaging the temples with cinnamon oil, a treatment for flu

Quantities
Take care that you always use the precise number of drops of oil advised under Ailments and remedies (pp.179-81). If you add more drops you can alter, or even reverse, an oil's effect and you may provoke an allergic reaction. For young children, use half the amount advised for adults; for babies, use only a minute amount – a drop highly diluted should generally be sufficient.

Bathing with oils
This is one of the easiest of treatments. Put just a few drops of an essential oil in a bath of warm water. If you have chosen the oil purely for its aroma, 6 drops should be ample. Close the doors and windows while you bathe, so that the air stays warm and aromatic, and relax in the bath for 10 minutes.

Inhalation with oils
Steam inhalations are particularly effective for respiratory problems. Add 1 or 2 drops of the appropriate oil to a bowl of steaming hot water. Put a towel over your head and around the bowl, and inhale for 10 minutes. This treatment may be repeated 3 times a day.

Massaging with oils
For massage, you use the oils diluted or neat, depending on the disorder you're treating. For a relaxing massage, use only 3 or 4 drops of your chosen oil to an eggcup of a carrier oil – soya or almond oil is recommended. (For relaxing massage strokes, see pp.245-6.) If you are treating a particular ailment, follow the instructions for dilution described under Ailments and remedies.

Oils are used neat on small troublesome areas. Massage them in gently with the fingertips, or, if the skin is broken, dab them on carefully using cottonwool.

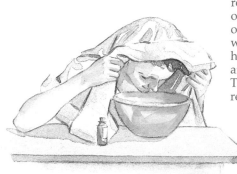

Steam inhalation

Ailments and remedies

Of the great range of aromatherapy oils those prescribed here are the most widely available, and generally the least expensive. In some cases there are several alternative treatments with slightly varying properties, allowing you to choose according to the scent that pleases you, and determine which of the oils suits you best.

Colds, flu, and sinusitis

Cinnamon Cinnamon oil is indicated for flu, for any flu-like condition which has developed from a chill, and for general debility. Add 6-8 drops to a warm bath; and rub neat cinnamon oil into the temples, as shown left, and into the sinus area and chest, 4 times a day. A steam inhalation also helps. Put 2 drops of oil into a bowl of hot water and inhale for a few minutes. Repeat 3 times a day, then once a day when you begin to feel better.

Eucalyptus Put 1 or 2 drops in a bowl of hot water. Inhale for 10 minutes, repeating a few times a day.

Hyssop A chesty type of cold responds well to a hyssop inhalation. For instructions see Coughs, below.

Lemon For a head cold (sore throat, or bleeding gums), add 4 drops of lemon to a cup of warm water and gargle for a few minutes. Repeat 3-4 times a day, then twice a day as the infection subsides.

Pine See Sore throats, below.

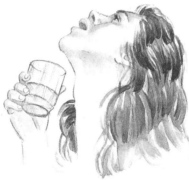

Gargling with diluted geranium

Sore throats, tonsillitis

Geranium This has a tonic and antiseptic effect. Add 3 drops to a cup of warm, boiled water, and gargle for a few minutes. Repeat a few times a day.

Lemon See Colds, above.

Pine This has a powerful antiseptic effect. Add 2 drops to a bowl of hot water and inhale a few times a day.

Coughs

Hyssop This eases coughs, helps expectoration, and has antiseptic and emollient (softening) properties. Add 2 drops to a bowl of hot water and inhale for 10 minutes. Repeat the treatment a few times a day, as necessary.

Bronchitis

Clove This acts as a stimulant and a mild analgesic (pain reducer). If you suffer from chronic bronchitis – or exhaustion – a few drops of clove oil rubbed into the chest 3 times a day will be helpful.

Eucalyptus See Colds, above.

Hyssop For acute or chronic bronchitis, add 3 drops of hyssop oil to an eggcup of almond oil, mix, and rub into your chest every day. See also Coughs, above.

Pine Add 4 drops of pine to a warm bath. See also Sore throats, above.

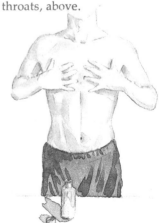

A clove oil chest massage for bronchitis

Indigestion
Garlic This is an excellent remedy for painful digestion or flatulence. Add 3 drops to an eggcup of soya oil and rub the mixture gently in to your stomach after a meal. (Garlic is specifically indicated for intestinal complaints.)

Flatulence
See indigestion, above.

Toothache
Cinnamon Rub a few drops of undiluted oil onto the affected area. Repeat a few times a day.

Bleeding gums
Sage This healing and astringent is helpful for the gums generally, and in cases of gingivitis. Add 3 drops of the oil to a cup of warm water, and gargle.

Lemon A gargle with lemon oil helps gingivitis. See Colds (p.179).

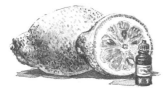

Lemon

Corns and warts
Garlic Every day, rub a few drops of the neat oil on to the corn or wart, and put a fresh dressing on it.

Boils and sores
Thyme This has an antiseptic effect and it helps scarring. Add 3 drops to a cup of warm water, and bathe, or apply gently with cotton wool to the affected area.

Acne, weeping eczema
Juniper Add 4 drops to an eggcup of almond oil, mix, and apply gently to problem areas, a few times a day.

Lavender This is a fine remedy for acne. Add 5 drops to an eggcup of almond oil, mix, and apply twice a day.

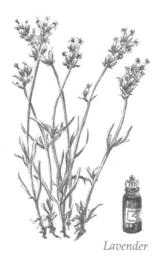

Lavender

Herpes, dry eczema
Geranium For facial herpes and dry eczema add 3 drops to an eggcup of almond oil, mix, and apply 3 times a day.

Hyssop This softens the skin, aids scarring, and has useful antiseptic properties, making it a good remedy for eczema, minor wounds and bruises. Mix a few drops of hyssop in an eggcup of soya oil and rub gently into affected areas.

Rheumatism, gout
Chamomile Add 6 drops to an eggcup of almond oil, mix, and rub into the affected areas after a warm bath. Repeat the treatment until the pain has gone.

Cypress For rheumatism, add 6-8 drops to a warm bath. After the bath you can rub the diluted oil (8 drops in an eggcup of almond oil) into the affected parts.

Eucalyptus Massage the rheumatic areas with a mixture of 3 drops of eucalyptus in an eggcup of almond oil. Take a warm bath with 6 drops of the oil.

Rosemary For rheumatism, mix 3 drops in an eggcup of soya oil and rub gently into the rheumatic areas.

Nervous disorders
Basil This is a stimulant and a tonic, especially good for the nerves. Take a warm bath twice a day with 6 drops.

Chamomile This is good for nervous depression, nervous crises, anxiety, and insomnia. Put 6 drops in a warm bath.

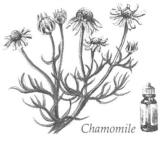

Chamomile

Orange blossom (Neroli) For anxiety, add 5 drops of the oil to a warm bath (or 2 drops for hyperactive children).

Insomnia
Chamomile or lavender Add 6 drops of either oil to a warm, relaxing bath.

Orange blossom (Neroli) Add 5 drops to a warm bath.

Neuralgia
Chamomile Facial neuralgia responds to a gentle massage with just a drop of the neat oil. Massage one area at a time for a few minutes around the temples, the sinus areas, and around the nape of the neck.

Irritability
Cypress Add 4 drops to an eggcup of soya oil, mix, and rub all over the body after a warm bath.

Chamomile Add 6 drops to a warm bath.

Palpitation
Basil Rub a few drops of neat oil into the chest.

Orange blossom (Neroli) Add 5 drops to a warm bath.

Bladder problems
Juniper Juniper has an astringent effect, reducing the secretion of body fluids. Its use is specially indicated for the urinary tract and for ailments like cystitis. Initially, add 6 drops of juniper to a warm bath. If the condition is chronic, mix 3 drops in an eggcup of soya oil and apply this to the lower part of the stomach and the sacral area.

Fluid retention
Caraway Put 6 drops in a warm bath. Caraway is a stimulant and a diuretic (it increases the flow of urine).

Cypress Add 6-8 drops to a warm bath.

Rosemary Add 3 drops to a warm bath. Relax for 10 minutes afterwards.

Loss of sex drive
Rosemary This oil has an aphrodisiac effect. Add 4 drops to an eggcup of soya oil, mix well, and rub into the sacral area.

Varicose veins
Lemon Lemon oil has a tonic effect on the veins and the arteries. Add 6 drops to your bath, and every day, rub a mixture of 3 drops of lemon oil in an eggcup of almond oil on the affected areas.

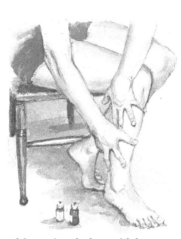

Massaging the legs with lemon oil

Menstrual problems
Basil For scanty periods, add 3 drops to an eggcup of soya oil, mix, and massage gently around stomach and sacrum.

Caraway For painful periods add 6 drops to a warm bath.

Vaginal infections
Sage Add 3 drops to a bowl of warm water, or a bidet, and wash the external area.

Menopausal problems
Cypress Add 4 drops to an eggcup of soya oil, mix, and rub all over the body after a warm bath.

Tiredness
Clove Add 6 drops to a warm bath. You can also rub a little clove in to the chest, a few times a day.

Cypress See Menopausal problems, above.

Garlic Add 3 drops to an eggcup of soya and rub this along the spinal column.

Lavender or lemon Add 6 drops of either oil to a warm bath and relax.

Peppermint Add 6 drops to a warm bath.

Sage or thyme Use 6 drops of either oil in a warm bath.

Body odors
Certain essential oils may be used purely to perfume the body (rose oil, though expensive, is a favourite). Others are known to help solve chronic problems of body odor.

Peppermint For bad breath add 2 drops of peppermint oil to a cup of warm water, and gargle for a few minutes. Repeat as often as necessary.

Cypress For sweaty feet, rub a few drops of neat cypress oil in to the soles of the feet and between the toes, once a day, until the condition improves.

Bach flower remedies

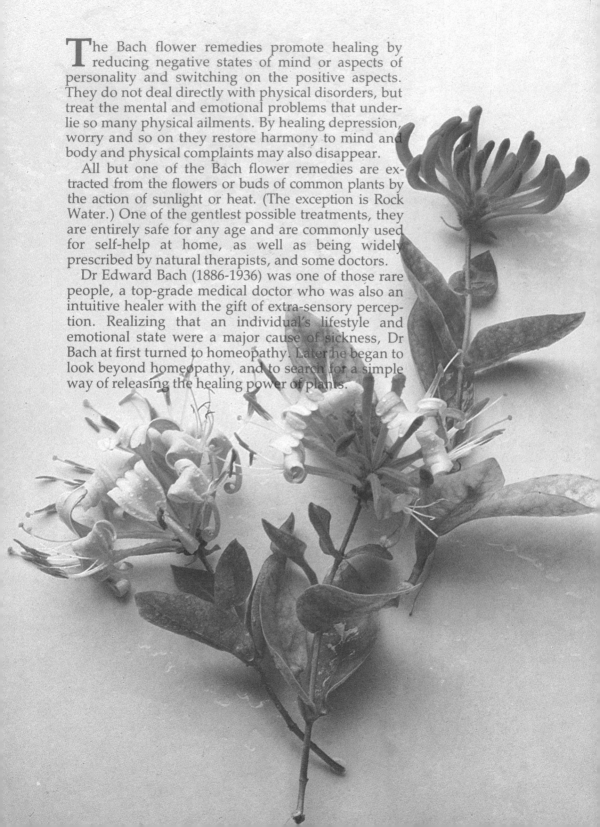

The Bach flower remedies promote healing by reducing negative states of mind or aspects of personality and switching on the positive aspects. They do not deal directly with physical disorders, but treat the mental and emotional problems that underlie so many physical ailments. By healing depression, worry and so on they restore harmony to mind and body and physical complaints may also disappear.

All but one of the Bach flower remedies are extracted from the flowers or buds of common plants by the action of sunlight or heat. (The exception is Rock Water.) One of the gentlest possible treatments, they are entirely safe for any age and are commonly used for self-help at home, as well as being widely prescribed by natural therapists, and some doctors.

Dr Edward Bach (1886-1936) was one of those rare people, a top-grade medical doctor who was also an intuitive healer with the gift of extra-sensory perception. Realizing that an individual's lifestyle and emotional state were a major cause of sickness, Dr Bach at first turned to homeopathy. Later he began to look beyond homeopathy, and to search for a simple way of releasing the healing power of plants.

Classifying people into twelve archetypes, each with a habitual negative emotional state indicated by a key-word, such as loneliness or fear, Dr Bach then set out to find the plants that made these states positive. He called them "The Twelve Healers", and eventually found 26 others – "The Helpers" – making 38 remedies in all.

The remedies at work

Nobody really knows how the remedies work. One possible explanation is that particular plants have patterns of vibration in their flowers or buds that are healing; and these patterns can be transmitted to water when you float the flower or buds in it and expose them to either sunlight (for the flowers) or heat (for the buds). Swallowing this water conveys healing vibrations to the body.

There is a lack of published scientific work on the Bach flower remedies, but there is no shortage of witnesses to their effectiveness. At the Plymouth General Hospital, UK, in 1976, two mixtures were made available for the nurses to give people suffering from emotional shock – the Rescue Remedy and a Grief Mix (p.187). They were soon in regular use, and by observing the results, successive groups of young doctors were persuaded to take them up. These remedies are invaluable for first aid at home (p.329).

Consulting a therapist

Self-prescription with the Bach flower remedies can work wonders, but it is essential for some people to go to a therapist, either because they can't see into themselves far enough or because they need other treatment. Consultations with a therapist will take from ten minutes to an hour, depending on individual needs. There are normally follow-up visits every month or six weeks.

The remedies work quickly with emotional problems, but more slowly with physical illnesses. They have an enviable safety record and combine effectively with other therapies, including orthodox medicine. Sometimes a patient will reject a remedy because it acts on an aspect of their personality that they cannot face at the time. Very rarely, a person may be sensitive to the alcohol in the brandy that preserves the remedies, but prior enquiry and advice will avoid these problems.

"There is no true healing unless there is a change in outlook, peace of mind, and inner happiness."
Dr Edward Bach

Using flower remedies

The 38 Bach flower remedies are made for self-treatment, and are readily available at homeopathic pharmacies or through the Dr Bach Memorial Centre (see Resources pp.342-4). To get the best results, always start by choosing two of the Twelve Healers: Rock Rose for terror; Mimulus for fear; Cerato for self-distrust; Scleranthus for indecision; Gentian for discouragement; Clematis for dreaminess; Water Violet for excessive self-sufficiency; Agrimony for concealed worry; Centaury for the inability to say no; Chicory for the tendency to take over; Impatiens for impatience; Vervain for over-enthusiasm. Use the fuller descriptions on pages 185-7 to guide you.

Take your two remedies for about a month, as explained below. If you feel better but find that some new problems have emerged, add not more than three new remedies for your most pressing negative feelings. Continue in this way, and stop taking the remedies once you have felt fine for a whole month. If you do not feel any improvement after your initial prescription, start again with different ones from among the Twelve Healers, or consult a therapist.

Storage and dosage

The remedies are supplied in 10 ml or 30 ml stock phials, each containing a single remedy. Sets of the 10 ml phials are available containing all the 38 remedies. Both sizes are of dark glass, with droppers attached to their caps. They should be stored in a cool dark place.

Once you have made up your personal mixture, or one of the combination remedies, as described on p.187, you take 4 drops in a little spring water, 4 times a day on an empty stomach. Sometimes it will be more convenient to take the 4 drops straight into your mouth from the dropper. Make sure the dropper does not touch your mouth since this will contaminate the remedy. Don't waste stock by consuming the remedies straight from the phials. They work better when diluted.

Making a personal mixture

Fill a small, dark, sterilized bottle (preferably one with a built-in dropper), three-quarters full of still spring water. Add 2 drops of each of your chosen remedies from the stock phials, then top the bottle up with brandy.

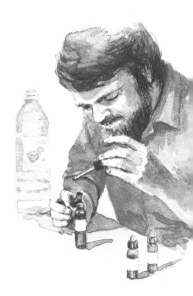

The 38 remedies

Each of the 38 Bach flower remedies acts on a negative emotional state to bring out its corresponding positive side. It is preferable to see these states as archetypes, with positive and negative sides.

Fear

Aspen Acts on fear of the unknown.

Red Chestnut Acts on excessive fear for the welfare of others.

Cherry Plum Acts on desperation arising from fear of losing control.

Rock Rose Acts on terror or panic, total self-involvement or self-abandonment. Brings the ability to act selflessly.

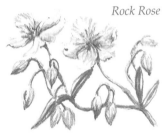

Rock Rose

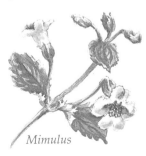

Mimulus Acts on fear of known things, shyness and speech impediments that arise from lack of trust in a divine pattern. Promotes faith and, with it, courage, acceptance and endurance.

Mimulus

Uncertainty

Gorse Acts on feelings of hopelessness.

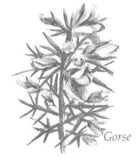

Gorse

Hornbeam Acts on tiredness caused by self-doubt.

Wild Oat Acts on lack of ambition and direction.

Cerato Acts on self-distrust and the tendency to seek advice from others. It promotes self-reliance, intuitiveness, and qualities of leadership.

Scleranthus Acts on indecision, mood swings and motion sickness. It promotes stability and decisiveness.

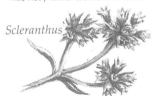

Scleranthus

Gentian Acts on discouragement and disappointments that produce "reactive depression". It promotes optimism and perseverance.

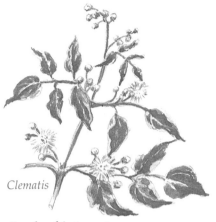

Clematis

Lack of interest
(in the present)

Clematis Acts on dreaminess, escapism and absent-mindedness. It promotes alertness, earthiness and intuitiveness.

Honeysuckle Acts on nostalgia and suffering from the loss of a person or object that you love.

Wild Rose Acts on resignation and feelings of apathy.

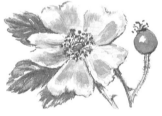

Wild Rose

Olive Acts on the effects of physical and mental stress.

White Chestnut Acts on a preoccupation with persistent, unwanted worrying thoughts.

Chestnut Bud Acts on the tendency to repeat mistakes, to be slow to learn from experience.

Loneliness

Water Violet Acts on excessive self-sufficiency. When negative the Water Violet type is proud, superior or aloof. When positive, this person is a sympathetic counsellor.

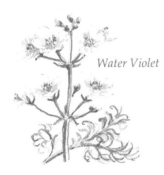

Water Violet

Heather Acts on excessive self-concern, talkativeness, a dislike of being alone, and a tendency to "buttonhole".

Impatiens Acts on impatience, instability and accident-proneness. When positive, these people are gentle and use their excessive energy creatively to help others.

Over-sensitivity
(to influence and ideas)

Walnut Acts on over-sensitivity to outside influences, and is helpful for the major changes in life (such as puberty and the menopause).

Holly Acts on anger or hatred – generally when they are directed against others but also when self-directed.

Agrimony Acts on worry or mental torment concealed by a mask of happiness or sociability. When positive, these people are the best of companions and partners.

Centaury Acts on an inability to say no, and an excessive anxiety to please. Those who need Centaury tend to bottle up anger (as in Holly) and depression (as in Gentian). Many cancer sufferers need these remedies, and they may also be useful for prevention.

Depression and anguish

Mustard Acts on sudden deep depression with no known cause.

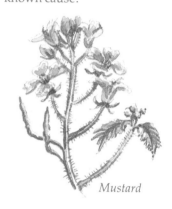

Mustard

Larch Acts on lack of confidence and fear of failure.

Pine Acts on guilt (both real and imagined), and the tendency to apologize needlessly.

Elm Acts on a sudden feeling of being overwhelmed by responsibility.

Sweet Chestnut Acts on extreme anguish and a feeling of total bereavement.

Star of Bethlehem Relieves the effects of any type of shock.

Willow Acts on resentment and bitterness.

Oak Acts on a tendency to relentless effort which can lead to a breakdown of mind or body, especially back problems.

Crab Apple Relieves feelings of uncleanness.

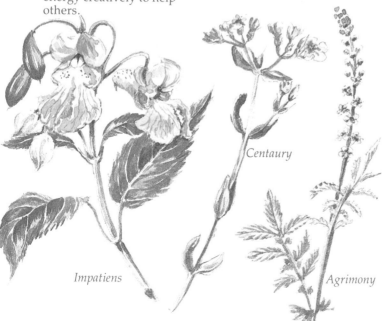

Impatiens

Centaury

Agrimony

Over concern
(for the welfare of others)
Chicory Acts on a tendency to "take over" people or situations. When negative, these people are emotional vampires, possessive, deceitful, strong-willed and easily hurt. When positive, they are selfless in their care and concern for other people.

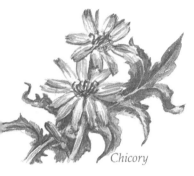
Chicory

Vervain Moderates extremes of energy, tension and enthusiasm.

Vine Corrects a tendency to extreme control – of yourself or of others, and excess will.

Beech Corrects a tendency to intolerance and criticism of others.

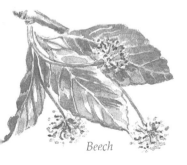
Beech

Rock Water Corrects excessive self-involvement, leading to mental rigidity.

Combination remedies
There are a number of composite remedies that are good for certain situations, as described below. You can make these mixtures up at home, following the instructions given on p.184, or get a supplier to make them up for you. The Rescue Remedy can be bought ready-made. Take the combinations, as described in Storage and dosage, p.184.

Rescue Remedy A mixture of Impatiens, Star of Bethlehem, Cherry Plum, Rock Rose, and Clematis is very effective in all forms of shock or emergency. Keep it handy, and take it as required – every 5 minutes if the condition is severe. It can also be used for animals, combined with another remedy if indicated by the animal's behaviour; 1 or 2 doses are usually sufficient. Rescue Remedy is useful too for plants after transplanting or for cuttings, mixed with Hornbeam, Olive and Vine. Repeat the dose at intervals where necessary.

Radiation Remedy A useful composite for people exposed to radiation, such as X-ray treatment, this mixture consists of Walnut, Wild Oat, Gentian, Cherry Plum, Star of Bethlehem, Rock Rose and Vine, plus the homeopathic remedies Mistletoe 6x and Silica 6x (p.146) in liquid form. Make up the combination in sea water or with 1 full teaspoon of sea salt in 100 ml of spring water.

Grief Mix This is a composite of Star of Bethlehem, Gentian, Honeysuckle and Sweet Chestnut. You can also add, as required, 2 drops of Pine, Holly, White Chestnut or Willow.

Star of Bethlehem

Gentian

Sweet Chestnut

Honeysuckle

Drug Detoxification Mix Combine Walnut, Crab Apple, Larch and Hornbeam and take this half-hourly until the condition improves, then 2-hourly for 48 hours.

Examination Mix This counteracts the panic that can incapacitate students at examination time. It is a basic combination of Larch, Clematis and Gentian, to which you can add 2 drops of Mimulus, Rock Rose or White Chestnut, according to your disposition.

Naturopathy

More than any other single method of treatment, naturopathy is a multi-disciplinary approach to illness and health. It comprises several systems of diagnosis and treatment, including hydrotherapy and various diet therapies. Its aim is to promote health rather than to confront disease and, where possible, to educate people toward improving their lifestyles in order to prevent further illness.

The individual symptoms by which an illness is classified – or the type of bacteria or virus which is rampant – are less important to a naturopath than the imbalances, physical, emotional, or biochemical, which may have caused the problem. It is largely the environment that we create within our bodies that controls our resistance to disease. If the body is burdened with impurities, invading micro-organisms may find it an agreeable home in which to multiply.

Naturopathic medicine is therefore directed toward restoring balance in our functions – by helping us to overcome negative emotions, teaching us ways of coping with stress, correcting physical obstacles to normal functioning, and providing nutrition of the best quality to sustain healthy body chemistry. By

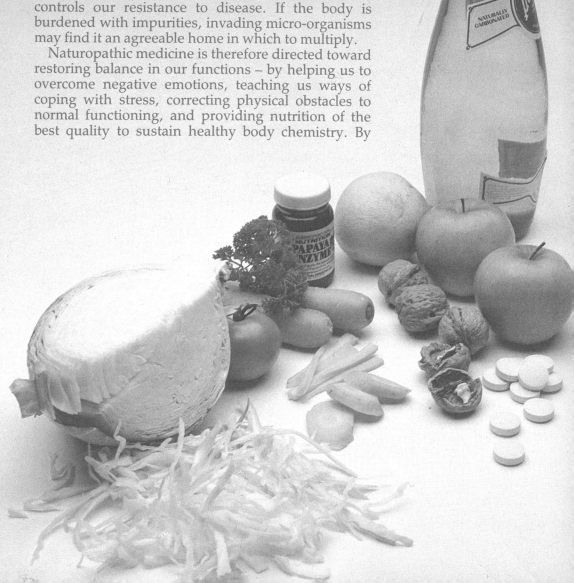

these means the homeostatic or self-regulatory mechanisms of the body are reinstated, so that it can heal itself or fight off the invading organisms.

The development of naturopathic methods

Naturopathy evolved empirically, by observation and application. Many of its principles developed through attentiveness to the workings of nature. Its origins can be observed in the instinctive behaviour of many animals – they stop eating when unwell, try to cool inflamed parts, or seek warmth when chilled. Early humans probably used the same instincts and gradually learned to use water, air, sunlight, and local plant life for the relief of aches and pains.

In ancient Greece, Hippocrates – the Father of Medicine – was one of the first to realize the importance of nature's own healing power. He described the basic rules of natural hygiene and also recognized the value of fevers as a manifestation of healing at work. The Romans made bathing for health into a science, establishing spas which, even now, serve a practical purpose in the relief of physical disorders such as arthritis.

Nearly 2,000 years later, in the 19th century, a number of people began to re-investigate these natural treatments and develop other simple measures to promote healing. A German farmer called Johannes Schroth noticed that his cart-horse ate only dry bran when it had strained a joint. This led him to develop the Schroth Cure, a dry-diet treatment still much used by naturopaths today for the relief of rheumatoid arthritis and other joint inflammations.

Iridology, the method of diagnosing physical or mental disorders from signs in the eye, was inaugurated by Ignatz von Peczely, a Prussian surgeon who observed changes in a particular part of his pet owl's iris when he accidentally fractured its leg. Also in the 19th century, in Germany, Vincent Priessnitz and Pastor Kneipp developed a more systematic approach to hydrotherapy.

The work of these pioneers was consolidated in the 20th century by Henry Lindlahr in the USA, James C. Thompson and Stanley Lief in the UK, and Dr Max Bircher-Benner, the creator of Muesli and the founder of a famous clinic in Zurich, Switzerland. It was Lindlahr who laid down the ground rules of naturopathic practice. He described as "healing crises" those aggravations of symptoms, such as fevers, colds, and discharges, which the body often undergoes in its natural sequence of recovery from ill health, distinguishing them from "disease crises" which occur when the body's vital reserve is no longer capable of overcoming disease.

Modern corroboration

The methods that naturopaths have found effective in promoting healing – especially the dietary measures – are now being confirmed and explained by modern research. Naturopaths, for example, have long advocated an adequate nutrient intake for the maintenance of not only physical but also mental and emotional well-being. It has now been established that both a deprivation of essential nutrients, such as certain proteins, and an excess of inappropriate foods, such as sugar, can create biochemical changes and imbalances in the metabolism which may result in a wide variety of symptoms, both mental and physical. Modern research has also confirmed the naturopath's belief in the healing functions of inflammation and fever. Hippocrates recorded his belief that these conditions served a constructive purpose, and naturopaths developed treatment with herbs and hydrotherapy that supported and encouraged the processes, for their role in eliminating toxins. Biochemists have now explained how the body defends itself against bacteria and viruses by setting its thermostat higher (a process that is controlled by pro- and anti-inflammatory hormones).

Consulting a professional

The first time you go to see a naturopath, he or she will start by taking a detailed case history. Flavor cravings, responses to climatic changes, and major crises in your life will all be noted since they may be important factors in your unique health profile. To this pattern will be added information gained from a careful physical examination and other special tests, such as examination of the spine for restrictions of mobility, or iridology. In addition, tests to determine your sensitivity to, or intolerance of, certain foods and environmental chemicals may form a part of the diagnostic procedure.

   As well as the usual blood or urine tests, a small amount of your hair may be sent away for an analysis

Iridology
Iris diagnosis is used by naturopaths and other therapists, particularly when an ordinary diagnosis is unclear. The iris charts below and on p.191 show just a few of the "reflex" areas of the iris zones which correspond to various parts of the body. The left iris relates to the left side of the body, the right iris to the right side.

Right iris

1 Physiological brain
2 Neck and shoulder
3 Lung and bronchials
4 Liver and gall bladder
5 Lower abdomen
6 Kidney and adrenal glands
7 Spine
8 Thyroid gland
9 Face and mouth
10 Psychological brain
11 Animation
12 Intestine
13 Stomach
14 Autonomic nerve wreath

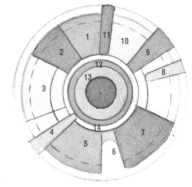

of the mineral levels which, in conjunction with other clinical findings, helps to assess your individual nutritional requirements. And sophisticated bio-electric equipment may be used to assess your vital reserves or your compatibility with particular foods, from a sample of blood, hair, or saliva.

Assessing individual needs

We are all unique in our biological needs. The variations in our physique, organ structure, and nutritional requirements mean that two people with the same illness may need quite different types of treatment. In one case of a cold, for instance, the inflammation and catarrhal discharge may be indicative of the body's attempt to rid itself of excess impurities, such as food chemicals or environmental toxins. In another case, the cold may be due primarily to lack of resistance, through lowered vitality as a result of nutritional deficiencies, poor breathing habits, and insufficient exercise.

The first case would require "catabolic" treatment, designed to assist the body's eliminative efforts and stimulate the breakdown of toxic deposits. The devitalized person, on the other hand, would need "anabolic" treatment to build up strength - including better nutrition, supplements of particular vitamins, and advice on correct breathing, gentle exercise, and sufficient rest and relaxation.

Having built up a picture of your constitution, vital reserves, hereditary tendencies, nutritional status, and mental outlook, the practitioner will be in a position to decide whether anabolic or catabolic treatment should be given and to advise you on what you can do to help yourself.

In most cases some basic advice on healthy eating will be given. Dietary analysis may lead to more specific recommendations: special vitamin or mineral requirements may be revealed and supplements prescribed. You may also be advised to carry out hydrotherapy at home – using compresses, sprays, packs, or special baths. The naturopath may recommend simple exercises and relaxation techniques, among other gentle introductions to a healthier lifestyle. Psychological counselling too is an important part of naturopathic practice, a vital ingredient of the triad of health – structural, biochemical and emotional well-being.

Left iris

1 Psychological brain
2 Face and mouth
3 Thyroid gland
4 Spine
5 Kidney and adrenal glands
6 Skin and circulation
7 Lower abdomen
8 Spleen
9 Lung and bronchials
10 Heart
11 Neck and Shoulder
12 Physiological brain
13 Animation
14 Intestines
15 Stomach
16 Autonomic nerve wreath

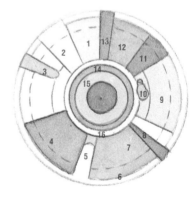

Naturopathic home treatments

Naturopaths prescribe a great variety of home treatments that can be used both to restore your health and to enhance it. The dietary and hydrotherapy techniques described here and on pages 194-5 play an important part both in curing and preventing common ailments (pp.196-207).

Diets for healing

In addition to the remedial diets outlined below, naturopaths also advise a basic health diet which establishes a balanced nutritional pattern. This daily menu is shown in the main Diet section on page 47. The fundamental principles are that your diet should be: low on animal fats, sugars and salt; high on raw fruit and vegetables; and low on alcohol, coffee and strong tea. Food should also be eaten as near as possible to its natural state.

Caution Strict diet control can sometimes cause unpleasant symptoms such as headaches or loose bowels. These symptoms are normal signs that the body is beginning to eliminate unwanted impurities. Generally they will be followed by a renewed sense of well-being. If these healing crisis symptoms recur some weeks later, return to the healing diet for a few days, and they should soon disappear.

Nutritional supplements
These form a major part of naturopathic treatment. Where specific vitamin or mineral supplements are recommended under Ailments and remedies (pp. 196-207), always use those prepared from natural ingredients – their benefit is far greater than that of chemical imitations.

Unless otherwise specified, follow the dosage prescribed on the bottle. Continue with treatment for a fortnight after symptoms have cleared up for acute disorders, 3-4 weeks after for chronic problems. Be sure that you use nutritional supplements as part of a basic health diet (p.47) – their benefit depends on an all-round good-quality nutritional programme.
Caution Do not use supplements while fasting.

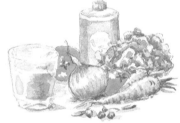

Raw food diet
This is beneficial for digestive troubles, for congestion, skin disorders, and many other complaints. However, it may not be well tolerated by people who have sensitive digestions, or those who are unaccustomed to raw food.

At each meal you should eat only uncooked vegetables and fruit. Select a reasonable amount of whatever is in season to satisfy your appetite. Garnish salads with nuts, seeds, natural yoghurt, and a little vegetable oil. Drink only pure fresh juices, herb teas, or mineral water. You can follow this diet for 1–7 days, or longer under professional supervision.

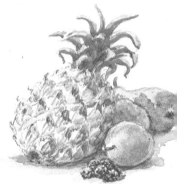

Raw fruit diet
This is a stricter version of the raw food diet in which you eat only fresh fruit at each meal. It encourages more elimination than the raw food diet and therefore helps to reduce skin rashes, mucus congestion, and rheumatic deposits. But it may not be suitable for the elderly and those with very sensitive digestions, unless the fruit is finely grated or puréed. Follow this diet for 1–7 days.

Light diet for sensitive digestions

This is an easily tolerated programme which rests the digestive tract to some extent and permits recovery without causing undue discomfort. It may be suitable for those who are unable to follow raw food diets. You may follow the regimen for 3-4 days, or a little longer, if you tolerate it well. Improvement is likely to be slower than with the stricter raw food diets.

On rising Peppermint tea or apple juice

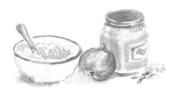

Breakfast Porridge with a little wheat germ, or puréed apple with yoghurt (use only a little honey to sweeten your food)

Mid-morning Peppermint tea or fruit juice (apple, grape, or pineapple)

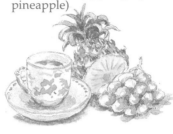

Lunch Steamed fish or savory rice with 2-3 cooked vegetables, or mixed vegetable broth (below)

Mixed vegetable broth
Make the broth with potatoes, beets, carrots, and celery, using about 50% potatoes. Use about 2 lb (1 kg) of vegetables to 3 pints (1.6 litres) of water. Slice the vegetables directly into the water (don't peel). Cook slowly until very soft (1-2 hours). Allow to stand for another ½ hour, strain, and serve warm.

Mid-afternoon Herb tea or fruit juice

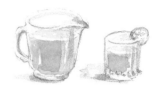

Evening Choose the alternative to your food at lunch – ie, a mixed vegetable broth or a savory brown rice or fish dish with vegetables.

As a second course, have puréed or soaked fruit, home-made fruit jelly, or tofu dessert (tofu flavoured with honey or fresh fruit).

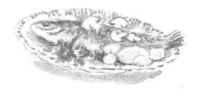

Fasting

This is complete abstinence from solid food. It rests the digestive tract, and allows the body to divert its energies to the elimination of toxic residues. It also affords relief from exposure to possible allergens in the diet.
Caution Fasting may not be suitable for the very frail or for those suffering from wasting diseases, or migraine. If you are in any doubt, consult a naturopath or your doctor.

How to fast Take only pure unsweetened fruit or vegetable juices and mineral water or herb tea. Juices must be free of coloring, sweeteners, or other additives. It is best to make them at home so you can be sure they are freshly prepared. Apples, grapes, pineapples, guava, oranges, carrots, beetroot, and celery, singly or in combinations, are all suitable. Take 1 tumbler 4 times a day and drink mineral water or herb teas at other times if you are thirsty. A 1-3

day fast is advisable – any longer fasting period *must* be supervised by a naturopath or a physician experienced in nutrition management.

After a fast Introduce solid food only gradually. The first day, the most appropriate diet would be plain yoghurt and fresh fruit, with perhaps a vegetable stew or salad in the evening. Gradually widen the menu with whole grains, legumes, nuts and seeds. Introduce milk and dairy products only after several days on solid food.

Naturopathic hydrotherapy

Many of the methods used in Hydrotherapy (pp.208-15) are common to naturopathic practice. They are all based on tried and tested principles. Hot or cold water on the body stimulates vital activity and relieves pain. Hot applications dilate the blood vessels, draw heat to the surface, and relax the muscles. Cold water drives the blood away from congested or inflamed tissues, speeding up the exchange of waste products and oxygen. Ice is only used in cases of extreme inflammation.

Compresses

Hot compresses are beneficial for stiff muscles, since they promote the dilatation of blood vessels. Cold compresses are used for any area of inflammation, such as an arthritic knee or a sore throat. Alternate hot and cold compresses are suitable for any stiff or painful condition.

Hot compresses Take a big flannel or a small towel, wring it out in hot water (tap-hot should be hot enough), and fold it to a convenient size. Apply this to the painful site. Leave it in place until it cools.

Cold compresses Follow the instructions for a hot compress, but wring out the flannel or towel in very cold water. Leave it in place for a few hours, or overnight (secure it with bandages).

Hot and cold compresses Place a hot compress on the painful site for 3 minutes, then replace it with a cold one, for 1 minute. Repeat the application for 20-30 minutes. You may need to make fresh compresses, since the temperatures even out.

Hot and cold bathing

For pain in the hands or feet, you will need 2 bowls, one containing hot water, the other cold. Place the hands or feet in the hot water for 3 minutes, then the cold for 1 minute. Repeat this process 3-4 times. Or you can spray the area with hot and cold water from a shower or tap.

Sitz baths

This contrast bath is good for back problems and genital and rectal complaints.

For a home sitz bath, you need 2 large bowls. Fill one with hot water, and the other with cold. Sit in the hot, with your feet in the cold, for about 3 minutes, then reverse your position for 1 minute, and repeat 2-3 times.

Friction rubs

These stimulate the skin and improve the circulation.

Take a loofah or a friction glove, dip it in cold water, and rub the skin vigorously. Work briskly from the extremities toward the heart, then over the front and back.

Steam inhalations

Inhaling steam is indicated for catarrhal congestion of the chest and sinuses. Half fill a bowl with freshly boiled water and add 2 or 3 drops of an aromatic oil – you can choose an appropriate oil from the Aromatherapy section (pp.176-81) or buy a blend of pure plant oils, such as clove, peppermint, eucalyptus and menthol, from a pharmacy. Put a towel over your head, making a tent to stop the steam escaping. Lean over the bowl and inhale deeply through the nose. Try to get the steam well back into your sinuses.

Aromatic steam inhalations help clear respiratory problems

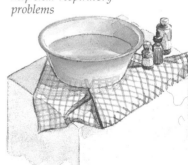

Abdominal packs

These are very beneficial for digestive disorders and constipation. Use the method described under Trunk packs, but cover only the lower half of the trunk, from waist to groin.

Epsom salts baths

These are beneficial for the early stages of chills and colds, or after exposure to cold and damp weather.

Fill a bath with enough hot water for you to lie immersed up to the neck. (It should be as hot as you can comfortably bear.) Dissolve 2 handfuls of unpurified Epsom salts in the water. Soak in this for 20 minutes with a cold compress placed on your forehead. Rise from the bath carefully, wrap yourself in a sheet and retire to a warm bed. This will encourage perspiration.

Hands or feet may be soaked in an Epsom salts solution. Use 1 heaped dessertspoon to a bowl of hot water and soak for 15 minutes.
Caution Not to be taken by the very young, the elderly, or those with high blood pressure.

Soothing bath solutions

There are a variety of other ingredients that can be used therapeutically in the bath. Add 2 tablespoons of sodium bicarbonate to bath water for irritating skin disorders. Bran, or hay-flowers (the flowers of wild hay) also have a soothing effect. Place 2 tablespoons of either in a muslin bag and infuse for 30 minutes in a saucepan of water. Discard the bag and add the infusion to the bath.

Trunk packs

A cold water pack applied to the trunk encourages the elimination of toxic residues. It is an excellent treatment for colds and flu, feverish disorders and skin complaints.

You will need a flannelette or heavy cotton sheet (a small one for a child), a plain cotton sheet, a blanket, and hot-water bottles.

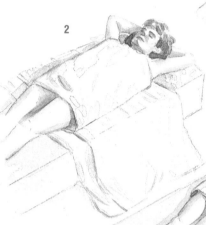

Making a trunk pack

Method Fold a blanket and a plain sheet into broad bands that will envelope the trunk from armpits to the top of the thighs. Place them across a bed with twice as much hanging over one side as the other. Soak a flannelette or heavy cotton sheet in cold water, and wring it out thoroughly, and fold it into another broad band. Place it over the dry sheet and blanket.

The patient should lie on top of the wet sheet, as shown above (1), and tuck the longer flap of the wet sheet around and under the body. The short flap is folded over next (2). The dry sheet is folded in the same way (3), then the blanket. You can secure the whole pack with safety pins. Put a hot-water bottle at the feet, and at the sides if necessary. Keep the pack on for a few hours or overnight.

Removing the pack When the pack is removed the body should be sponged with cool or tepid water, and dried briskly with a rough towel.
Caution If within an hour the trunk pack has not warmed up, it should be removed, and the body sponged and dried as described above.

Ailments and remedies

For most common ailments, naturopaths advise three levels of treatment, which are practiced simultaneously – general (which is also preventive), local, and supplementary treatment. Remedies for first aid purposes are given on pages 324-30.

Coughs

General Follow first a raw food or raw fruit diet (p.192) and then the basic health diet (p.47), excluding mucus-forming foods (see Catarrh). Do breathing exercises (pp.58-9) and give yourself friction rubs (p.194).

Local Apply hot and cold compresses (p.194) to the chest and upper back and take steam inhalations (p.194).

Supplementary Take the following: 1-3 g bioflavonoids a day; and 3 garlic tablets at night. If you suffer from throat catarrh, gargle with red sage solution (see below).

Sore throats

General Apply an abdominal pack with a cold throat compress (pp.194-5) to balance the circulation and encourage elimination. Follow the basic health diet (p.47) and reduce your intake of mucus-forming foods (see Catarrh).

Local Apply a cold compress (p.194) and gargle with red sage solution (see below).

Supplementary Take the following: vitamin B complex; 1-2 g bioflavonoids a day; and 3 garlic tablets at night.

Colds and flu

General At the first stage (chilly, aching muscles, sore throat) take an Epsom salts bath (p.195). When a feverish cold or flu is established, fast (p.193) for 1-3 days or follow the raw food or raw fruit diet (p.192). Apply a trunk pack (p.195). At the catarrhal stage adopt a raw food or light (pp.192-3) diet – see advice for Catarrh. Give yourself friction rubs (p.194).

Local You may benefit from steam inhalations (p.194) and hot and cold spraying or sponging on the face and over the sinuses. Start with hot water for 3 minutes, then cold for 1 minute, and repeat 3-4 times. Mind your eyes with the hot water.

Supplementary Take the following: 1-4 g bioflavonoids (vitamin C compound) a day; 3-4 garlic tablets at night; and a compound mineral supplement. Gargle with red sage solution (see below) 2-3 times a day.

Catarrh

General Fast (p.193) for 1-3 days, then follow the raw food or raw fruit diet (p.192). The catarrh should gradually loosen and become clearer. Return to the basic health diet (p.47), excluding all mucus-forming foods, notably milk products, sugar, and refined carbohydrates. Give yourself friction rubs (p.194).

Local See advice for Colds.

Supplementary Take the following: vitamin B complex; 1-3 g bioflavonoids a day; and 3-4 garlic tablets at night. Gargle 2-3 times a day with red sage solution (see below).

Red sage solution
Mix 1 teaspoon of red sage extract in a cup of warm water and gargle, or use an infusion (p.164) of sage.

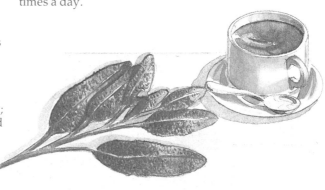

Tonsillitis

General Start by fasting (p.193) for a couple of days, then adopt the raw food or light diet (pp.192-3).

Local Apply cold compresses (p.194) to the throat overnight and gargle 3 times a day with red sage solution (p.196). Apply an abdominal pack (p.195) to promote general elimination. Friction rubs (p.194) may help.

Supplementary Take the following: vitamin B complex; 1 g bioflavonoids a day; and 3 garlic tablets at night.

Bronchitis

General Follow the basic health diet (p.47). For acute bronchitis, adopt the raw food or raw fruit diet (p.192) or fast for 24-48 hours (p.193). Cut out all milk products, sugar and refined carbohydrates to reduce the catarrh. Do breathing exercises (pp.58-9).

Local Give yourself hot and cold compresses and steam inhalations (p.194). Try postural drainage, below.

Supplementary Take the following: vitamin B complex; 1-3 g bioflavonoids a day; 3-4 garlic tablets at night.

Asthma

General Do regular breathing exercises (pp.58-9) and follow a relaxation routine (p.63). Adopt the basic health diet (p.47) and exclude mucus-forming foods (see Catarrh). If you have nasal or chest catarrh you may follow the raw food or raw fruit diet (p.192) for short spells but it is advisable to seek professional advice.

Local During an attack, apply hot compresses to the chest and back to ease lung congestion (p.194). Steam inhalations are also helpful (p.194). If you do not suffer from skin sensitivity, rub your chest with aromatic warming oils, such as wintergreen, juniper, or eucalyptus.

Supplementary Take the following: 5,000-10,000 IU of vitamin A a day; vitamin B complex; 1-3 g bioflavonoids a day; and a compound mineral supplement.
Caution Asthma can be life-threatening so do not attempt to reduce any prescribed anti-spasmodic drugs without professional advice.

Voice loss

General Follow the basic health diet (p.47) and avoid mucus-forming foods (see Catarrh) and stimulants, such as coffee, tea, and alcohol. Take cold drinks only. Give yourself friction rubs (p.194) and follow a rest and relaxation routine (p.204). Exercise your voice by light humming projected into the sinuses ("Mmmmeeeee. . . .").

Local Apply cold compresses (p.194) to the throat and gargle 3-4 times a day with red sage (p.196).

Supplementary Take the following: vitamin B complex; 1-3 g bioflavonoids a day; and a compound mineral supplement.

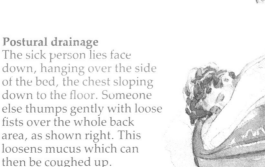

Postural drainage
The sick person lies face down, hanging over the side of the bed, the chest sloping down to the floor. Someone else thumps gently with loose fists over the whole back area, as shown right. This loosens mucus which can then be coughed up.

Diarrhea

General Begin by fasting (p.193) for 24-48 hours (ideally with apple or carrot juice), then for a further 24-48 hours introduce finely grated or puréed apple and plain yoghurt. Build up to a light diet (p.193). Lactic fermented products such as yoghurt and lacto-fermented vegetable juices help to re-establish intestinal flora. Avoid stimulants such as coffee, strong tea, and alcohol. Apply hot and cold compresses (p.194) to the abdomen.

Supplementary Take the following: vitamin B complex; a compound mineral supplement; and slippery elm powder as a gruel at or before each meal.

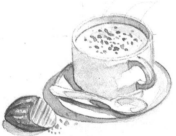

Emergency In case of prolonged diarrhea sip a cup of hot milk with 1 teaspoon of grated nutmeg sprinkled on the top.

Haemorrhoids

General Follow the basic health diet (p.47). Adopt a raw food or light (p.192) diet for up to 1 week. Twice a day do the abdominal tone exercise (see below).

If constipation is an accompanying problem, follow the general and supplementary treatments advised under constipation and the local treatment described below.

Congestion of the veins in the rectum may be the result of back pressure from a congested liver, so you should refer also to the treatment for nausea (p.199).

Local Spray or splash the rectum with cold water for 5 minutes twice a day and, if possible, after passing stools. Hot and cold sitz baths (p.194) are also beneficial.

Supplementary Take the following: vitamin B complex; and 100 IU of vitamin E, 3 times a day.

Abdominal tone exercise
Lie on your back with your feet flat on the floor close to your buttocks, as shown below left. Lift your hips off the floor, drawing your abdominal muscles up and in as you do so, as shown below right. Lower yourself to the floor and repeat 6 times.

Constipation

General Follow the basic health diet (p.47), making sure that you get plenty of fiber from brown rice, jacket potatoes, wholemeal bread, and raw vegetables. If this doesn't help, fast for 48 hours, then follow the raw food diet (p.192) for up to 1 week. Apply hot and cold compresses to the abdomen or take hot and cold sitz baths (p.194).

Twice a day do the abdominal tone exercise (shown below). Regular brisk exercise is also beneficial.

Supplementary Take 3 garlic tablets at night. Herbal laxatives should be of the "bulk-action" type which encourage the muscular function of the colon and re-educate the bowels.

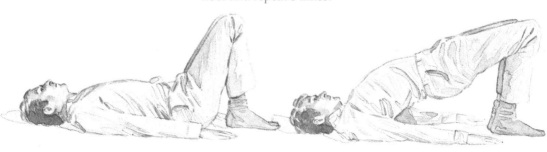

Nausea

General Fast (p.193) for 48 hours to clear inadequately digested matter, then for 24 hours eat puréed or finely grated apple and yoghurt before returning to a light diet (p.193). Exclude animal fats, coffee, strong tea, sugar, and alcohol.

Local Apply hot and cold compresses (p.194) to the upper abdomen.

Supplementary Take 2 capsules lecithin, 3 times a day, and a compound mineral supplement.

Indigestion, stomach ache

General For indigestion and stomach ache, fast (p.193) for 1-3 days, then take puréed or finely grated apples and yoghurt, or mixed vegetable broth for 24-48 hours before adopting a light diet (p.193). Avoid eating fruit in the same meal as starchy foods or protein, and limit your intake of carbohydrates (p.39). Follow a relaxation routine (p.204) and try to have your meals in a calm unhurried atmosphere.

Local Apply hot compresses or alternating hot and cold compresses (p.194).

Supplementary Take the following: vitamin B complex; an enzyme preparation made from pawpaw (papain), with each meal; and slippery elm powder made up as a gruel before each meal.

Flatulence, colic

General Fast for 24-48 hours to clear inadequately digested matter, then follow a light diet (p.193). Limit carbohydrates (sugars, starches, and raw vegetables) and do not mix starchy food with protein or fruit in the same meal (eg, avoid pastry with fruit, bread or potatoes with meat or nuts). Exclude coffee, strong tea, and sugar and do not drink at mealtimes. Excessive quantities of legumes, especially soya products, may also increase flatulence.

Local Apply alternate hot and cold compresses (p.194) or hot abdominal compresses (see below).

Supplementary With each meal take papain (an enzyme preparation made from the tropical fruit pawpaw). *Caution* Flatulence may be a sign of a more serious disorder. If it persists, obtain professional advice.

Abdominal compress
A hot compress (p.194) relaxes stiff muscles. Applied to the stomach, as shown right, it is good for abdominal colic or indigestion.

Bleeding gums

General This complaint may be a signal of a disorder elsewhere in the body and certainly implies some degree of nutritional deficiency. Consult a professional, and ask your dentist for advice on oral management.

Follow the basic health diet (p.47) initially. As a cleansing programme introduce the raw food or raw fruit diet (p.192), or, in the case of underlying digestive disorders, a light diet (p.193).

Local Clean your teeth with herbal medicinal toothpaste, massaging a small amount into the gums where you may leave it without rinsing. After dental care, rinse your mouth well with red sage solution (see p.196).

Supplementary Take the following: vitamin B complex; 1 g bioflavonoids a day; 3 garlic tablets at night; and a compound mineral supplement.

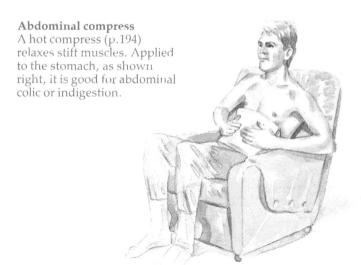

Abscesses

General You may hasten the healing by a short fast (p.193), or a raw fruit or raw food diet (p.192), which encourages detoxification.

Local If the abscess is on the trunk or upper legs, take Epsom salts baths (p.194) to help to draw it out. Treat abscesses in other areas with hot and cold compresses (p.194).

Supplementary Take the following: 10,000 IU of vitamin A a day; 1-2 g bioflavonoids a day; and 3-4 garlic tablets at night.

Boils

General Fast (p.193) for 1-3 days, then adopt a raw food or raw fruit diet (p.192) for up to a week. After that, stick to the basic health diet (p.47), to prevent recurrence of the boils. Friction rubs (p.194) to unaffected areas promote elimination.

Local Encase some finely chopped or grated raw cabbage leaves in a piece of gauze to make a poultice and place it over the boil. Secure it with bandages or sticking plaster. This will gradually draw out the pus; apply a fresh poultice each day until the boil heals.

Supplementary Take the following: vitamin B complex; 4,000-10,000 IU of vitamin A a day; 1-2 g bioflavonoids a day; and a compound mineral supplement.

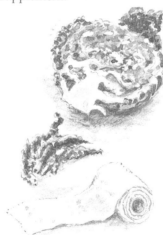

Natural poultices
Cabbages make an excellent poultice (see also p.327).

Acne

General Adopt the basic health diet (p.47) and cut out all sugar and refined carbohydrates. Regular short fasts (p.193) and a raw food diet (p.192) will help cleanse the blood. Give yourself daily friction rubs (p.194) on unaffected areas and a trunk pack (p.195) twice a week to promote skin metabolism generally. If the problem is persistent, you should consult a naturopath for advice on the treatment of underlying causes and for herbal remedies to promote general cleansing.

Local Cleanse sore or bleeding spots with warm water containing sea salt or a few drops of tincture of calendula. You may also apply calendula ointment.

Supplementary Take the following: vitamin B complex; 1-2 g bioflavonoids a day; 3 garlic tablets at night; and a compound mineral supplement.

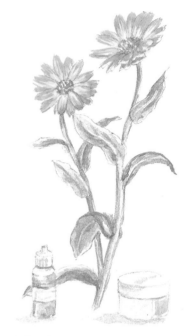

Calendula (marigold) Acne, chilblains and burns and bruises (see First aid pp.324-6) are soothed and healed by calendula.

Chilblains

General Take regular exercise, and follow the basic health diet (p.47).

Local Try hot and cold foot baths (p.194). If the skin is sore use calendula.

Supplementary Take the following: 1 g bioflavonoids a day; two 100 IU vitamin E capsules 3 times a day; two kelp tablets 3 times a day; and a compound mineral supplement.

Eczema

General Adopt the basic health diet (p.47) and exclude milk products, sugar, and citrus fruits. You may also follow the raw food or raw fruit diet (p.192) in preparation for a short fast (p.193). Eczema is linked with asthmatic tendencies and often has an allergic basis. If this is the case, follow the general treatment prescribed under Allergies (p.206). You should seek professional advice in all but the mildest cases.

Local Take sodium bicarbonate baths (p.195) to relieve irritation.

Supplementary Take the following: 5,000-10,000 IU of vitamin A a day; vitamin B complex; and a compound mineral supplement.

Impetigo

General Although impetigo is regarded as contagious, there is invariably an underlying toxic encumbrance or nutritional deficiency which allows the condition to become established. Good dietary habits are essential to prevention and recovery. Fast (p.193) for 48 hours, then follow the raw food or raw fruit diet (p.192) for 1 week before returning to the basic health diet (p.47). Continue to avoid sugar, coffee, and refined foods.

Supplementary Take 5,000-10,000 IU of vitamin A a day, vitamin B complex, 1-2 g bioflavonoids a day, and a compound mineral supplement.

Earache

General If the earache is associated with catarrhal congestion follow the treatment for Catarrh (p.196). Fast for 24-48 hours (p.193) and then adopt the raw food or raw fruit diet (p.192). Return to the basic health diet (p.47) with the exclusion of milk products, sugar, and starchy foods. It is very important to treat earache promptly, paying special attention to your diet.

Local Put a few drops of warm vegetable oil into the external passage of the ear and then plug the ear with cotton wool. Alternatively, place 3-4 tablespoons of salt in a muslin bag and warm it up in the oven. When it is sufficiently warm, place it against the affected ear to ease the pain and draw out any matter which may have accumulated.

Supplementary Take the following: vitamin B complex (must be yeast-free); 1-2 g bioflavonoids a day; and 3 garlic tablets at night.

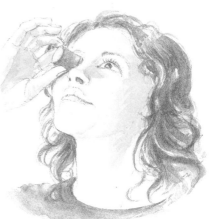

Styes

General Follow the raw food or raw fruit diet (p.192). If your case is severe, fast (p.193) for 24-48 hours.

Local Irrigate the eye with a weak solution of sea salt, or an infusion of eyebright; or take homeopathic Euphrasia.

Supplementary Take 5,000-10,000 IU of vitamin A a day, vitamin B complex, 1-2 g bioflavonoids a day, and a compound mineral supplement.

Eyebright (*Euphrasia officinalis*) This is an excellent remedy for eye problems. Use the dried herb (p.164, and p.170) for an infusion to bathe the eye, or take homeopathic Euphrasia (p.146).

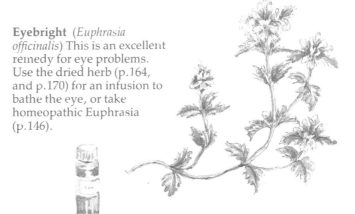

Backache

General Rest on a firm flat surface, eg, a mattress on the floor, to minimize the strain on affected joints. Follow a relaxation routine (p.204) to reduce muscle tension.

This may give you relief from the discomfort of back pain, but the causes must be corrected by professional manipulation and exercise. Consult an osteopath or a chiropractor (pp.228-41).

Local Apply alternate hot and cold compresses (p.194) to the affected areas 2-3 times a day and whenever pain is acute. Take sitz baths with Epsom salts (p.195).

Supplementary Take 1-2 g bioflavonoids a day; and a compound mineral supplement.

Lower spine stretching Lie flat on a soft but firm surface (eg, a rug on the floor), and draw your knees up to your chest . With your hands clasped around them, pull the knees toward you in a wide rotating action which stretches and loosens the base of the spine. Rotate 6 times towards the left and 6 toward the right, as shown below.

Rheumatism

General Follow the basic health diet (p.47) and reduce your intake of meat, eggs, sugar, and stimulants (coffee, strong tea, and alcohol). Periodically adopting a raw food or raw fruit diet (p.192) will also be therapeutic. A relaxation routine (p.204) is also beneficial.

Local Apply hot and cold compresses (p.194) to the affected joints or muscles. Take Epsom salts baths (p.194) for the relief of general stiffness or bathe the affected joint in an Epsom salts solution.

Supplementary Take the following: vitamin B complex; 1-2 g bioflavonoids a day; 3 garlic tablets a night; 2 kelp tablets 3 times a day; and a compound mineral supplement.

Lumbago

General Follow the advice for Backache, above, and regularly perform the spine stretching exercise shown below (or a similar one).

Local Give yourself hot and cold compresses and Epsom salts baths (pp.194-5).

Fibrositis

General Adopt the basic health diet (p.47) and reduce your intake of meat, eggs, and sugar. Follow a relaxation routine (p.204).

Local Apply hot and cold compresses (p.194) several times a day if the pain is acute. Take Epsom salts baths (p.195) 2-3 times a week. *Caution* This complaint can be caused by displaced vertebrae and should always be checked professionally.

Sciatica

General Seek osteopathic or chiropractic attention (see pp.228-41). Diet is also important, since poor nourishment of surrounding tissues will hinder progress.

Rest, lying on a firm surface, with a pillow beneath the knees if necessary. Do not attempt to exercise. Adopt the basic health diet (p.47).

Local Apply hot and cold compresses (p.194) to the lower back area.

Supplementary Take the following: vitamin B complex; 1-3 g bioflavonoids a day; 2 dolomite tablets 3 times a day; and a compound mineral supplement.

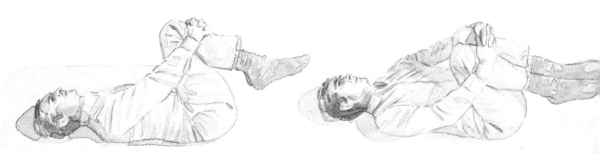

Arthritis

General In osteoarthritis (OA), the cartilage is worn away in the major weight-bearing joints (eg, knees and hips), impairing the joints' normal smooth movement and causing stiffness and pain. A considerable thickening around the margins of the joints may also occur – the body's attempt to protect the bones from undue friction.

Rheumatoid arthritis (RA) affects the entire body and destroys the cartilage and tissues in and around the joints as well. The joints become swollen and painful and the tendons and muscles also become sore, and often waste away through lack of proper use.

The arthritis syndrome is complex, requiring attention at various levels, so you should obtain professional naturopathic advice. Adopt the basic health diet (p.47) and limit your consumption of meat, eggs, and citrus fruits. You may also benefit by occasionally adopting the raw food diet (p.192) for up to 1 week. Follow a relaxation routine (p.204) to reduce muscle tension – stress often aggravates arthritis.

Local For OA, apply hot and cold compresses (p.194) to the affected joint or area of the back, to aid circulation and ease the stiffness. Give either the affected area or the whole body Epsom salts baths (p.195). To relieve RA, keep cold compresses (p.194) on the affected joints overnight. Alternate hot and cold compresses may help larger areas of the body.

Supplementary Take the following: 1-3 g bioflavonoids a day (especially for RA); a compound mineral supplement; and dolomite tablets (calcium and magnesium).

Raw diets
Raw food and raw fruit diets (p.192) benefit several musculoskeletal problems.

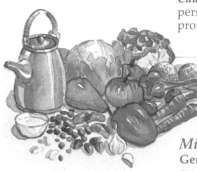

Stiff neck

General Gently roll your head from the front round to the back and forward again, if the movement does not aggravate the pain. Repeat several times in both directions. Follow a relaxation routine (p.204).

Local Apply hot and cold compresses (p.194) to the neck and across the shoulders. With your fingertips, knead gently in circular movements from the back of the skull, moving down the sides of the neck to the shoulders.
Caution If the problem is persistent, be sure to seek professional advice.

Headache

General Adopt the basic health diet (p.47), exclude all sweet foods, and make sure of a regular intake of protein. Relaxation (p.204) will help.

Local Apply cold compresses (p.194) to the forehead and back of the neck, or hot and cold compresses on the back of the neck and the shoulders.
Caution If you suffer from persistent headaches, seek professional advice.

Migraines

General Migraines have many causes and may need attention at a variety of levels – emotional, structural, and nutritional. You should seek professional attention for possible food intolerance, metabolic imbalances, or restriction of the neck and cranial bones.

Adopt the basic health diet (p.47), and cut out all sugar and caffeine. Make sure your mealtimes are regular and if possible take extra protein snacks between meals – migraine is often aggravated by low blood sugar (see Sugars, p.44).

Emergency Rest in a darkened room. Attempt a relaxation routine (p.204). Apply cold compresses to the forehead and the back of the neck (p.194).

Neuralgia

General Following a relaxation routine, as shown below, may reduce the intensity of the pain and divert your attention.

Local Apply hot and cold compresses (p.194) to the painful area, or the source of the affected nerve if this can be traced.

Supplementary Take vitamin B complex.

Insomnia

General Spray the lower legs and feet with cold water, or paddle in cold water, for 5 minutes before retiring. A short walk in the fresh air before bed will help to quieten your mind. Avoid over-stimulation just before going to bed (eg, from reading, work, TV, friends, coffee, or strong tea). Practice relaxation, as shown below, when you are in bed.

Relaxation routine
Adequate rest and relaxation are essential for nervous tension problems. Practice this routine in bed (before sleep or on rising), or during the day at any time when you can switch off for 10 minutes.
   Lying down on your back, as shown right, try to imitate a cat when it rouses itself from sleep, stretching a little at a time, gradually increasing circulation to the muscles. Slowly stretch your arms and legs and breathe a little more deeply as you circulate more oxygen. You will now feel rested, and calmer (and you may feel you have more energy).

Nervous stress

General Try to discover the cause of your tension. Follow a relaxation routine, as shown below. Adopt the basic health diet (p.47), increase your protein intake, and between meals have snacks of nuts or seeds to sustain your energy.

Supplementary Take vitamin B complex; 1 g bioflavonoids a day; two 100 IU capsules vitamin E, and 2 dolomite tablets, 3 times a day; and a compound mineral supplement.

Anxiety

General Use a relaxation technique, see below, to reduce tension. Adopt the basic health diet (p.47) and ensure extra protein intake.

Supplementary Take the following: vitamin B complex; 1 g bioflavonoids a day; two 100 IU capsules vitamin E, and 2 dolomite tablets, 3 times a day; and a compound mineral supplement.

High blood pressure

General Adopt the basic health diet (p.47). Cut out salt, sugar, and stimulants (coffee, alcohol, and tobacco). You will benefit from periodic fasts (p.193) or raw food diets (p.192). Take twice daily hot and cold foot baths (p.194) and follow a daily relaxation routine, as shown below. Regular and gentle non-competitive exercise is helpful, eg, yoga, t'ai chi, or walking.

Supplementary Take the following: one 100 IU capsule of vitamin E, 2-3 times a day; 2 lecithin capsules 3 times a day; and 3 garlic tablets at night to reduce blood fats. *Caution* If you suffer from high blood pressure, you should seek professional advice and regular monitoring of your blood pressure.

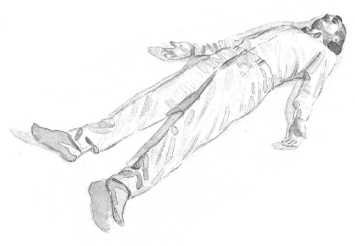

Low blood pressure

General Assist your general vitality by adopting the basic health diet (p.47). Make sure you take regular meals and have an adequate balance of rest and exercise. Exercise promotes the secretion of adrenal hormones which raise the blood pressure, but the heart must have adequate nutrition to sustain the increased work. Take mixed vegetable broth (p.193) 2-3 times a week and avoid artificial stimulants which speed up the metabolism without providing nourishment.

Supplementary Take the following: two 100 IU capsules of vitamin E, 3 times a day; and a compound mineral supplement.

Varicose veins

General Take regular brisk walks, with your leg veins firmly supported by elasticated stockings. Adopt the basic health diet (p.47) to make sure you have an adequate intake of fiber and to maintain the health of your liver, which may be the source of back pressure in the veins. Avoid weight gain.

Local Gently sponge or spray your legs with cold water, as shown right. Rest with your feet up when possible during the day to help drainage.

Supplementary Take the following: 1 g bioflavonoids a day; two 100 IU capsules of vitamin E, 3 times a day; and a compound mineral supplement.

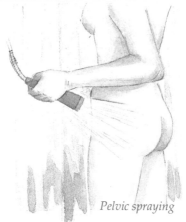

Pelvic spraying

Cystitis

General Cut out meat, eggs, and citrus fruits. Fast for 48 hours (p.193), then follow a raw food or light diet (p.192).

Local Hot and cold spraying to the pelvic area (3 minutes hot then 1 minute cold, repeated 3-4 times), or hot and cold sitz baths (p.194), may give you relief.

Vaginal infection

General A fungal disorder is often due to an excess of a rogue yeast called *Candida albicans*.

Follow a 48-hour fast (p.193) with a diet which excludes yeast-containing foods, such as bread, stock cubes, blue cheeses and wine, and sweet foods, which encourage yeasts to multiply. Obtain professional advice on anti-*Candida* management.

Local You may relieve some infections by applying pure goats' milk yoghurt or an acidic gel.

Supplementary Take the following: vitamin B complex (must be yeast-free); 1-2 g bioflavonoids daily; and 3 garlic tablets at night.

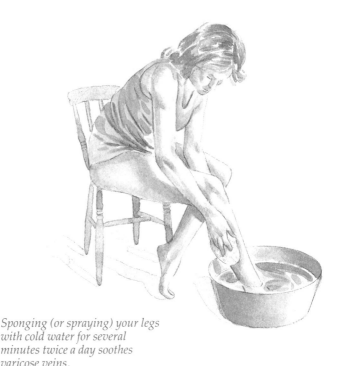

Sponging (or spraying) your legs with cold water for several minutes twice a day soothes varicose veins.

Tiredness

General Make sure you get adequate sleep (see Insomnia, p.204). Practice a regular relaxation routine (p.204). Adopt the basic health diet (p.47), and reduce your intake of sugars and stimulants. Eat regularly, taking light protein snacks halfway between main meals. Seek professional advice and investigation for possible causes such as anemia, low blood sugar, or poor digestive function.

Supplementary Take the following: vitamin B complex; 1 g bioflavonoids a day; two 100 IU capsules of vitamin E, 3 times a day; a compound mineral supplement; and 2 kelp tablets 3 times a day.

Feeling faint

General Recurrent feelings of faintness or lightheaded-ness may be associated with low blood sugar. Adopt the basic health diet (p.47) and cut out all sugars and honey as well as caffeine and other stimulants. Ensure that you eat regular meals and take a light protein snack (eg, nuts or seeds) halfway between meals. Seek professional help for possible causes, such as low blood pressure, anemia, or displaced neck bones.

Hay fever

General Avoid the irritant whenever possible, but also aim to reduce your sensitivity and increase your resistance. Fast (p.193) for 48 hours to reduce the inflammation and sensitivity, then revert to the raw food or raw fruit diet (p.192) and then the basic health diet (p.47), excluding mucus-forming foods (see Catarrh, general treatment, p.196). Do breathing exercises (pp.58-9).

Local Hot and cold bathing or sponging of the face and sinus areas may help. Use hot water for 3 minutes, cold for 1 minute, and repeat 3-4 times. If acute, use cold water only. Splash it on or use a sponge.
   You may obtain temporary relief by inhaling cold water through your nostrils and then expelling it again.

Supplementary Take the following: 5,000 IU of vitamin A a day; 1 g bioflavonoids a day; and 3 garlic tablets at night. See also the advice on Allergies, below.

Allergies

General Avoid allergens by all means, but the underlying imbalance which causes the sensitivity must be corrected. Seek professional advice. Adopt the basic health diet (p.47), and fast (p.193) or follow the raw food diet (p.192) to relieve acute symptoms and reduce toxic irritants.
   Allergies may be due to low blood sugar, so cut out all sweet foods (sugar, honey, chocolates, etc) and stimulants (such as coffee and strong tea) which disturb the metabolism and lower energy reserves. Make sure you take regular meals and protein snacks (eg, nuts or seeds) every 2-3 hours.

Local This depends on the form of the allergy. For skin troubles, see Acne and Eczema (pp.200-201), for catarrhal symptoms, see Catarrh (p.196).

Supplementary Take the following: 5,000 IU of vitamin A a day; 1-2 g bioflavonoids a day; and a compound mineral supplement.

Eating to avoid allergies
Allergic sensitivity can be reduced by cutting out sugar and stimulants and taking protein snacks. Dandelion coffee can replace ordinary coffee; carob is a naturally sweet substitute for chocolate.

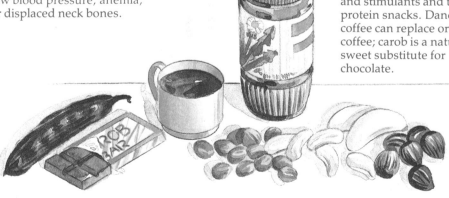

Food allergies

General A true food allergy is not as common as may be supposed. Most symptoms attributed to food are due to an intolerance which may be caused by a pharmacological reaction (to caffeine, for example) or by metabolic sensitivity to an excessive intake (of sugar, for example). You should seek professional advice to determine possible causes.

You can often reduce your sensitivity by excluding all sugars and adopting the basic health diet (p.47). A fast of 3 days (p.193). followed by a gradual re-introduction of foods (starting with the raw food diet, p.192), should cleanse the system, may relieve acute symptoms and help you to identify foods to which you have a particular sensitivity.

Supplementary Take the following: 1-2 g bioflavonoids a day; and a compound mineral supplement.

Addictions

General Cravings for stimulants such as tobacco and alcohol may be associated with the low blood sugar syndrome. Cut out sugar, honey, and other sweet foods and make sure that you get regular protein in the context of the basic health diet (p.47). Fast (p.193) for 24-48 hours to clear the toxins of the addictive substance. Follow a relaxation routine (p.204). Give yourself a daily friction rub (p.194) and take brisk exercise to tone your metabolism generally.

Supplementary Take the following: vitamin B complex; 1-2 g bioflavonoids a day; and a compound mineral supplement.

Cooling a fever

Sponging the face, neck, arms, and legs of a feverish child helps reduce a high temperature. Keep the torso covered to prevent the child becoming chilled.

Childhood diseases

General Children have a high level of vitality and a fast metabolism. They develop acute feverish conditions which sometimes last for only a few hours while the body burns up the toxic waste.

For most feverish disorders, such as measles, chickenpox, and flu, you can allow or encourage the child to fast, and try packs and compresses (see Fever below).

Local To relieve the irritation of rashes in measles or chicken-pox use sodium bicarbonate or bran baths (p.194).

Fever

General Withhold solid food. Fruit and vegetable juices may be taken (1 tumbler 4-6 times a day). If the sufferer is frail, but has an appetite, he or she may take mixed vegetable broth (p.193). As the fever reduces and the appetite returns, re-introduce solid food such as fresh fruit and/or yoghurt.

Local For adults and older children, apply a trunk pack or abdominal pack (p.195) for 3 hours or overnight. If this is too extreme, or the child is under the age of 5, use tepid sponging every 2-3 hours, unless the patient is very debilitated. Apply cold compresses (p.194) to the forehead.

Hydrotherapy

Hydrotherapy, or "water healing" as it is literally translated, is one of the oldest, cheapest, and safest methods of treating many common ailments. We instinctively recognize the therapeutic benefits of water in our everyday lives. At home, for example, we take baths and showers not only to cleanse the body, but also, after gardening or strenuous exercise, to help relieve fatigue and prevent stiffness.

The healing properties of natural hot and cold springs were recognized in many ancient civilizations. The Greek physician Hippocrates was already prescribing bathing and drinking spring waters for therapeutic effect in the 4th century BC. The Romans were firm believers in the value of hot springs and became the most outstanding builders of communal baths. It was not, however, until the 16th century that water "cures" as such developed in Europe around mineral springs or wells, with practitioners imposing a strict regime of drinking and bathing. In the 18th and 19th centuries, as hydrotherapy became more popular, the repertoire of treatments expanded. Hundreds of European towns and cities became famous for their waters. The cold water cures of

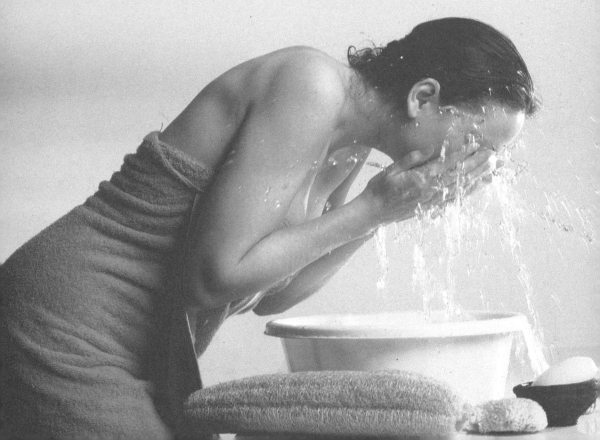

Vincent Priessnitz and the hot-and-cold treatments of Pastor Kneipp – developed in Europe in the 19th century – are still standard practice in hydrotherapy. Dr J.H. Kellogg of Philadelphia produced a comprehensive tome, *Rational Hydrotherapy* (1900), which described in great detail the effects of a huge number of douches, sprays, packs, inhalations, and baths.

Today, hydrotherapy is widely available in city hospitals all over the world. In Europe its use is mainly concentrated in spa towns, where people flock not only for treatment but also for prophylaxis. As a professional treatment, it is most frequently prescribed for patients suffering from orthopedic, rheumatic or neurological conditions, and consists of a series of special exercises performed in warm therapeutic pools. For the disabled or physically handicapped, hydrotherapy is especially beneficial, since the natural buoyancy of water allows a greatly increased range of movement.

There is a wide variety of hydrotherapy practices commonly used for self-help treatment. In the form of whirlpools, jacuzzis, saunas, hot tubs or other special baths, hydrotherapy is now widely available in health farms, sports clubs, fitness centers, and in some hotels and homes. In New Zealand, Iceland, the USA, and other parts of the world, natural hot springs too are frequented for their therapeutic value.

Pool treatment

If you consult your doctor with a musculoskeletal problem, hydrotherapy may well be recommended. If so, the treatment will be given in the therapeutic pool of the nearest hospital or perhaps at a local spa. The pool itself is very much like a small swimming pool but with much warmer water – usually 92-97°F (33-36°C). (Research has recently confirmed this as the optimum temperature range for increasing blood flow.) At your first visit, the therapist will make sure that there are no contra-indications to your receiving treatment, such as known heart problems, that you do not have either very high or low blood pressure or any breathing difficulties, and that you do not have any infection that could be spread to other users of the hydrotherapy pool.

Treatment consists of a series of exercises suitable to your condition. The water needs to come up at least as far as your waist to give you sufficient support for friction-free exercise. It is this quality that therapists make use of to re-educate and strengthen weak or damaged muscles and to loosen up stiff joints. You will find that some movements that are normally impossible or painful cause you no problem in the water.

At the completion of the session, which usually lasts for between 15 and 30 minutes, you must have a rest period of about 20 minutes, to allow time for your blood pressure, heart rate, and respiration to return to normal. The length of a complete course of treatment will vary according to the nature and severity of your problem. If you have found the therapy helpful, you will be advised to continue by yourself with recreational swimming and exercises in your own or a public pool. The exercises described on page 213 represent a small selection of those prescribed for general stiffness or debility.

Other hydrotherapy treatments
Other forms of treatment you may be given, or advised to use at home, involve the application of heat, cold, or alternate heat and cold to specific parts of your body (pp.211-12) in the form of baths, showers, packs, or compresses.

The application of heat is soothing. Muscle tension is reduced and pain relieved. Heat also causes nearby blood vessels to dilate, thus improving circulation, enhancing the body's self-healing ability and, through the increased blood flow, speeding up the removal of waste products.

The application of cold can be either stimulating or soothing. Skin temperature is initially reduced due to constriction of the superficial blood vessels, causing a correspondingly increased flow in the deeper blood vessels. After the cold water or pack is removed, the vessels once more dilate, flooding the site with blood.

The application of alternate hot and cold is intended to stimulate circulation. The alternate dilatation and contraction of the blood vessels forces an increased flow through problem sites.

Some courses of treatment, especially at spas, include drinking various mineralized waters. Ionized calcium, nitrogen, and sulphur, present in many spa waters, are widely recognized for their importance in maintaining metabolic function and are believed to benefit rheumatic disorders in particular.

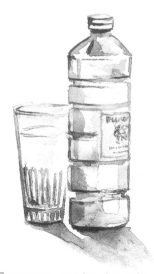

European spa treatments
The term "spa" derives from a Belgian town of that name whose mineral waters have long been known for their therapeutic value. Many European spas became famous for their waters, including Vichy in France, Malvern in England, Baden Baden in West Germany, and Marienbad in Czechoslovakia. Several different treatment regimes emerged, notably thalassotherapy (salt-water treatment), and the Kneipp water cure (based on water, sunshine, fresh air and regular activity), which remains very popular in European spa centers.

Hydrotherapy treatment

Home treatment with hydrotherapy revolves around a variety of simple techniques involving the application of heat or cold to the body. They can be used to treat a variety of common ailments (pp.214-15).

Baths, showers, and sitz baths

Baths and showers are used for ailments that require whole body treatments. Baths need to be deep enough to get your shoulders under the water. Showers are used to give an added stimulus to the skin. Be sure to use the precise temperature ranges given below, as these have been proven most effective. Sitz baths are designed to accommodate only the bottom, hips, and lower abdomen. They are used particularly for ailments affecting the abdomen and the reproductive system.

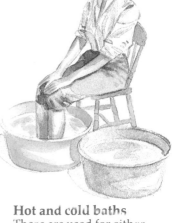

Sitz baths
You can have an improvised sitz bath at home, using a large basin or baby's bath.
Hot 99-108°F (37-42°C) You need to immerse your bottom and hips in the water. The water should come up to your waist. Start with 2 minutes on the first day, and increase a little each day until a maximum of 10 minutes is reached.
Cold 59 68°F (15-20°C) Follow the procedure above.
Contrast Use 2 large basins, one with hot water, the other cold. Sit in the hot water, with your feet in the cold for 3 minutes, then vice versa for 1 minute. Repeat this routine 2-3 times.

Standard baths and showers
Hot 99-108°F (37-42°C) Don't stay in a hot bath longer than 20 minutes – otherwise you may become dizzy or light-headed when you get out because of the fall in blood pressure.
Tepid 92-97°F (33-36°C) You can stay in a tepid bath for up to an hour.
Cold 59-68°F (15-20°C) Take a quick bath or shower only, then towel briskly.

Hot and cold baths
These are used for either hands or feet. The hot water must be as hot as you can stand it, and the cold as cold as you can get it – use ice if possible. For hands, you need 2 bowls, big enough to get both hands and wrists under water. For feet, you need 2 deep containers, as shown above.

Put your hands or feet in the hot water for 1 minute, then plunge them into the cold for 20 seconds, then back into the hot and so on for about 10 minutes. Finish with a quick plunge in the cold.

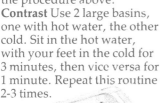

Sitz bath

Packs, friction rubs, and compresses

Hot dry packs are used when you need more prolonged heat on a part of the body. Water packs, hot or cold, are used to treat large areas. Ice packs are excellent for numbing pain and helping to reduce swelling. Friction rubs stimulate the skin and improve circulation. They are usually done in the bath or shower. For injuries or ailments that need heat or cold applied to a small area only, use a compress.

Water packs

Hot Wring out a piece of towelling in hot (not boiling) water and fold it to match the size of the area to be treated. Put the pack in place, using another towel to cover it, and leave it there until it cools.
Cold Use some thin sheeting wrung out in cold water and placed over the affected area.
Trunk Wrap the cold wet sheeting tightly around the body, covered with a woollen blanket. It *must* start to warm up within 10 minutes (poke your fingers between the pack and the body to check). If it does not, take it off and dry the body vigorously with a rough towel. If the pack does warm up quickly, it can be kept in place for at least 3 hours or even overnight. When you remove it, sponge with cool or lukewarm water, then towel briskly to warm up.
Hot dry pack Buy a ready-made hot dry pack. Place the pack in boiling water and simmer it for 10 minutes. Let it drain well and wrap it in a thick towel so that there are several layers between the pack and your body. Steam will seep through to your skin. Cover the pack with something waterproof, such as plastic sheeting, and leave it in place until it cools.

Ice packs

Crushed ice wrapped in a damp towel, a plastic pack of frozen peas, or a plastic freezer sachet (the malleable sort used to keep food cold on picnics) all make excellent ice packs. Put a little vegetable oil on your skin first to protect it from possible frostbite, and a single layer of damp towelling between the pack and your skin. Never leave an ice pack in place for more than 10 minutes.
Caution Ice packs should not be used by anyone suffering from a heart condition.

Friction rubs

Stand in the bath or shower with the cold water running, and use a bath brush, loofah, or string glove to scrub your skin with water. Work briskly, starting with one foot and going up to the hip, then doing the other leg, followed by one arm and then the other. Once you become used to frictions, do your trunk as well, front and back. End by towelling yourself quickly and thoroughly, until you achieve a pleasant glow.

Compresses

Hot Wring a small towel out in very hot water. Fold it into the appropriate shape and size and hold it in place until it cools down.
Cold Wring a small towel out in very cold water. Fold it, bind it in place with a bandage and leave it on for several hours or overnight.
Alternate hot and cold It is usual to start with a hot compress and finish with cold. You should keep the hot towel in place for 3 minutes, the cold one for 1 minute, and alternate them a few times. Repeat as necessary. If you treat two areas simultaneously, apply each compress for 1 minute, then swap them. Continue for about 10-20 minutes.

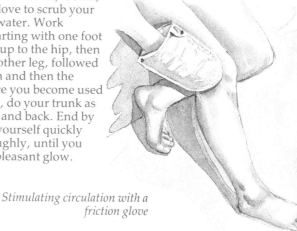

Stimulating circulation with a friction glove

Pool exercises

The following simple routines are good for stiff joints and weakened muscles. Practice them regularly in a shallow warm-water pool, preferably one that has a handrail, with the water about halfway between your waist and your armpits.

1 Feet and ankles

Stand sideways to the edge of the pool. If there is a handrail hold on to it with one hand. Put your feet together. Stand on your toes and then back on your heels, getting as much ankle movement as possible. Repeat 10 times.

2 Hip joints

Stand on one leg and swing the other back and forth. Start with a gentle swing then gradually increase the range, swinging as far in each direction as you can. Do this 10 times with each leg, keeping your trunk upright.

3 Spine

Face the edge of the pool, with both hands on the handrail. Starting a short step away from the wall, pull yourself forward so that your back arches, keeping your head well back. Then push backward, rounding out your spine, head forward and stomach tight. Repeat 10 times keeping your hands on the rail.

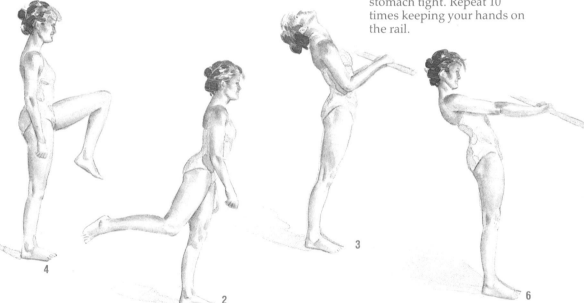

4 Knees and thighs

Begin by marching on the spot and gradually quicken your pace, bringing your knees up higher, until you are almost running. Do 20 running steps, then do another 20 kicking your heels up behind you.

5 Waist

Standing with feet apart, hands on hips, twist around first to the left, then to the right, as far as you can. Repeat 10 times.

6 Arms and shoulders

Step close to the side of the pool, and hold the handrail, as shown above. Now push your body backward and pull it forward again, keeping your back straight. Repeat 10 times, without letting go of the rail.

Ailments and treatments

The following ailments may be treated at home using the self-help methods described on pp.211-12. It is important to follow the advice on temperatures. *Caution* In cases of severe, unremitting pain, don't attempt to treat yourself before consulting a professional.

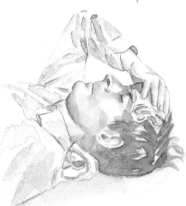

Soothing a headache with alternate hot and cold compresses

Respiratory ailments

Colds, flu, and fever Take strong, hot blackcurrant tea on going to bed and apply a cold water pack to your trunk. It can stay on overnight, but it *must* warm up within the first 10 minutes. **Catarrh and sinusitis** Alternate hot and cold compresses on the base of the skull and the forehead give almost instant relief. A cold sitz bath daily is good, or alternate hot and cold foot baths. **Bronchitis** Apply a cold water pack to the chest. Put a hot pack between the shoulderblades to ease coughing. **Asthma** Swimming, particularly breast-stroke, is helpful.

Skin problems

Chapping and chilblains Use alternate hot and cold hand or foot baths daily. Hands benefit if you use hot and cold compresses between the shoulderblades and the root of your neck. For your feet use alternate hot and cold compresses applied to your lower back, and foot baths. This stimulates circulation. **Psoriasis** Take a tepid (coolish) bath, with either 2 lb (0.9 kg) of salt dissolved in it, or 2 oz (56 g) of coal tar.

Conjunctivitis

Use a clean eyebath to bathe your eyes in tepid, boiled water with a little added salt. Blink several times into the water. A cold compress over closed eyes is also soothing.

Clearing congestion with a cold face plunge

Hay fever

Plunge your face into cold water and give your body a cold friction every morning. A cold sitz bath will act as a decongestant.

Cramp

If this is caused by poor circulation, use alternate hot and cold baths and give yourself cold frictions daily.

Headaches

For headaches and migraine, use alternate hot and cold compresses. Start with the cold compress held to your forehead, and the hot one at the base of the skull. Swap them round 6 times, finishing off with hot at the front and cold at the back.

Nervous tension

Anxiety, insomnia For relaxation, take a long tepid bath. If there is tension at the base of your skull, use alternate hot and cold compresses to this area. Try daily cold frictions in the morning. **Tiredness** Cold water frictions are stimulating.

Urino-genital problems

Cystitis and menstrual problems Take contrast sitz baths daily. **Impotence** Cold baths, cold showers, or cold sitz baths with daily cold frictions will all be stimulating.

Arthritis

Arthritis means inflammation in one or more joints, accompanied by pain and stiffness.

Use hot packs to relieve pain, unless you already have a hot, swollen joint, in which case use a cold water pack or ice pack. When the pain subsides do some exercises to keep your joints supple. Take long hot baths and exercise in a warm pool. Treat hands and feet with alternate hot and cold baths.

Fibrositis, rheumatism

These terms are used to cover non-specific muscular aching and stiffness – rheumatism can affect the whole body, while fibrositis usually occurs around the back of the neck and shoulders.

A variety of remedies are helpful: hot packs, hot baths, hot showers, or alternate hot and cold compresses over the kidneys. Try them all and stay with the one that helps most. Complete your self-help treatment with gentle exercise, deep breathing (p.59), and relaxation (pp.62-3).

Backache, lumbago, sciatica

For backache, lumbago, and sciatica, it is best to get a professional diagnosis, since there are numerous possible causes. Swimming and general exercise in a warm pool are beneficial. Also, for any back problems, think about your posture (p.232). For sciatica, place a hot water pack on your lower back. To stimulate circulation, use hot and cold foot baths.

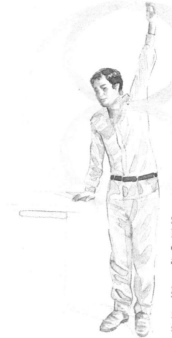

Standing shoulder exercise

Stiff shoulder

This complaint usually progresses through 3 stages: pain; stiffness; and recovery. If the shoulder is painful, use cold or ice packs. Don't, however, put ice on the left shoulder because of connections with the heart.

Try to prevent stiffness developing by exercising the area, either standing or sitting down. During recovery, you will find that hot packs and hot showers will be most helpful, and swimming too is excellent.

Sitting exercises
Sit in front of a mirror, to check that your shoulders are level. Practice these exercises 6 times.
1 Turn your head slowly to the right, then left.
2 Bend your head down on each side. **3** Shrug your

Standing exercise
Put your hand on the edge of a table, as shown above, to steady yourself.

Swing your free arm in a gradually increasing circle. Then change to a big figure-of-eight movement, so that you are crossing through the original circle, backward and forward. Then change the direction of the swing, so that your arm moves across the body and outward. Repeat with the other arm.

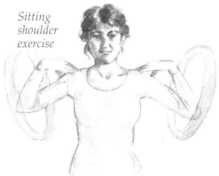

Sitting shoulder exercise

shoulders, right up and down. **4** Circle your elbows, forward then backward, as shown above. **5** Raise both hands above your head. **6** Put your hands behind your neck, and then behind your back.

Traditional medicine

Traditional or folk medicine is a term loosely applied to a great variety of curative substances or practices, generally used by lay people as a means of self-help. Evolved through the ages, and passed down from one generation to the next, it continues to occupy a cardinal position in the health care of millions of people all over the world. For even today, as countless surveys have shown, it is to traditional remedies that most people turn first when they are sick, to the care that family and friends variously have to offer and recommend. And it is only if their traditional approach proves ineffectual that recourse is made to another form of care, whether lay or professional, orthodox or complementary.

Indigenous medicine and folk wisdom

By definition, traditional medicine includes both indigenous medical systems such as the Indian Ayurvedic medicine and Chinese herbal medicine, and the trance healing, spells, and charms of priests and shamans, as well as the body of practices that constitute the storehouse of "domestic" medicine and that characterize the traditional approach in most

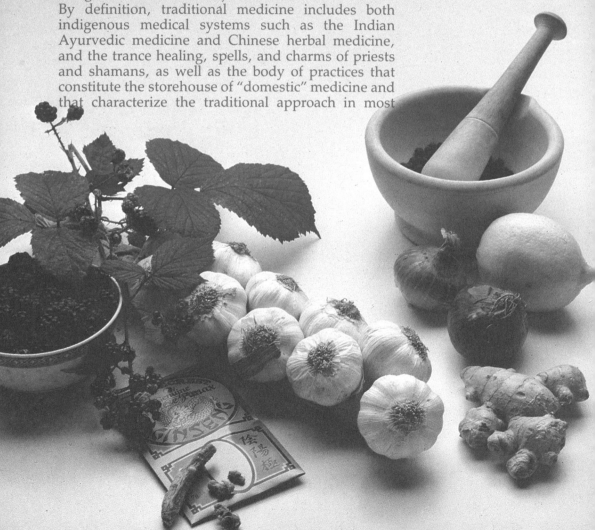

people's eyes. Unlike many other medical practices, traditional medicine makes use of common, inexpensive substances that can be found and used quickly at the first sign of illness. It also consists mainly of remedies that have stood the test of time, and that have been effectively used by an older relative or friend. Many traditional remedies are taken both to prevent ill health and to treat specific disorders – apples, garlic, and onions are familiar examples.

Origins and development

Most people assume that traditional medicine consists of old wives' tales, left over from the days of pre-scientific medicine. In fact, however, its scope is far broader and many practices were discovered or recommended by the physicians, alchemists, and other "experts" of ancient times. The use of peony, for example, which today is a popular folk remedy for epilepsy, has been traced back to Pliny, the Roman natural historian, who pointed out that the plant takes its name from Paion - a healer who appears in the Iliad. The use of amulets and stones in medicine has a similarly long history. Accounts exist of Queen Mary of Scotland sending her brother two stones to safeguard his health on the day of her death in 1587, and 11th-century manuscripts have been found which recommend amethyst for alcoholics, amber for fevers, and so on. There is even evidence that stones were used for health in prehistoric times. The modern herbal repertoire (see Herbalism, pp.160–75) provides several examples of remedies that have been in use for many centuries. The common names of these herbs often reflect their ancient use in folk medicine – pilewort, for example, was traditionally used for treating piles (hemorrhoids), eyebright for soothing irritated eyes, wormwood for dispelling infestations of worms.

Not only do traditional remedies withstand the test of time, however, they also migrate across traditions and cultures. Thus, for example, Latin American folk medicine today contains much that is found in the medicine of Galen, the 2nd-century Greek physician, whose influence lasted until the period of the European Renaissance. And folk medicine in the United States has learnt much from the wisdom of the North American Indian, in particular the value of excellent plant remedies, such as witch hazel.

Traditional medicine and modern pharmacology

Serious attention to the intrinsic value of traditional medicine for health care is sadly lacking among the orthodox medical professionals. There is, however, a certain amount of research taking place in the area of pharmacology. A number of age-old folk medicines and treatments are now achieving medical recognition as their action on the body begins to be understood. Probably the most colorful recent example of this is the use of leeches, which most of us associate with the Dark Ages of medicine. They are now, however, back in use in orthodox medicine as an adjunct to microsurgical techniques, for instance in plastic surgery. Among numerous other examples, willow bark and cooked cranberries, both traditional remedies for rheumatism, have been found to contain salicylates which have anti-inflammatory properties. Then there is garlic, whose anti-bacterial, anti-fungal and anti-thrombotic properties have recently been ascribed to the sulphur compounds that underlie its powerful smell. Finally, mention must be made of a class of folk remedies that has only recently been identified – the "adaptogens". These work not by killing off disease but by nourishing the body to help it to cope with stress. Royal jelly, the substance which honeybees excrete and feed to the queen larvae, has been classed as an adaptogen, and so has the ancient eastern remedy, ginseng.

The value of folk medicine

Given our current state of knowledge, it is not possible to assign a precise value to traditional curative practices. Perhaps more than anything their usefulness may be said to lie in their familiarity and simplicity and the fact that they are easily administered by the lay person. Certainly, no matter what their real therapeutic value may be, our health care systems would be quite unable to cope if they had to expand to take over the entire management of everyday ailments and minor illnesses for which traditional medicine is currently used.

As with any other type of medicine – both natural and orthodox – the same commonsense cautions should be observed. If, for example, an unexpected or adverse reaction occurs after administering a traditional remedy, it should be stopped immediately and a trained medical practitioner consulted.

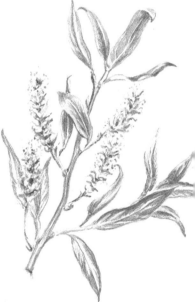

White willow bark has been used for centuries to ease fevers and pain. Its active ingredient, salicin, is very similar to the compound salicylic acid, which combined with acetic acid, forms the modern drug aspirin.

Traditional remedies

It's safest to use traditional remedies for mild disorders only. Some of the remedies involve making herbal infusions or decoctions (p.164), others require hot or cold compresses, which are described in the Hydrotherapy section, on p.212. If a symptom continues to get worse, or if a person becomes seriously ill (for danger signs see p.115), discontinue the treatment and seek professional advice. If the problem is persistent (though still mild) continue with the remedy for about a week – that will be long enough to find out whether it works for you. A selection of traditional remedies for first aid is included in First aid, pages 320-37.

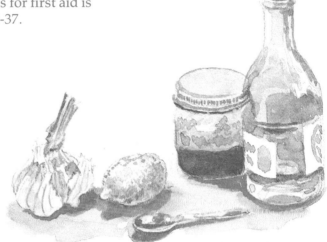

Garlic, lemon, honey, cider vinegar

Colds

Garlic Raw garlic, because of its antibiotic properties, is thought to help stem a cold in the early stages. Eat 3 or 4 raw cloves. Garlic oil capsules or tablets are a popular, odorless, alternative.

Mustard Mustard baths can be helpful. For instructions, see Coughs (p.220).

Citrus fruit This is amongst the best-established modern "folk" remedies for colds, though its usefulness is contested by orthodox medicine. Take up to 6 glasses of fresh citrus juice a day, or eat 2 or 3 large oranges.

Cold water A remedy used by Eskimos and Icelanders, this involves immersing the nose in cold water or snow. This causes the swollen membranes in the nose to shrink, expelling excess mucus.

Sore throats

Lemon juice A gargle made of the juice of a quarter lemon with ¼ pint (140 ml) of warm water is antiseptic and reduces inflammation. It may be alternated hourly with a gargle of a non-herbal tea. Continue gargling at regular intervals for about 2 days.

For a stronger medicine drink the juice of a lemon with a pulped clove of garlic in it. Tastier soothing drinks can be made from lemon juice, honey and hot water, or barley water (see Fever, p.226) with lemon juice.

Cider vinegar Make a soothing drink with hot water, honey, and a scant tablespoon of cider vinegar.

Malt vinegar Gargle with a mixture of vinegar and salt in warm water, or sodium bicarbonate in water.

Alternatively, inhale the steam from vinegar diluted with 4 times the volume of boiling water.

Coughs

Licorice For a soothing cough medicine simmer 1 teaspoon of licorice root in a large cup of water for about 10 minutes. Strain, and drink while still hot.

Lemon and olive oil Mix together an equal volume of lemon juice and olive oil. Sip small quantities as required.

Mustard Mustard powder is excellent for coughs, colds, flu and general debilitation. Prepare a hot bath. Mix a tablespoon of mustard powder into a paste, add this to the bath and stir. You can either immerse yourself or just soak your feet in the hot mustard tub. You can also dip towels in the water, wring them out, and wrap them round the chest as hot compresses.

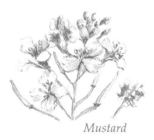

Mustard

Asthma

Cranberries Cranberries contain a bronchial anti-spasmodic which eases breathing during an asthma attack. Mash 1 or 2 teaspoons of the berries in a cup of warm water. Or cook the berries, mash them, and store in the refrigerator; then, whenever required, take a teaspoon mixed into a cup of warm water.

Catarrh

Juniper berries Make a tea by infusing ¼ oz (7 g) each of juniper berries, root ginger, angelica, and peppermint, in 1 pint (560 ml) of freshly boiled water.

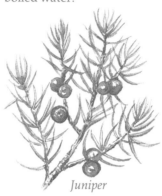

Juniper

Olbas oil Several essential oils relieve nasal congestion when their vapour is inhaled. Olbas oil is a mixture of eucalyptus, peppermint, cajuput, juniper, winter-green, clove and menthol. Put a few drops into a bowl of freshly boiled water, cover your head with a towel, and inhale the pungent steam for a few minutes.

Cranberries Follow the procedure described under Asthma.

Stomach ache

Cinnamon Cinnamon has been used in the East as a cure for stomach pains for hundreds of years. Mix about half a teaspoon of powdered cinnamon in a glass of milk or water. Take this at regular intervals until the pain goes.

Diarrhea

Cider vinegar Before each meal drink 2 teaspoons of cider vinegar diluted in a glass of water.

Arrowroot Prepare a gruel using 2 teaspoons of arrowroot mixed in 1 pint (560 ml) of milk or water. You can flavor this gruel with honey, fruit juice, or cinnamon, all of which add to its effectiveness.

Blackberries These are held to be a powerful antidote to diarrhea. Take a heaped teaspoon of blackberry jam. Or make an infusion from the berries and the leaves: steep 3 oz (84 g) of blackberry fruit and leaves in 1 pint (560 ml) of freshly boiled water for 10 minutes.

A good medicinal syrup can be made by boiling together 2 pints (1.1 litres) of blackberry juice, a tablespoon each of allspice, cinnamon and nutmeg, and a cup of honey. To this add a ½ pint (280 ml) of rum or brandy. Take a tablespoon before each meal. Sip it slowly.

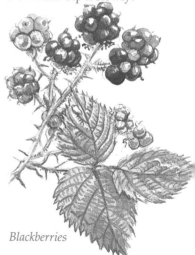

Blackberries

Constipation

Prunes Drink the juice from 5 or 6 stewed prunes each morning. The prunes themselves should be eaten late at night. Figs, pears, and rhubarb are also good natural laxatives.

Molasses This is an effective and harmless laxative. Take 1 teaspoon daily.

Bran Eat a tablespoon of bran with buttermilk or yoghurt each morning. In trials, a high-fiber diet including bran was found to solve many patients' digestive problems. But beware that bran can also produce wind and a bloated feeling in some people. *Caution* Avoid castor oil and senna as remedies for constipation. Recent research indicates potential dangers in their use.

Indigestion

Lemon juice or cider vinegar A tablespoon of either taken in a cup of hot water before meals is surprisingly effective for acid indigestion.

Herbal teas Various herbal teas are helpful, including parsley, mint, raspberry, chamomile, and blackberry. The standard method is to infuse 3 oz (84 g) of fresh leaves in 1 pint (560 ml) of freshly boiled water for 10 minutes. Mint tea can also be made by adding a handful of the leaves to a large pot of hot, weak, black tea.

Bran and oatmeal Soak a tablespoon each of bran and oatmeal in 1 pint (560 ml) of water. Strain and drink a cupful before meals.

Juniper berries Infuse 1 oz (28 g) of crushed juniper berries in 1 pint (560 ml) of freshly boiled water. Allow to stand for 15-20 minutes. Strain, and drink a cup before meals. This is a time-honored remedy.

Angelica See Flatulence, below.

Flatulence

Angelica An infusion of angelica root is a classic remedy for indigestion accompanied by flatulence. Pour 1 pint (560 ml) of boiling water on to 1 oz (28 g) of the cut root and leave to steep for about 10 minutes. Take 2 tablespoons before meals, 3 times a day. Alternatively, the leaves or root may be chewed raw.

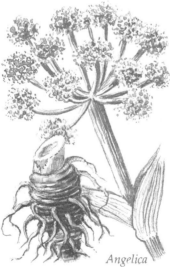

Angelica

Mustard seeds A few mustard seeds chewed with plenty of water on an empty stomach are helpful.

Hemorrhoids

Pilewort (Lesser celandine) Some herbal or health food stores stock suppositories containing this herb. As the name implies, this is an ancient cure.

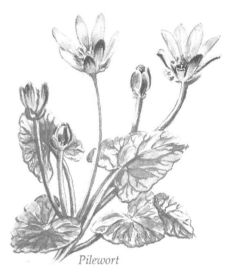

Pilewort

Canadian pine The fluid extract of Canadian pine is a powerful astringent, contracting tissues and reducing secretions. Apply a few drops 3 times a day, and take up to 10 drops in a little water at meal times.

Golden seal This is astringent and antiseptic. Half a teaspoon of the finely powdered herb is mixed with a few drops of tincture of myrrh for application.

Toothache

Cloves Even quite severe toothache can be alleviated by chewing a clove or rubbing a few drops of oil of cloves onto the gums.

Worms
Pumpkin seeds Fresh pumpkin seeds have long been used as a remedy for threadworms and tapeworms.

Wormwood An infusion of wormwood leaves is a traditional remedy for worm infestation. Pour a cup of freshly boiled water on to a teaspoon of the dried herb and leave to stand for 10 minutes. Strain, and drink a cup 3 times a day.

Wormwood

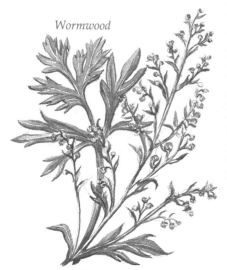

Gallstones
Olive oil and lemon Mix half a cup of olive oil with half a cup of lemon (or grapefruit) juice. Stir vigorously and drink the whole cupful at once. This helps gallstones to pass out of the body painlessly, but you should retire to bed immediately after the treatment as it is likely to induce nausea.

Cod liver oil and apple It is claimed that a mixture of cod liver oil and apple juice can dissolve gallstones.

Boils
Poultices One of the commonest boil remedies is the poultice, which is usually made by preparing a hot, moist mixture of some natural substance, wrapping it in gauze and binding it to the boil. The poultice draws out the pus and helps the wound to heal. All the following poultices should be changed every 3-4 hours.
　For a fig poultice, mash a fresh fig in a quarter of a cup of milk. Heat it, wrap it in gauze and allow it to drain. Apply while still hot. Or split the fig and apply it cold. Bread also makes an excellent poultice. Crumble a slice into a little freshly boiled milk or water, wrap it in gauze, drain and apply while hot. Grated raw potato bandaged in position is another effective remedy. Some naturopaths use raw cabbage for a cleansing poultice (see p.200).

Herpes
Potatoes Large quantities of potato in the daily diet can help to clear up facial herpes (cold sores). This remedy was traditionally used by Irish and Russian peasants.

Athlete's foot
Honey A piece of cotton wool impregnated with honey and bound to the sores overnight is soothing and helps the healing process.

Cider vinegar This may be used in the same way as honey, see above, but it will sting at first.

Skin irritations
Calamine lotion Applied with cotton wool and left to dry on the skin, this lotion is very soothing. It helps reduce the irritation from itchy spots (such as chickenpox), and heat rash, and it soothes sunburned skin.

Corns
Lemon Bind a fresh slice of lemon round the corn and leave it on overnight. Repeat this treatment nightly. The corn should soften and eventually disappear.

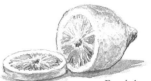

Fresh lemon

Turpentine Soak a small strip of cloth in turpentine, then wring it out. Bind it to the corn and leave it on overnight to soften it. Repeat until the corn disappears.
Caution Never use turpentine on broken skin.

Ingrowing toenails
Lemon Ingrowing toenails respond to the same treatment as corns, see above. The lemon softens the nails, which can then be eased out of the flesh and trimmed.

Chilblains, chapping
Myrrh Massage the problem areas with tincture of myrrh.

Friars' balsam Apply this to unbroken chilblains before going to bed.

Nappy rash
Cornstarch Both as a preventive and remedial measure, cornstarch can be invaluable. Dust it on danger spots or affected areas, but watch out for possible allergic reactions and discontinue at once if there are any signs.

Dandruff
Rosemary After washing the hair, massage the scalp with oil of rosemary, or rinse the hair using ½ pint (280 ml) of water in which a sprig of rosemary has been boiled.

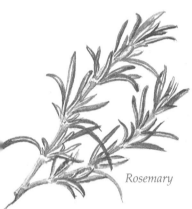

Rosemary

Witch hazel and eau de Cologne One of the problems associated with dandruff is poor scalp circulation. A mixture of witch hazel and eau de Cologne may be used as a tonic, rubbed vigorously into the scalp twice a day.

Hair loss
Bay rum and jaborandi A ready-made hair restoring lotion containing bay rum and jaborandi is available. Follow the manufacturer's instructions.

Castor oil Once or twice a week, massage the scalp with castor oil at night. Shampoo the following morning.

Eyestrain
Salt water Bathe eyes in sea water. If this is not possible, use a weak salt solution.

Honey Boil a teaspoon of honey in ½ pint (280 ml) of water. Leave this until it is cool. Use for an eyebath, or place pads soaked in the solution over the eyes.

Eyebright Make an infusion from 1 oz (28g) of the dried herb in 1 pint (560 ml) of freshly boiled water. Leave until cold. This can be taken internally (3 small cups each day), or used for an eyebath.

Earache
Salt Hold a hot salt bag to the ear. For instructions, see Rheumatism, p.224.

Oils Put a few drops of olive or castor oil in the inflamed ear.

Gout and sciatica
Potato Drink raw potato juice mixed with other raw vegetable juices.

Turpentine compress Drip turpentine on to a hot towel and wrap it around the site. **Caution** Never use turpentine on broken skin.

Olive oil Sciatica may respond to a massage with warm olive oil.

Aches and pains
Tiger Balm For the relief of minor muscular aches and pains, rub the affected area with this pungent ointment.

Arthritis
Flannel compresses A variation on the standard hot compress (see p.212) is to wrap painful joints in pieces of heated flannel which have been sprinkled with powdered sulphur.

Cod liver oil and orange Add 1 tablespoon of cod liver oil to 2 tablespoons of fresh orange juice. Mix well, and take it before breakfast or last thing at night.

Camphor and cayenne pepper Massage painful joints with a mixture of olive oil, camphor, and cayenne pepper. Use 1 part cayenne to 4 parts olive oil and 8 parts spirit of camphor.

Honey and cider vinegar Cider vinegar (a dessert-spoon in a glass of hot water), flavoured with a teaspoon of honey, taken twice a day, is a cleansing medicine.

Dandelion roots Boil 2 or 3 dandelion roots (preferably picked in spring) in 2 pints (1.1 litres) of water for 1 hour. Drink a glass of the tonic before each meal.

Copper For centuries arthritis sufferers have used copper bracelets, on the wrists or on the ankles, to ward off arthritic pains.

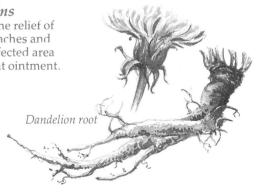

Dandelion root

Rheumatism

Salt Heat salt in the oven and place in a cloth bag. Hold the bag to the painful joint for at least 30 minutes.

Salt compresses Swollen joints can be treated using hot compresses. Add a cup of salt and a teaspoon of cayenne pepper to 1 pint (560 ml) of boiling water. Soak a cloth in this solution, wring it out, and apply to the problem area. Cover with a towel to keep the heat in and leave for about an hour.
   Alternatively, the affected parts may be bathed in the hot solution.

Asparagus Make a tea by boiling a handful of asparagus roots in 1 pint (560 ml) of water for an hour or more. Sweeten the drink with molasses.

Herbal teas Traditional soothing teas include ginger, mint, hops, rosemary, chamomile, or lavender. Use a teaspoon of the dried herb (or a teaspoon of grated fresh ginger root) to a cup of freshly boiled water. Allow to steep for about 5 minutes.

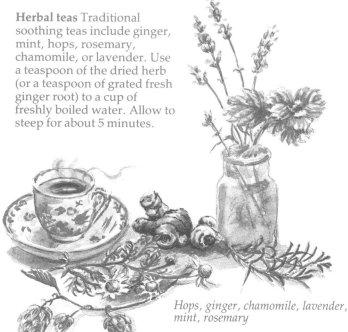

Hops, ginger, chamomile, lavender, mint, rosemary

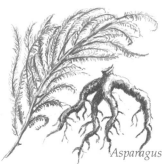

Asparagus

Headaches

Onion poultice Apply shredded, raw onion wrapped in gauze to the back of the neck. Remove after 20 minutes and place a warm towel on the same spot.

Aromatic massage Massage the temples with a few drops of peppermint oil or menthol, or rub the skin gently with lemon peel.

Malt vinegar and brown paper This folk remedy is celebrated by an old nursery rhyme. Soak a folded brown paper bag in malt vinegar and hold it against your forehead.

Malt vinegar Inhale the steam from boiling water mixed with an equal quantity of vinegar, putting a towel over your head to stop the steam escaping.

Insomnia

Honey This is highly recommended in Japan: take 2 tablespoons of honey followed by a glass of hot water.

Garlic An old-fashioned remedy for a child who often wakes in the night frightened by bad dreams, is to rub garlic on the soles of the feet.

Hops Pillows stuffed with hop flowers have been used as a remedy for sleepless-ness for many centuries.

Skullcap For a relaxing medicine, pour a cup of freshly boiled water on to a teaspoonful of the dried herb, and allow this to stand for 10 minutes. This may be combined with a standard infusion of valerian (p.172).

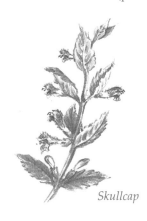

Skullcap

Varicose veins

Witch hazel Apply compresses made by soaking cloths or towels in distilled witch hazel, and take a glass of water mixed with 2 or 3 drops of the distilled extract, at mealtimes.

Calendula To relieve aching varicose veins, make a cold compress (p.212) with tincture of calendula and cold water.

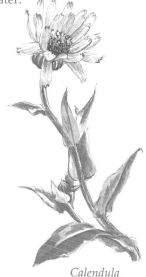

Calendula

Hay-flowers Boil hay-flowers in a pan of water. Soak towels in this water, wring out, and wrap a towel round each leg at night.

Cider vinegar Apply neat cider vinegar to the swollen veins, once in the morning, and once at night. Allow the vinegar to dry on the skin.

Menstrual problems, labor pains

Beetroot Syrup of beetroot is an old-fashioned medicine for a delayed menstruation. Boil fresh beets until soft. Remove the beets from the pot and continue to boil the liquid until it turns syrupy. Drink a cup of this syrup 4 times a day.

Mustard Soaking for a few minutes in a hot mustard bath may help to bring on menstruation (and to combat colds and flu). Make a paste with about 1 tablespoon of mustard powder and a little water, then dissolve this in the bath water.

Raspberry leaf tea Menstrual cramps and labor pains are eased by drinking raspberry leaf tea. Put about 1 oz (28 g) of leaves in a small pan with 1 pint (560 ml) of water, bring to the boil, take off the heat, and allow to stand for 10 minutes. For cramps treatment should be started several days before the onset of menstruation. As a preventive treatment for labor pains, the tea should be taken regularly in the late stages of pregnancy.

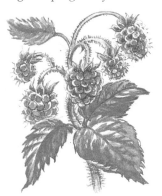

Raspberry leaves

Loss of sex drive

Ginseng The ginseng root is believed to be one of nature's greatest cures for loss of sex drive, and general debility. The root is available in various forms – dried, in a tincture, in tablets, or in tea mixtures. Follow the manufacturer's recommendations for dosage.

Cold water A daily bath in cold water is an old remedy, for impotence.

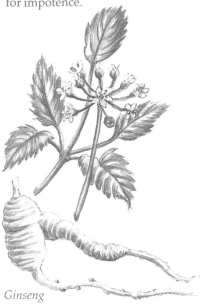

Ginseng

Tiredness

Ginseng The restorative capacities of ginseng are justly famous. It counteracts fatigue and depression, improves bodily functions in general and brings renewed vitality. The herb is available in many forms. Follow the manufacturer's instructions for dosage.

Fever

Chicken soup "Soup from a fat hen" was considered therapeutic as long ago as the 12th century. The Chinese add a little ginseng to it.

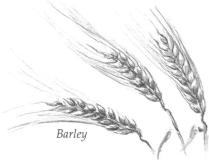

Barley

Lemon barley water Home-made barley water is good in feverish cases. Put 2 oz (56 g) of well-washed barley in 4 pints (2.2 litres) of water, boil to reduce by half, strain, and add honey and lemon juice.

Hay fever

Honeycomb Use small lumps of honeycomb as a medicinal chewing gum throughout the spring and winter. Local honeycomb is said to help the body to develop immunity to specific, local irritants.

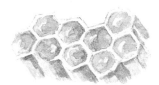

Honeycomb

Brewers' yeast Take brewers' yeast tablets for several weeks before the onset of the hay fever season. Follow the manufacturer's recommended dosage.

Onion Drink a glass of water in which a sliced raw onion has been soaked for several hours. Or place a bowl of sliced onions beside the bed at night to ease breathing while asleep.

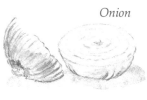

Onion

Comfrey Some hay fever sufferers have found lasting relief from comfrey. The fresh leaves can be eaten (1 a day) or made into a tea (2 teaspoonsful of chopped leaves steeped in a cup of freshly boiled water). **Caution** Avoid the young leaves of comfrey. Daily consumption could, over time, be dangerous.

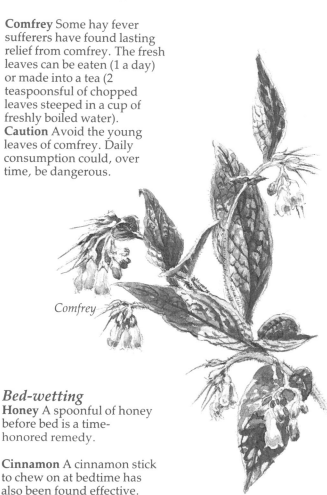

Comfrey

Bed-wetting

Honey A spoonful of honey before bed is a time-honored remedy.

Cinnamon A cinnamon stick to chew on at bedtime has also been found effective.

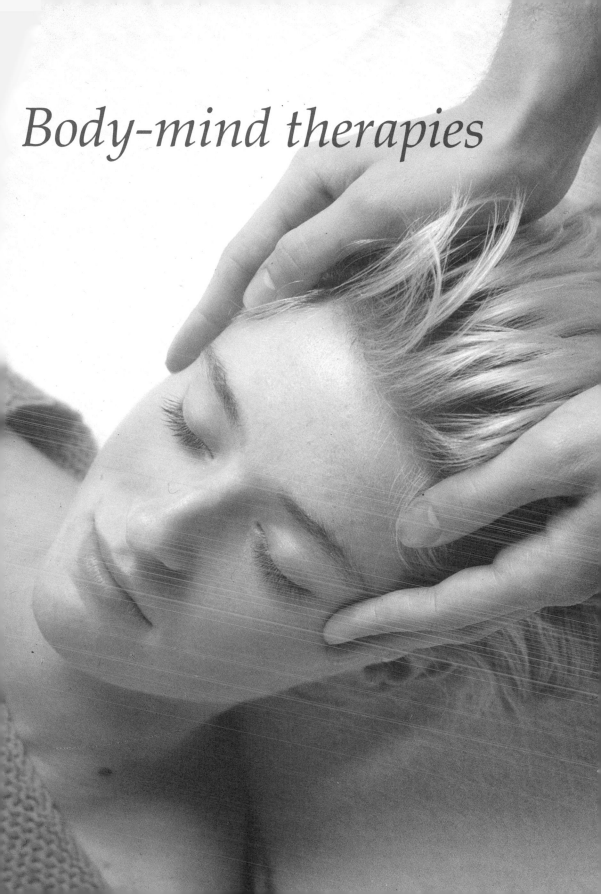

Body-mind therapies

Osteopathy

Osteopathy is a system of manual medicine, which is concerned with the structural and mechanical problems of the body. It deals not only with the spine but with the body's whole framework – its bones, joints, muscles, ligaments, and other supportive soft tissues. Its aim is to restore proper movement and functioning to this system by means of gentle manual pressure and articulation.

One of the main factors that predisposes the human body to structural problems, osteopaths believe, is our biped stance itself. While we stand upright, gravity exerts a continual strain on our structure, particularly on the joints of the spine and the cushioning intervertebral discs between them. The joints and discs are all weight-bearing, and have to support the whole body. Our abdominal and pelvic organs also have to struggle against a continual downward pull. Add to this the gradually accumulating effects of poor posture, and our stressful lifestyles, and mechanical faults can quickly develop.

Osteopathy was founded by Dr Andrew Still in Kirksville, Missouri, USA. Dr Still's instinct was to look for treatments that would stimulate the body's

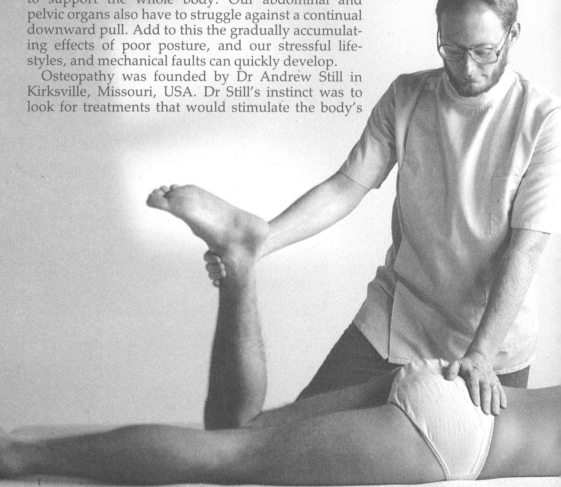

own healing mechanisms, rather than trying to destroy or suppress a particular disease process. He also realized that the body had a much better chance of functioning well if it was structurally and mechanically sound. His breakthrough came during an epidemic of dysentery in the summer of 1874 when he successfully treated a child suffering from the disease by easing tension in the contracted back muscles and restoring movement to the joints of the spine. Dr Still went on to treat 17 further cases, all of whom recovered.

The essence of modern osteopathy

Modern osteopathic philosophy and practice are founded on the concept that a person's normal state of being is health. Diagnosis and treatment are based on three fundamental principles. First, that the body's natural tendency is to heal itself. Its ability to maintain proper functioning in a continually changing environment is dependent, however, on its complex communications networks – the circulatory, hormonal, and nervous systems. Second, that there is an intimate interrelationship between structure and function, between the gross movement of a joint and the workings of the smallest cell. And third, that the body has a better chance of functioning properly on all levels if it is structurally and mechanically sound. Thus osteopathic treatment of musculoskeletal abnormalities is often followed by clinical improvement in a patient's overall condition.

This is because of the relationship between the spine and the nervous control of the organs and other structures of the body. When a mechanical fault exists in the spine, spasm of the surrounding muscles sends irritating nervous impulses to the local area of the spinal cord. The nerves from this part of the cord become over-sensitive, and then bombard other related structures with abnormal nervous stimulation. This often has the effect of reducing proper blood flow to the organ, thus reducing its efficiency and weakening its defences. In addition, therefore, to the various structural problems such as joint pains, arthritis, neuritis, and sports injuries, osteopathy is also successfully used to treat a wide range of functional conditions – that is conditions where there is no major change or breakdown in the tissues concerned. These include asthma and several other respiratory problems, headaches, irritable bowel syndrome and other digestive disorders, period pain, palpitation, and circulatory problems.

Today osteopathy is an established part of American primary health care; there are 15 osteopathic medical schools, 210 osteopathic hospitals, and over 20,000 osteopathic physicians practicing in the USA. In Europe, however, it is less well-established, except in the UK where there are two full-time undergraduate osteopathic schools, as well as several specialist osteopathic clinics for sports people, children, and for pregnant women.

Research findings

The majority of modern research into osteopathy is being carried out in the USA, where the effect of osteopathy on a wide range of conditions, including myocardial (heart muscle) infection, coronary artery diseases, neck pain, lower back pain after childbirth, pneumonia, and migraine, is under investigation. It has even been demonstrated at an osteopathic hospital in Michigan that osteopathic treatment applied to women while in childbirth significantly lowers pain levels in the majority of cases.

In a research trial in Britain, published in the *British Medical Journal* in 1975, 450 backache sufferers were divided into four groups and each group was then treated exclusively either by the standard combination of painkilling drugs and rest, by wearing back-immobilizing corsets, by orthodox physiotherapy, or, finally, by osteopathy. The results showed that the group treated by the osteopath had, in fact, shown slightly more improvement than the other groups. Furthermore, out of a total of 70 from all groups who failed to finish the experiment, more than 25 subjects who were treated osteopathically stated that their condition had improved to the point where they felt that they no longer needed any additional therapy.

Consulting an osteopath

When you first visit an osteopath complaining of, for example, pain in your lower back, a full and detailed case history will be taken. The osteopath then conducts a careful structural examination, observing you standing, moving, and sitting down. Orthodox orthopedic and neurological tests, such as testing reflexes with a percussion hammer, are also performed. In some cases, an X-ray may be taken, particularly if you have recently had an accident or a major health crisis, but this is not routine procedure.

A detailed assessment of the range of movement and the mechanical stresses in the tissues surrounding particular joints is normally carried out with the patient lying down. At the end of this examination the osteopath will decide whether or not your condition is likely to respond to osteopathic treatment – and if not, whether medical or surgical treatment would be advisable.

In osteopathy, treatment is geared to the needs of each individual patient and guided by the moment-to-moment changes within his or her tissues. Osteopaths use their trained, highly developed sense of touch to detect minute stresses within the body's structure and to release them gently. The popular conception of osteopaths is that they make joints "click", but in reality the clicking or mobilizing of a joint is only a small part of their technique.

A typical osteopathic treatment for lower back pain, for example, would consist of small rhythmical movements to the lower spine in order to stretch contracted tissues. Gentle pressure would then be applied to painful muscles to aid their relaxation. If a particular joint had lost some of its freedom of mobility it might be necessary to "gap" the joint surfaces gently. This is performed by taking the joint quickly and painlessly through its normal movement which often produces the famous "click". For other problems such as head or facial pain, the osteopath may simply apply very gentle pressure to the head and upper neck. He or she will be feeling for very subtle stress patterns within the tissues, then holding them painlessly at a point of tension until they release. This sort of approach can be applied to any mechanical problem, and is especially suitable for infants, children, and the elderly.

A treatment session usually lasts about 20 to 30 minutes (perhaps longer the first time), and most people find it an enjoyable and relaxing experience – some even fall asleep! The length of a course of treatment varies enormously. It depends on the type of condition and how long you have had it, on age (younger people respond more quickly), on attitude to health, and general environmental conditions.

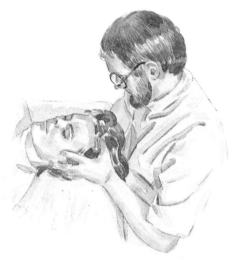

Cranial osteopathy
This technique is sometimes used as an alternative to standard osteopathic treatment. A trained practitioner feels for the body's subtle cranio-sacral rhythm, caused by the ebb and flow of cerebrospinal fluid around the brain and spinal cord.

Abnormal stresses within this mechanism can impair the rhythm and give rise to disorders such as head pain, earache and sinus problems. The treatment consists of very gentle pressure on the patient's head, as shown above, to remove the stress patterns and to restore mobility.

Osteopathy: preventive care

Since osteopathy is largely a manipulative therapy, treatment is usually given by a professional. But special exercises and other self-help measures are normally prescribed as an adjunct to professional treatment and are often essential to its success. For home treatment, you should practice the exercises described below regularly, and be sure to observe the general preventive measures too.

In many cases, the conditions described are related to incorrect posture, and poor muscle tone. Yoga (pp.284-93) and the Alexander technique (pp.294-7) are excellent preventive therapies.

Combating morning stiffness

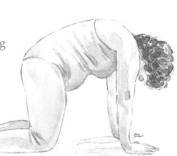

Backache

About 50% of the problems presented to osteopaths are concerned with back pain, and their record for effective treatment is exceptional. There are, however, several self-help measures you can use at home to relieve backache and, more importantly, a number of basic things you can do to prevent back problems occurring (see also p.234). If your problem is chronic or incapacitating, you should consult a registered osteopath.

General exercises for backs
1 Practice stretching exercises such as yoga. This will tone and strengthen your body, sparing you a lot of back pain. The morning stiffness routine, shown right, and the lower back exercise, shown on p.233, will also increase your general mobility.

2 Go swimming as often as possible (backstroke is particularly good for back muscles). Or start a program of fast, rhythmic walking (p.53) – this has many of the advantages of jogging, but without the dangers of leg, foot, and back injury. Don't play squash if your back is at all vulnerable – it can cause serious damage to muscles and joints (badminton is better).

Yoga exercises
The salute to the sun shown on pp.54-5, and the simple sequence of asanas shown on pp.288-9, include several excellent back exercises which give the spine a gentle forward, backward and lateral stretching. They are practiced in a set order so as to counterbalance one another. In the pelvic lift, shown below (described on p.293), the spine receives a gentle workout, encouraging strength and suppleness without imposing any excessive strain.

Pelvic lift

Morning stiffness routine
This is a useful exercise for an aching back, particularly if it is stiff in the morning. Lie on your back, clasping your hands around your knees. Then, keeping your legs and hips relaxed, very slowly pull your knees into your chest. Hold them there for about 10 seconds and very slowly let them down again. This whole exercise takes about a minute.

Lower back exercise

This is a useful exercise for a back that is worse when standing still or sitting.

Sit on the edge of an upright chair with your feet on the floor. Spread your legs so that your head and arms can pass between them. Starting at the top of your neck, begin to bend your spine forward, slowly. Let your shoulders drop between your knees with your arms hanging down loosely: Stay in this position for about 5 seconds, and then slowly return to an upright position. If, as you are bending forward, you feel pain, do not carry on. You should, however, feel a gentle stretch on your lower back. Ideally you should do this exercise once or twice every half hour.

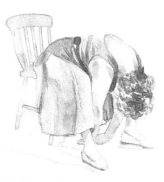

Lower back exercise

Posture exercise

Maintaining a good posture is the best way to prevent or relieve backache. It means standing and moving in a way that doesn't put excessive strain on muscles and joints. You can improve your posture by practicing this exercise frequently.

Stand tall against a flat wall and imagine that you are being suspended by a string attached to the top of your head. Place a hand between the hollow of your lower back and the wall. Now, keeping head, shoulders, buttocks, and heels in contact with the wall, tighten your abdominal and buttock muscles so that the front of your pelvis tilts upward and slightly forward. This should cause the hollow of your back to flatten and press your hand against the wall. With practice you will be able to assume the posture without the help of the wall.

Hydrotherapy treatment

If back pain has been caused by simple back strain, this easy home hydrotherapy technique can be very helpful. It is safe to use this treatment as often as it is required.

Fill a hotwater bottle with cold water and put it in the freezer until it is just on the point of turning to ice. Fill another hotwater bottle with hot, but not boiling, water. Place the cold bottle, well wrapped in a thin towel, across the painful area and hold it there for about 1 minute. After a minute replace the cold bottle with the hot one (wrapped in a thin towel). Leave the hot bottle in position for about 2 minutes before replacing it with the cold again. Repeat this procedure for about 15-20 minutes, ending with the cold bottle. You can do this by yourself, in a sitting position; otherwise, lie flat on your stomach and have someone else apply the hotwater bottles.

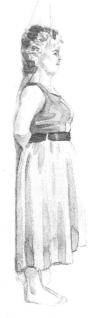

Posture exercise

Preventing backache

Try to avoid backache by observing the following basic preventive measures, by practicing a specific posture exercise (p.233), or by taking up a sport that helps improve posture (p.50).

1 If you lift anything, do it with a straight back, bending from the knees, and keeping the load close to your body. Try to use your legs to take the strain. Never twist while lifting.

2 When carrying suitcases or heavy shopping, try to divide the load equally between both arms. If you carry a shoulderbag, swap shoulder from time to time.

3 When driving, make sure your back is supported properly. If necessary, use a small cushion or blanket behind the lower back.

4 Avoid any activity or exercise that involves twisting while bending forward.

5 Avoid spending too long in any one position. Move about as much as possible.

6 Try to position worktops at a height that does not involve hunching your shoulders or stooping. If your work is sedentary, you should adjust your chair according to your work surface, or choose a comfortable chair that is specially designed to prevent backache (p.71). Don't make do with inadequate office chairs – people with sedentary jobs are particularly at risk from back problems.

7 At home, use high-backed chairs which support the length of your spine. Try not to slump. Place a cushion in the small of your back to allow you to relax without slouching.

8 Don't stand with your weight on one leg and, when you are sitting, avoid crossing your legs. Either of these positions can distort the spine and pelvis.

9 Some people find that sagging mattresses provoke backache. Sleep on a firm bed (p.71).

10 High heels contribute to backache since the heels force you to lean backward. The best rule is not to wear them except, if you must, on special occasions.

Pelvic congestion

Many digestive ailments and lower back problems are the result of muscle weakness in the abdominal region. Much of the abdominal contents is supported from above by the diaphragm, and it is essential that this large muscle functions correctly. If the diaphragm sags and abdominal tone is poor, the abdominal and pelvic contents are compressed downward, which produces pelvic congestion, with a tendency for sluggish bowel movement and associated constipation. There is also a long-term risk of hemorrhoids, and varicose veins.

Diaphragm exercise

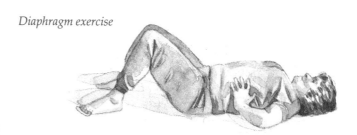

Diaphragm exercise

The simple exercise shown above will tone both the abdominal muscles and the diaphragm and it will gently massage the abdominal organs.

Lie on your back with your knees bent and place the palms of your hands on the sides of your chest over the lower ribs. Then slowly inhale and attempt to fill the bottom of your lungs. Your hands should be pushed outward. Once you have fully inhaled, purse your lips as if to whistle and steadily but forcefully exhale. Breathe normally for a few moments and then repeat the exercise. Continue for 3-5 minutes, stopping if you feel dizzy.

Abdominal tone exercise

This exercises all of the abdominal muscles with minimal strain, whereas if you perform a full sit-up, you risk straining your neck and lower back.

Lie on your back with your knees bent, and clasp your hands behind your neck, as shown below left. Then, without putting strain on the neck, gently begin to sit up, as shown below right. You need rise up only about 2-3 inches (5-7.5 cm), just so that your shoulder blades are off the floor. Hold this position for 5 seconds, then slowly lie back down. Repeat, taking a breath between each movement. You can do this exercise as often as you like, but when your muscles ache, it is time to stop.

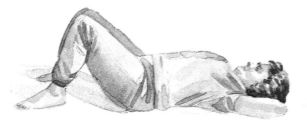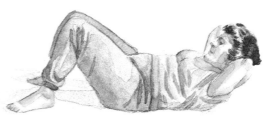

Abdominal tone exercise

Abdominal rocking

Another strengthening exercise involves kneeling down on all fours, but with the top half of your body supported on your elbows, as shown right. In this position, rock yourself rhythmically and gently backward and forward for 5-10 minutes. This counters general sagging of the abdominal and pelvic organs. (Don't do abdominal rocking too soon after eating.)

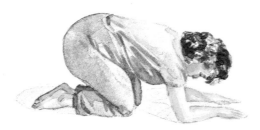

Abdominal rocking

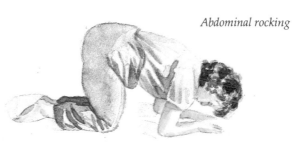

Preventing congestion

Apart from regularly practicing the exercises described on pp.232-3, there are some general measures you can take to help prevent pelvic congestion and its attendant ailments.

1 Make sure that you eat a diet that is high in fiber (see the basic health diet, p.47), and avoid refined and processed foods.

2 Drink plenty of plain water every day.

3 Don't sit for too long, and don't strain on the lavatory.

Chiropractic

Chiropractic is aimed at treating mechanical disorders of the joints, especially the spinal joints. The word comes from the Greek, meaning "treatment by manipulation". If your back fails you in Melbourne, or your neck locks in Geneva, or you need to know quickly why you have developed unusual leg pains, it is a chiropractor who is likely to be recommended. Although the conditions most often treated are rarely life-threatening, they make up some of the commonest causes of pain and disability in the modern world. Many of the problems are closely related to today's style of living, resulting above all from sitting for long periods, at desks or in cars, on unsuitable seating, as well as from bad bending and lifting habits.

The treatment given by a skilled practitioner is gentle and painless, and is much safer than taking drugs to suppress pain, or carrying on as normal, ignoring your complaints. Today, there are an estimated 36,000 chiropractors at work worldwide, giving many millions of consultations each year. All qualified chiropractors undergo intensive training, and often work within state health care systems.

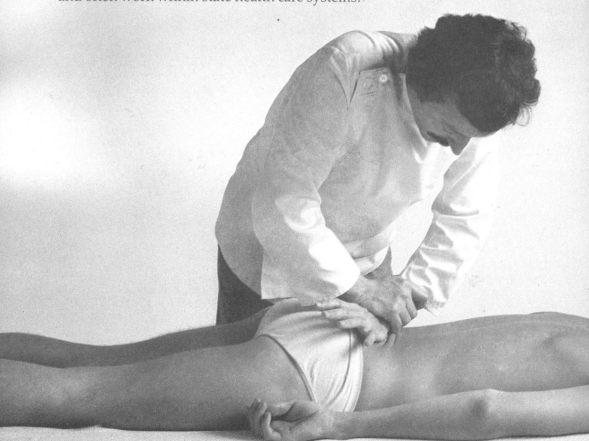

It is clear from the origins of the therapy (see below) that it is closely allied to osteopathy (pp.228-35). Both practices are manipulative and concerned with joint disorders, and both involve an element of preventive care. In treatment methods also, the differences between the two are quite subtle – a chiropractor tends to use less leverage but will manipulate directly over a joint, in a precise direction, whereas an osteopath normally uses more leverage but makes the adjustment further away from the joint which is being worked. But therapists of either profession often borrow the other's techniques.

The origins of chiropractic

In bygone years, serious musculoskeletal problems crippled many people permanently; there was little choice of treatment, and "orthodox" medicine was ill-equipped to help. Some sufferers, however, were treated with startling effectiveness by backwoods "bonesetters" and medicine men – lay healers who used intuitive skills to help mend sprains, strains, breaks, and related disorders. They lacked understanding of the body's complex functioning, and undoubtedly they also harmed people through their ignorance. But these lay manipulators established a strong tradition of non-medical treatment in the field, which certainly encouraged the birth of new therapeutic disciplines for musculoskeletal disorders, foremost among them osteopathy and chiropractic.

Chiropractic entered the scene in 1895, independent of mainstream medicine. It was developed by a talented US healer, David Daniel Palmer (1845-1913). Palmer's breakthrough came when he discovered the power of spinal manipulation. By adjusting vertebrae in the neck area he treated one patient for chronic deafness, and another for heart disease. Convinced that the basis of disease was in the spine, he developed the theory that "subluxed" or displaced vertebrae restricted the spinal nerves, interfering with the flow of nervous energy through the body. Though some of Palmer's views corresponded with contemporary medical research into the spine and nerves, and their relationship to proper organ functioning, his theories were rejected by orthodox medicine. Today, the profession no longer holds Palmer's original ideas as gospel, though chiropractors are still primarily spinal experts.

Research

As a large but independent branch of medicine, chiropractic has often been challenged, indeed hounded, to prove its worth. Chiropractors have long maintained various theories of skeletal function and malfunction that, until very recently, were hotly dismissed by doctors. For instance, they contend that bad movement and weight-bearing speed up degeneration of the body's framework; and that spinal discs can be treated by manipulation. These beliefs have since been supported by detailed medical research.

Other clinical trials and research studies have confirmed the therapy's effectiveness. The simplest evaluations were based on American workmen's compensation studies, which compared records of employees whose problems were taken to chiropractors, with those of people who had been medically treated. These studies showed that chiropractic treatment produced results twice as fast as orthodox medical procedures, and in general left patients feeling more satisfied that their problems had been explained. In another study chiropractic treatment was found to increase tolerance to pain – although the mechanisms are complex. Further research in different countries has revealed the same pattern of success. In 1978 the New Zealand government made a comprehensive investigation into the therapy. Its commission concluded that, for common mechanical joint disorders, chiropractic was likely to be the most effective treatment. Various clinical trials are continuing, to evaluate chiropractic's success in the management of common musculoskeletal problems.

Suitable cases for treatment

Most chiropractic patients are active adults in their middle years, but children and the elderly are also treated. Approximately half the adults have back pain and most of the rest have some other type of spinal problem. People suffering from general joint problems, lumbago, neuralgia, strains, slipped discs, and generalized back pain often respond well to chiropractic. Other complaints that have occasionally proved suitable for treatment include arthritis and rheumatism, migraine, headaches, asthma, and some types of chest pain. A professional diagnosis is always essential for sudden or unidentified pain, especially since some problems may require urgent hospital treatment. The cause of pain may be organic – heart disease, for example. Any injury to the neck, especially if followed by vomiting, speech difficulties, or problems with swallowing, and any neck pain which spreads to the legs when the person moves the neck or coughs, requires urgent professional attention. Anyone who has lower back pain and is unable to empty his or her bladder must be treated as an emergency. Severe head and neck pain which makes looking downward intolerable is another danger sign. Some other symptoms are less urgent but still need careful diagnosis, for example when there is constant pain, particularly in the night. Finally, cramp and restless legs in bed are common in older people, but leg cramp on walking may be a problem of narrowed or blocked arteries.

Consulting a chiropractor

It has been said that for an unorthodox medicine, chiropractic methods seem surprisingly clinical. In fact, in several countries, it is widely accepted and practiced by doctors. On your initial visit to a chiropractor, he or she will take a thorough case history and give you a full physical examination. Your blood pressure may be tested and blood or urine specimens sent for analysis. The practitioner will frequently feel the spinal column to reveal where movement is restricted or excessive, as well as possibly testing mobility in other joints. X-rays are taken, if necessary. They will usually be done with you standing up, so that the condition of your spine can be assessed when it is bearing weight.

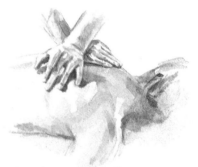

Gentle manipulation
Manipulation of the spine by a fully qualified chiropractor can alleviate discomfort due to such conditions as osteoarthritis, curvature of the spine, poor posture, or a previous injury. A specially designed couch moves through 180° to allow for a variety of treatment positions.

The aim of the treatment that follows is to restore mechanical integrity to the locomotor system. The main work is to adjust the strains on specific joints, using manual pressure. A special treatment couch may be used to place you in the best position for each manipulation. Sometimes the joints make noises during treatment, as if they are "slotting" back into place. But in fact, the noise is usually caused by bubbles of nitrogen inside the joint cavities forming and dispersing in response to the movement. Soft-tissue techniques may also be given, in the form of pressure on the ligaments or massage of muscles, to alleviate muscular pain and prepare a joint for manipulation. Treatment is backed up by advice on special exercises, and other preventive measures.

Chiropractic: preventive care

Chiropractic techniques of manipulation are not suitable for home use by novices, since manipulation is a precise art, and requires a long period of supervised instruction. There are, however, certain steps you can take to ensure that musculoskeletal and related problems are less likely to occur, and to relieve minor pains and discomfort. An enormous number of musculoskeletal problems are the product of everyday activities such as carrying heavy shopping, gardening, lifting children, sitting at a desk for long periods, and driving long distances. Keeping active and changing your position frequently are important to a healthy spine.

Caution If you are ever in acute pain, or if less severe symptoms don't abate in a few days, consult a specialist without delay. And be alert to warning signs of serious injury (see Suitable cases for treatment, p.238).

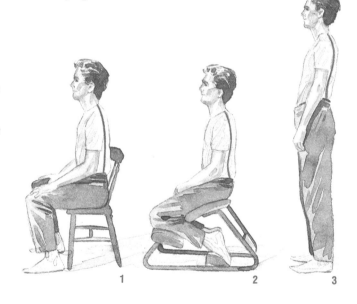

Sitting comfortably
Sitting is commonly accepted as a resting state, but as far as the base of the spine is concerned, it is very much like bending. The lower spine loses its natural hollow, and ligaments across the back tighten. Research has shown that pressure inside the disc is higher when sitting than when standing, and other studies have revealed a relationship between ruptured discs and long-distance driving. People who get backache during or after sitting may eventually rupture a lower spinal disc, unless they take care to adjust their posture.

The best method of prevention is to pay full attention to healthy seating at home, at work (p.71), and when driving. A car seat should offer good lumbar support, and it should be reclined to produce a wide thigh-to-trunk angle. And a carefully positioned head support is vital, to prevent possible whiplash effects.

Disc pressures In the position shown above (1), the lower spine is straightened. A few discs take all the weight, as shown right (A), and their centers tend to be forced backward. Chairs that are designed to protect backs (2) encourage the normal spinal curve of a good standing position (3). In this position the discs share the weight with the bony joints behind them (B).

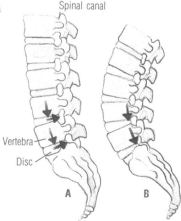

Spinal canal

Vertebra

Disc

A   B

Soothing inflammation

Beware of hot baths – they may temporarily soothe aching muscles, but many skeletal problems involve at least some inflammation, and this may worsen with heat. This is because the chemicals involved with inflammation accumulate when the heart slows down during rest. Heat can heighten this effect, if applied before rest. A small ice pack (p.212), however, will often prove effective in reducing local inflammation.

Remedial exercise

The golden rules of exercise for a healthy spine are: keep active; get adequate rest; know your limits, and if a movement hurts, stop it.

If you already have a back problem, exercises should be prescribed only by somebody who understands your individual problem fully. Like heat, injudicious exercise can relieve symptoms temporarily, but it may make them worse the next day.

It is also important to avoid over-stretching. Research has shown that ligaments (especially those of the lower spine) lose some of their elasticity after the teenage years. Excessive toe-touching work, sit-ups, and other back-stretching activities, can make them vulnerable to damage in later years.

Easy lifting techniques

If you suffer occasional back pain, take extra care when you are lifting heavy objects. Think of your spine, and try to use your arm and leg muscles to reduce strain on it. The rule is, if it hurts, find another way.

For example, if you are lifting a heavy case, start by kneeling (as shown below, left), with one foot flat on the floor and the shin vertical. Use your free hand to push up against your bent knee. Alternatively, try using the pressure of your free arm against the surface of a table or a firm chair to lever yourself upward (as shown below right).

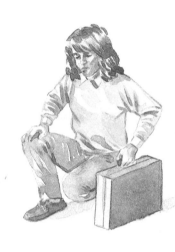
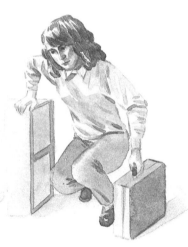

Resting a backache

If you are suffering from back-related problems, such as pain or discomfort in the lower back when you cough or sneeze, or numbness or pins and needles in a leg when you raise it from a resting position, you may be in danger of seriously damaging a disc. Don't carry on as normal. It is important that you rest your back as much as possible, by lying down on a firm surface. Use cushions to support your head, the small of your back, and your knees, as shown below. Make sure that your bed is giving you firm support too (p.71). If this does not relieve pain, get specialist help.

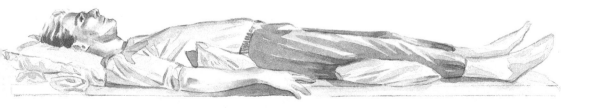

Massage

First and foremost, massage is a way of using touch to create a rapport between practitioner and receiver and to encourage and restore balance on a physical, mental and spiritual level. Through stroking, pressure and kneading, massage relaxes, stimulates or tones the body, affecting not only the skin but also the musculoskeletal system, the circulation, and the meridians or energy channels (p.271).

Along with its technical qualities, massage is an opportunity simply to experience touch. The sense of touching and being touched, so greatly ignored in modern society, is an essential part of well-being. By using caring and sensitive hands, the practitioner can bring about in us a sense of wholeness from which our own healing energies can be released.

Massage, past and present

The origins of massage are as old as humankind, for touch is the most instinctive response to soreness, pain, and debility. As a studied therapy, however, it is said to have been born in China over 5,000 years ago, coming from the same tradition as acupuncture (pp.268-73) and taoism. But while the East continued

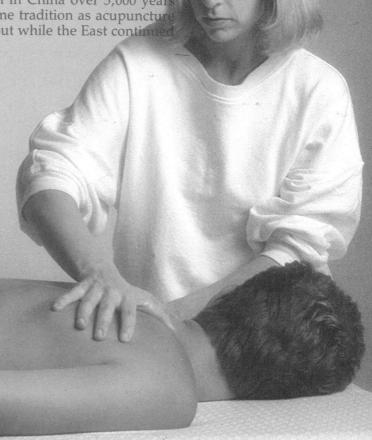

its use of massage, the West lost touch with it during the Middle Ages. It was not until the 16th century that a French doctor, Ambroise Paré, renewed interest in the subject with his more anatomical and physiological approach. Then, early in the 19th century a Swede, Per Henrik Ling, developed a method of massage and gymnastics known as Swedish Movement Treatment or, more simply, Swedish massage. From that time, many schools of massage have sprung up, and to the present day different methods continue to develop.

The effects of massage

As babies, touch is essential to our growth, both physically and mentally. In a recent experimental study on premature babies, Dr Ruth Diane Rice, a US psychologist, nurse, and specialist in early childhood development, demonstrated that massage from the mothers increased nerve and brain cell development, accelerated weight gain, and generally increased hormonal functioning and cell activity.

One of the prime benefits of massage is to the muscular system. Muscles may be loosened and relaxed, if they are tight or knotty, or toned, if they are found to be too loose or lacking in tone, according to whether the strokes used are relaxing or stimulating. In restoring a balanced tone to the muscles, massage also aids the circulation of blood and lymph.

Fundamental to an understanding of the effects of massage is the relationship between the surface and the interior of the body. In the East, the body's organs and systems are affected by treating points on the meridians with acupuncture or shiatsu (pp.274-83). This interaction between the inner and outer body has been researched in the West too, chiefly by the English neurologist Sir Henry Head and by Elizabeth Dicke, the German founder of Bindegewebsmassage, who found that stimulating specific areas of the body by touch could in time produce definite changes in certain organs and body systems. Further research has revealed a possible cause of this "reflex effect". Massaging the skin appears to stimulate receptor nerves that transmit a response via the spinal cord to the brain from where it returns to produce effects in zones of the body supplied by nerves from the same part of the spinal cord. These effects include the stimulation and relaxation of voluntary muscles, the opening and closing of blood capillaries and, possibly, the sedation of nerve sensors, resulting in pain relief.

Massage not only affects a person physically, however; it can also produce profound emotional and mental changes. It will relieve stress and anxiety and is therefore of great benefit to people suffering from any stress-related disorders. The masseur allows people to become aware of tensions they are holding through his or her touch and, in releasing the physical tensions, can dispel the worry, anxiety, sadness or irritability that go with them.

A professional massage session

When you go for professional treatment, it is advisable to avoid eating for two to three hours beforehand, and to avoid alcohol on the same day. The practitioner you choose may have been trained in any one of the various schools of massage, but there are certain procedures you can always expect to be followed. In the treatment room you should find a massage table or couch, clean linen, and a place where you can undress in privacy. Massage is most efficiently performed in direct contact with the skin. Some practitioners use a drape or towel, so that only the part of your body being worked on is exposed, while others may work without a drape, so as not to break the continuity of the massage. A suitable lubricant will generally be used – such as an oil (vegetable or mineral), talc, or cream.

The exact procedure will depend on your problem. Treatment may be extremely localized, with the masseur working solely on the back, for example, if you have a severe back complaint, or you may be given a complete body massage, including the feet and face. Length of treatment varies, but a session is normally 45 minutes to an hour long. If your problem is longstanding, you may need a series of treatments.

Working on chronically stiff muscles is not always comfortable. A sensitive practitioner, however, will only work to a level that is tolerable to you. When deep massage is carried out you may feel stiff in the affected areas the next day, but this should pass by the following day. Lying in a warm to hot bath for about half an hour followed by a 30-second brisk towelling or cold shower on the evening of the massage will help to prevent any soreness.

Areas for gliding

Upward strokes ⟶

Light returning strokes ⟶

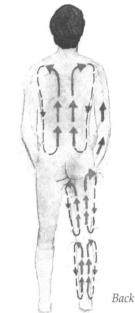

Back

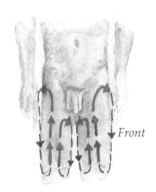

Front

Home massage treatment

Massage is a natural part of everyday life, beneficial for the receiver as well as the giver, and everybody should be able to do it. Relaxation is central to the benefits – the more you can do to help your partner feel comfortable and at peace, the more effective the massage will be. Since he or she will be either partly or wholly naked you should ensure that the room is warm. Cold air and draughts are unrelaxing.

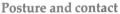

Working surface
You will need a firm surface to work on (a table or the floor), covered with foam and a large towel to make it comfortable. When working on the calves, support the ankles with a cushion; when working on the front of the legs support under the knees similarly. When working on the back and shoulders, try placing a cushion under the chest to accentuate the curve and make tension points more accessible.

The lubricant
Keep the oil, cream or talc you use to lubricate your hands close beside you during the massage. Warm it with your hands, and then spread it on the receiver's body. In a whole body massage, apply lubricant to each area before you work on it – don't lubricate the body all at once.

Posture and contact
Make sure that your own body posture is relaxed and comfortable. If working on a table, keep your knees slightly "broken" – this will keep your lower back more relaxed and reduce the tendency to lean too far over.

Gliding
This is the commonest of massage strokes. It is used to apply lubricant to each part of the body, and it is good on long stretches of muscle.

Extend your hands and close the gaps between your fingers. Leave your hands relaxed but not limp, as shown right. Glide along the length of the muscle in the direction of the heart, as shown on the gliding zones diagrams on p.244, allowing your hands to be moulded by the contours of the body. The longer the stroke is, the lighter it will be; the shorter it is, the deeper it will be. Faster strokes are stimulating, slower ones more sedating.

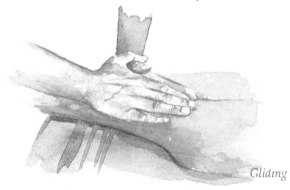

Gliding

By putting more pressure on the upward stroke and returning with your fingertips only, you will reinforce the return flow of blood to the heart.

Arms are massaged using your active hand in a C shape and running up the arm from the wrist to the shoulder, while the other hand firmly holds just above the wrist.

Gliding strokes relax and stretch the muscles in preparation for the kneading strokes (p.246).

Kneading

This is a deeper stroke than gliding. It milks the muscles of toxic waste products and helps to separate bunched muscle fibers. It is most useful on the legs, buttocks, back, and upper chest, as shown on the kneading zone diagrams, right.

Place the heels of your hands on the mid-line of the area to be worked, leaving the fingers outstretched and relaxed. Push with the heel and palm of each hand alternately in the direction of the fingers, as shown below. Don't pull the fingers up or you will pinch the skin. Use sufficient pressure to loosen the muscle, but always keep the comfort of the receiver in mind. Avoid putting pressure on the back of the knees and on any bony areas.

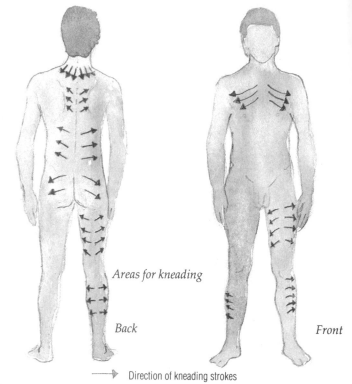

Areas for kneading

Back

Front

⟶ Direction of kneading strokes

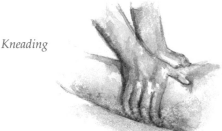

Kneading

Friction

This deep-tissue stroke should be used with discretion and with the person's tolerance level in mind. It is mainly used on the back (see the Zones for friction diagram, p.247).

Using the pad of your thumb or index finger, slowly apply pressure to the point, as shown right. Then rotate the pad very slightly for 10-15 seconds before releasing it slowly. With a sore point it may be helpful simply to increase the pressure as the person breathes out, releasing it gradually with the in-breath. Friction can also be used anywhere on the back where you find a knot or stiffness. The pressure will help release the knot. At most, repeat friction on a point only two or three times. Always follow friction with relaxing gliding strokes.

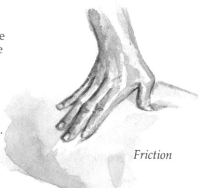

Friction

Zones for friction

Like the feet and the hands (see Reflexology, pp.256-63), the back has several reflex zones relating to different organs of the body, as shown right. While any type of massage on a zone will affect the relevant organ, friction has the most powerful effect. The points to apply it to are situated three-quarters of the way up the ridge of muscle on either side of the spine, level with the tip of each vertebra.

Percussion

These brisk rhythmic strokes are difficult to perform properly and are best learned from a professional. They are used to stimulate soft-tissue areas, such as buttocks or thighs, as indicated on the percussion zones diagram, right. They should not be used with everybody, as many people require relaxation rather than stimulation. Use these strokes only after you have first warmed the muscles up by kneading them.

Chopping Also known as hacking, this involves contacting the skin with the outer edge of the palms and little fingers, striking it first with one hand and then the other, as shown above right. Relax your fingers, hands and wrists and don't raise your hands more than 2-4 inches (5-10 cm). Chopping is best used on the calves, upper legs, and buttocks. Never use it on bony areas.

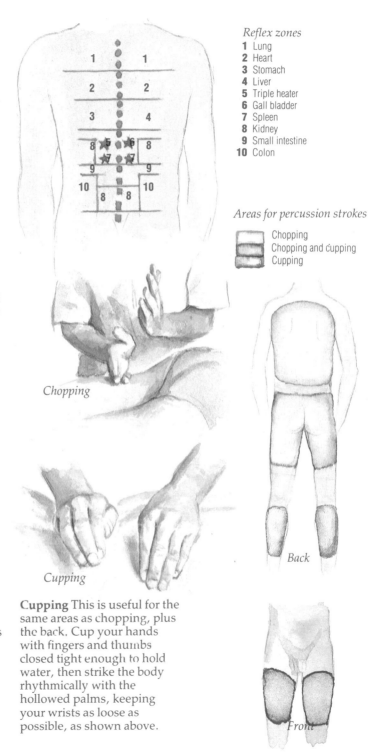

Reflex zones
1 Lung
2 Heart
3 Stomach
4 Liver
5 Triple heater
6 Gall bladder
7 Spleen
8 Kidney
9 Small intestine
10 Colon

Chopping

Areas for percussion strokes

Chopping
Chopping and cupping
Cupping

Back

Cupping

Cupping This is useful for the same areas as chopping, plus the back. Cup your hands with fingers and thumbs closed tight enough to hold water, then strike the body rhythmically with the hollowed palms, keeping your wrists as loose as possible, as shown above.

Front

Ailments and remedies

The techniques described on pages 245-7 can be used to alleviate many common ailments, but muscular disorders respond particularly well. If the ailment is longstanding, a series of treatments may be required.

Although problem areas can be massaged separately with great benefit, it is always good to treat the whole body where possible. Start on the back, working up the body from the legs, to assist the flow of blood back to the heart. Then ask the receiver to turn over slowly, and massage the front of the body, again working up from feet to head. Finish the massage with some long relaxing strokes, to link all parts of the body and give the receiver a feeling of connectedness. Always maintain contact with the body between different strokes, when moving from one area to another, and even when putting more oil on your hands.

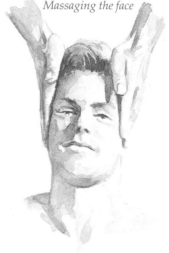
Massaging the face

Asthma, coughs

Work generally on the upper and middle portion of the back to release tension in the muscles forming the chest cavity, and use friction on the lung zone points (p.247). Use gliding strokes on the back, knead around the shoulders, and then use cupping strokes over the entire upper middle back, as shown below right. If the cupping is done with the receiver lying at a slant, with the head lower than the feet, catarrh in the lungs will be released. You can also knead the muscles of the upper chest, from the sternum toward the shoulder joints, and "drag" your fingers gently along the grooves between the ribs. This helps to stretch tense muscles, improving the receiver's capacity to breathe.

Headaches

Headaches are often the result of tension in the neck and shoulders, so you should concentrate on these areas first. Finish by massaging the face, as shown above right, especially the forehead and temple areas.

Colds

Colds are nature's way of eliminating toxins from the body and so symptoms should not be suppressed. Instead, give a general, invigorating massage, using gliding, kneading, and percussion strokes, and then let nature take its course.

Facial massage
Use standard gliding and kneading strokes, but work in miniature and use gentle pressure only. Be sure to use upward strokes, and avoid touching the delicate skin below the eyes.

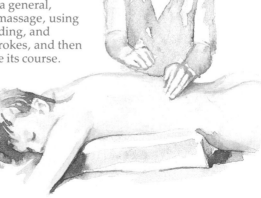

Cupping the back

Digestive problems

Constipation, flatulence, stomach aches, and menstrual cramps and irregularities will benefit from various massage techniques. First, always treat any tensions in the back zone corresponding with the problem. Stomach problems are often due to a general digestive disorder. Where this is the case, massage can help by aiding the eliminative process. A self-help tip for massaging the colon is to take a tennis ball and roll it firmly up the right side of the abdomen, across the bottom of the ribcage, then down the left side. You can do this at any time, but it is particularly effective first thing in the morning before rising.

Otherwise, massage the abdominal or pelvic area, using an open hand in a clockwise stroking motion on the belly, then gentle cupping on the belly and along the colon to invigorate these areas.

Menstrual problems

See Digestive problems, left.

Backache

Treat the whole of the back and spine, not just the sore spot. Use gliding strokes to relax the area and kneading strokes to break down stiffness in the shoulders and in the sore area. Apply friction down the back muscles on either side of the spine and finish off with some cupping strokes to leave the area invigorated.

Cramp

Work on the whole area, not just the part that has cramp. If, for example, the cramp is in the foot, then work on the entire leg. Use your hands to stretch the area in cramp. Use gliding and then kneading strokes until you feel the cramp loosening. To help the blood supply in the affected area, end with some chopping strokes.

Arthritis, rheumatism

For these complaints, and for shoulder stiffness and fibrositis as well, a general body massage is advised, spending most time on the affected joints, using lots of soothing gliding strokes. Knead the muscles above and below the affected joint, where this is possible. With a stiff or frozen shoulder, the muscle will often need extra work. After gliding and kneading, apply friction if the patient is not too sore. Massage the upper arm below the frozen shoulder, bringing your hands up high enough to include the muscle "capping" the shoulder joint.

Sciatica

Massage as if for backache, but also use gliding strokes down the legs, and knead any muscles that are tight. Have the patient take a hot bath before the massage to help relax the muscles.

Caution Before you try massage on anyone who is ill, you must be aware that it could do serious damage if used inappropriately.

Don't give massage at all to people with undiagnosed lumps or bumps, with undiagnosed or weepy skin conditions, sudden swellings or pains of unknown origin, raised temperature, septic conditions, high or low blood pressure, thrombosis, cancer, epilepsy or severe mental or emotional states (unless you have permission from a professionally qualified person and have been given instructions as to how you should proceed).

Do not work at all on or near any injured, infected, scarred or otherwise damaged areas of the body. Do not work near bone fractures within six months of the injury (after which use gentle gliding strokes).

Work only very lightly on pregnant women. Heavy work on the abdomen or lower back should be totally avoided. Varicose veins may be massaged with light gliding strokes, provided that this does not cause pain.

Applied kinesiology

Applied kinesiology is a method of diagnosis and treatment that uses muscle testing to discover and correct imbalances in muscles and other body functions. The self-help therapy which was developed from it, touch for health, uses some of the same muscle tests, in conjunction with light touching techniques designed to restore bodily balance.

One of the major premises on which applied kinesiology is based is the belief that the body has an innate knowledge of itself – it "knows" what is wrong – and that this knowledge can be accessed by testing certain muscles. Muscle tests can be used to discover energy excesses or deficiencies due to either mental, physical, biochemical, or energy stressors which impair normal physiological activity. Both the diagnostic and treatment methods are entirely safe, and often achieve rapid results with musculoskeletal problems, especially headaches, neck and back pain, and with problems related to stress, hypertension, and fatigue. The techniques are now used by many health professionals, including chiropractors, osteopaths, dentists, homeopaths, and acupuncturists as an adjunct to their own special skills.

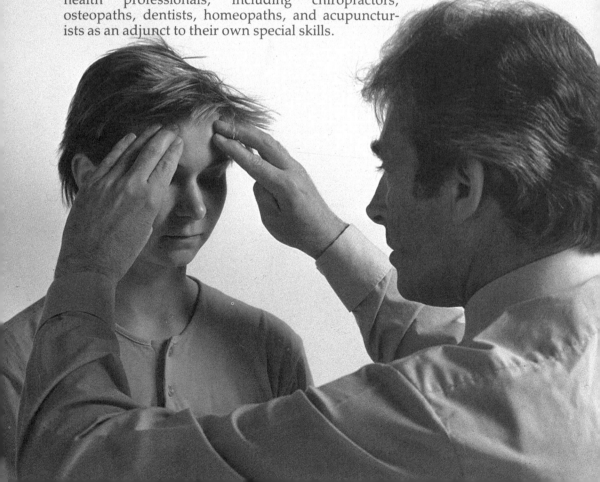

Kinesiology discovered

Applied kinesiology was developed by Dr George Goodheart, an American chiropractor. Dr Goodheart had been in practice for over 20 years when, in 1964, he observed in one of his patients a change in muscle strength after massaging tender spots on the fascia lata muscle (a long muscle running from the hip to below the knee). This led him to further research, during which he found that massaging the neuro-lymphatic reflexes (known to improve lymphatic flow), strengthened weak muscles. Painstakingly, he discovered the links between each reflex and each muscle group. Other discoveries followed that became the basis of kinesiology – methods of improving blood supply, nutrition, and energy flow, linking the best of eastern and western physiology.

Dr Goodheart's early workshops for fellow chiropractors drew, among others, Dr John Thie, who became the founding chairman of the International College of Applied Kinesiology, Kansas, USA, and subsequently went on to devise touch for health.

Consulting an applied kinesiologist

An initial visit to a practitioner may take up to an hour, but subsequent visits will last only 10 to 15 minutes each. First, a complete history of your health problems will be taken. The kinesiological part of the examination involves testing many different muscle groups and analysing your posture. The practitioner may also use standard diagnosis methods, such as X-rays, blood chemistry tests, and electro-cardiograms, depending on your complaint. From these tests, the kinesiologist discovers in which parts of your body the natural energy flow is disturbed. Imbalances are corrected by massaging specific reflex points, by touching acupuncture points, or by using electro-stimulation. As a patient you may be asked to help the process by touching various places on your body while the practitioner tests the related muscles – a process known as therapy localization. Your need for nutritional support will also be assessed by placing various nutrients in your mouth and testing previously weak muscles to see if they are made stronger or weaker. As a result of this, you may be asked to add certain foods to your diet, to take appropriate supplements and to avoid any foods that have been found to weaken the muscles.

Touch for health

Dr John Thie developed touch for health as a lay program, in order to offer some of the simpler and more basic techniques of applied kinesiology to the public as a system of self-help. His synthesis of kinesiological methods with techniques based on the meridian system has now been taught to tens of thousands of people all over the world. It has been of notable benefit to sports' coaches and trainers.

Unlike kinesiology, touch for health is intended primarily as a preventive technique. It sees malfunctions as the result of some muscles being weak or inhibited, which in turn causes other muscles to do more than their share of work, making them tight or contracted. In the basic touch for health course, which is usually completed after about 16 hours' instruction, people learn to find minor imbalances or weaknesses by testing 14 muscles – each one corresponding to one of the 14 meridians (pp.254-5). Imbalances are discovered when a muscle under test fails to "lock" properly when gentle pressure is applied to it while it is contracted. Any muscle that is found to be weak or inhibited can then be corrected using the strengthening techniques taught during the course. In the process, the tight overworked muscles also let go and relax. When all the weak muscles have been corrected, the person is said to have been "balanced". The course also teaches simple manual treatments (pp.253-5) which can be used by anybody, with or without a partner, to enhance well-being. (It does seem to be true, however, that the massaging of points and reflexes by another person results in the most effective and long-lasting treatment.) The standard textbook contains valuable information, including advice on the strengthening and weakening effects of various foods, and suggestions for sensible adjustments to the daily dietary pattern.

Even somebody in good health may experience more energy, and an enhanced sense of well-being after treatment. Those who are regularly "balanced" report an improved overall state of health and fewer colds and general aches and pains. It must be emphasized, however, that it is important to consult a health professional if symptoms persist. Touch for health does not suggest itself as an alternative to professional help, but clearly it does promote health, reducing the need for costly medical care.

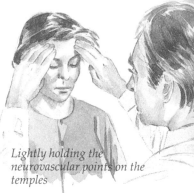

Lightly holding the neurovascular points on the temples

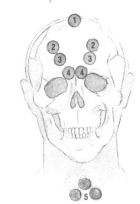

Neurovascular points (frontal)
1 Supraspinatus, subscapularis, anterior deltoid, anterior serratus
2 Pectoralis major sternal
3 Pectoralis major clavicular, peroneus
4 Peroneus
5 Teres minor

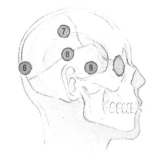

Neurovascular points (lateral)
6 Psoas
7 Quadriceps, gluteus medius, fascia lata
8 Latissimus dorsi
9 Teres major, teres minor

Touch for health techniques

To get full benefit from touch for health and to learn muscle testing, you should enrol in a basic course. There are, however, some invaluable techniques for beginners. It is possible to correct the cause of muscle inhibition by touching two series of reflexes or points on the body. Pressing the neurolymphatic points improves the flow of lymph, which feeds and cleans the cells of the body. Lightly holding the neurovascular points on the head enhances the blood supply to the related muscles and organs.

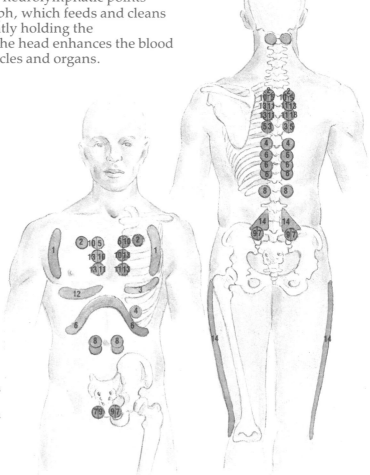

Neurovascular points

The neurovascular points shown on p. 252 need only the lightest possible finger pressure. Benefit usually comes after 20 or 30 seconds, although you will not do any damage by holding them for longer. Initially, you may feel an irregular pulse, which smooths out once the point is balanced.

Neurolymphatic points

Press these points quite firmly with your fingertips, in order to stimulate them. Those needing most attention will usually be tender to the touch, but any tenderness should lessen after 15 to 20 seconds. For the longer reflexes, such as those at the sides of the chest, work along the line, pressing for a few seconds then moving on to the next part. If you are pressing your own points, you can, with a little ingenuity, a tennis ball, and a wall, even treat the points on your back.

Neurolymphatic points

1 Supraspinatus
2 Teres major
3 Pectoralis major clavicular
4 Latissimus dorsi
5 Subscapularis
6 Quadriceps
7 Peroneus
8 Psoas
9 Gluteus medius
10 Teres minor
11 Anterior deltoid
12 Pectoralis major sternal
13 Anterior serratus
14 Fascia lata

The meridians

The meridians are channels of energy which govern the functioning of the body's organs and muscles (p.271). This energy can be affected by energy flowing from your own or another person's hand, if you "run" or trace lightly along the meridians. Apart from the Central and Governing meridians (also known as the Conception and Governing Vessels) which run up the front and back midlines of the body, all the meridians are bilateral, so you should trace their course on both sides of the body. You can "run" just one meridian, or all 14, but if you decide to "run" all of them, be sure to observe the order shown here. Tracing the meridians produces a great energy boost when you are tired and is extremely relaxing.

Stimulating a meridian

To stimulate a meridian lightly brush the skin with your fingers in the direction shown. Start at the beginning of the meridian and move smoothly along its pathway, following the arrow. You may do this fairly quickly, taking 4-5 seconds or less for an arm meridian, but it is important to cover the precise beginning, surface line, and end point of the meridian. Note that the start of the next meridian is often close to where the last one finishes, facilitating a smooth transition from one to the other.

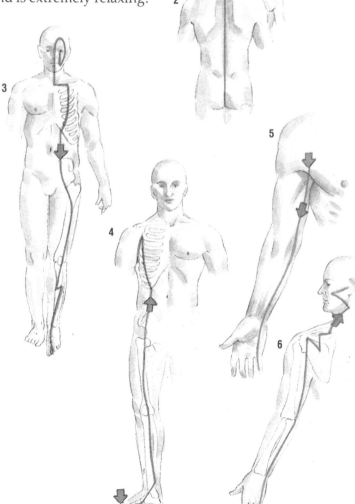

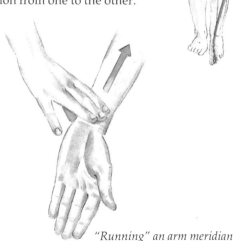

"Running" an arm meridian

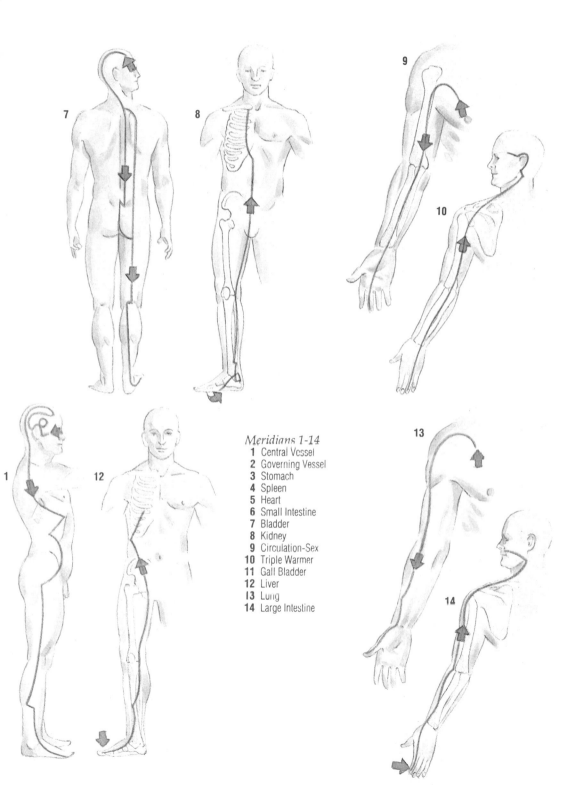

Meridians 1-14
1 Central Vessel
2 Governing Vessel
3 Stomach
4 Spleen
5 Heart
6 Small Intestine
7 Bladder
8 Kidney
9 Circulation-Sex
10 Triple Warmer
11 Gall Bladder
12 Liver
13 Lung
14 Large Intestine

Reflexology

Reflexology works on the principle that there are "reflexes" or "responsive zones" in the feet and hands corresponding to each and every part and organ of the body. Working on these reflexes systematically with pressure and manipulation has three main effects: it brings about normal functioning of all the organs and glands in the body, improves nerve function and blood supply, and finally and very importantly, induces a state of relaxation. The reflexes are arranged in such a way as to form a map of the body on the hands and feet (pp.259–60) – the right foot relating to the left side, and vice versa.

When giving treatment, professional reflexologists use only their fingers, thumbs and hands, never any of the massaging implements which can prove both painful and harmful to the feet. The full spectrum of techniques can be taught only at special training seminars, but some can be practiced by novices with complete safety if carried out with care (pp.259-63).

Since modern research has indicated that as much as 75 percent of all diseases are stress-related, a therapy such as reflexology, whose principal effect is relaxation, can be of immense value. Apart from

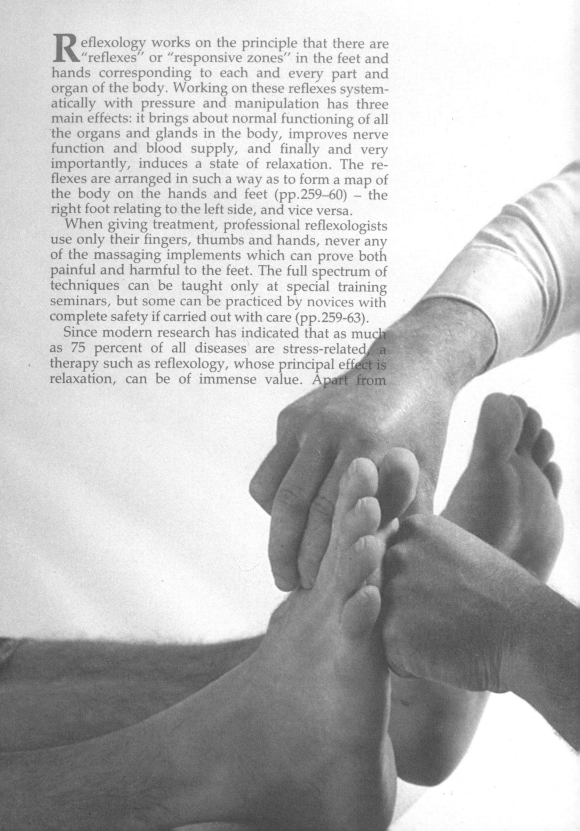

inducing a general state of relaxation, it also aids lymphatic and venous circulation. It has been found beneficial for a wide range of disorders, from back pain to migraines, sinusitis, and digestive problems. Reflexology is also extremely effective for the alleviation of pain. Though little clinical research has been undertaken, it seems probable that its analgesic properties stem from the same origin as those of acupuncture. One explanation for these properties is that during various acupuncture techniques a group of chemicals, known as endorphins, are released into the bloodstream. Endorphins are opiates which act like morphine and are able to block pain. Though it has yet to be confirmed, the likelihood is that reflexology treatment can also elevate the level of endorphins in the bloodstream.

The origins of reflexology

The roots of reflexology can be traced in many countries, including Egypt, Persia, and, to an extent, in China and Japan. It may even have emerged before acupuncture, which is said to have originated about 5,000 years ago (p.269), and it certainly shares many fundamental principles with oriental philosophy. In India and in some parts of Africa, the therapeutic value of reflexology has long been recognized and today it is practised in many parts, by children as young as 13 or 14 years old, as well as by adults.

Western reflexology, however, dates only from the early 20th century when an American physician, Dr William Fitzgerald, discovered the existence of ten zones of communication passing vertically through the body (p.258) from the head to the fingertips and toes. Fitzgerald found that by applying pressure to certain areas of the fingers he could induce anesthesia in areas of the head and face so completely that he was able to carry out surgery on those areas.

In the 1930s, another American doctor, Shelby Riley, read of Fitzgerald's findings and became interested in pursuing them. But it was his physical therapist, a young woman by the name of Eunice Ingham, who really took up the banner and started extensive research into the therapy we now know as reflexology. By researching, and working on thousands of pairs of feet, Ingham was able to confirm Dr Fitzgerald's findings – that where painful reflexes existed, the parts of the body that these related to were in a congestive state. And, further, by working on those painful sites over a period of several treatments, a state of normal function could usually be restored. In order to draw wider attention to reflexology, Eunice Ingham published her findings in *Stories the Feet can Tell* (1938), and proceeded to found the National Institute of Reflexology in order to take care of the enormous number of enquiries she received. She began to lecture to various medical schools, and within a few years she was teaching the therapy across the United States and in Canada.

The International Institute of Reflexology was established in 1973 to promote her technique, now known as the Ingham method. Since then, reflexology has become one of the fastest growing natural therapies. In Denmark, treatment is now available on the national health service, if prescribed by a doctor.

Consulting a professional

A typical treatment session lasts about 30-40 minutes. To receive treatment, you either lie on a massage couch or sit in a reclining chair, with your knees supported, and the soles of your feet facing the therapist. He or she will work systematically over each foot and ankle, seeking out and treating any painful areas with a compression technique. This is a caterpillar-like movement, performed mainly by either thumbs or index fingers, and it clears congestion in those parts of the body corresponding to the painful reflexes, by improving lymphatic, nerve, and blood circulation. Any pain you experience while the reflexologist treats these areas should be pleasant, not unbearable. The compression technique is interspersed with a variety of relaxation movements.

The number of treatments you will need depends on the condition being treated and how you respond. Two treatments a week for three weeks is the average time it takes before you begin to feel a change; for a complete return to normal health, as many as 30 visits may be necessary. During a course of treatment your body undergoes a detoxifying process, and this may manifest itself in, for example, cold, aching joints, a sore throat, diarrhea, or increased urination. This healing response depends on the amount of toxicity in your body and on your level of vitality. It may not occur, but if it does, it will not last long and should be regarded as a good sign.

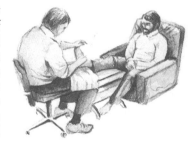

Position for treatment
Both therapist and receiver should be comfortable. The receiver's feet need to be level with, not lower than, the therapist's lap. A reclining chair is ideal, since it offers firm support for the knees. If a normal armchair is used, the receiver's knees should rest on a stool.

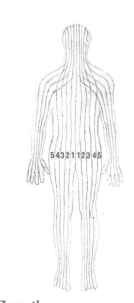

Zone theory
Ten zones or channels of energy run vertically up from feet to head. The reflex for any part of the body that lies within a specific zone will be found in the corresponding zone of hands or feet.

Reflexology treatment

As well as being an effective treatment for many different types of ailment, reflexology may also be used preventively. If possible you should try to learn the treatment techniques at a special teaching seminar, as here we can give only basic instructions (p.260). But first you should understand some of the principles on which the science is based – especially the zone theory (see opposite) and the charts of reflexes (see below, and p.260). This will enable you to relax specific parts of the body by working on the corresponding reflexes.

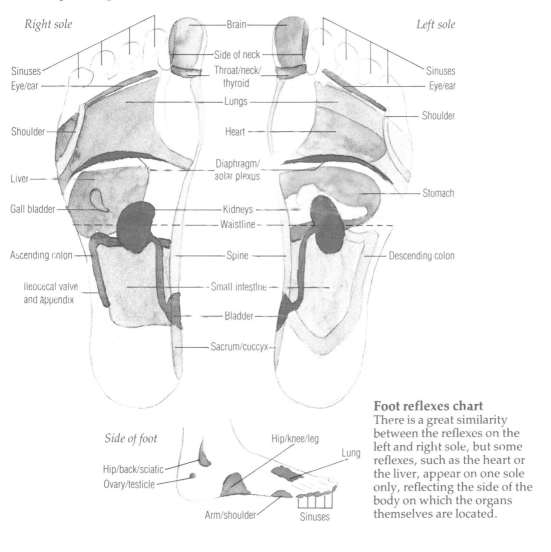

Right sole

- Sinuses
- Eye/ear
- Shoulder
- Liver
- Gall bladder
- Ascending colon
- Ileocecal valve and appendix

- Brain
- Side of neck
- Throat/neck/ thyroid
- Lungs
- Heart
- Diaphragm/ solar plexus
- Kidneys
- Waistline
- Spine
- Small intestine
- Bladder
- Sacrum/coccyx

Left sole

- Sinuses
- Eye/ear
- Shoulder
- Stomach
- Descending colon

Side of foot

- Hip/back/sciatic
- Ovary/testicle
- Hip/knee/leg
- Lung
- Arm/shoulder
- Sinuses

Foot reflexes chart
There is a great similarity between the reflexes on the left and right sole, but some reflexes, such as the heart or the liver, appear on one sole only, reflecting the side of the body on which the organs themselves are located.

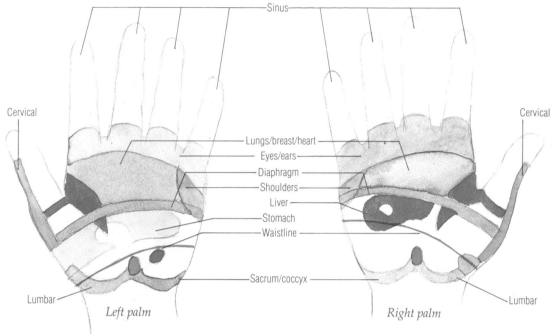

Sinus

Cervical — — Cervical

Lungs/breast/heart
Eyes/ears
Diaphragm
Shoulders
Liver
Stomach
Waistline

Sacrum/coccyx

Lumbar — — Lumbar

Left palm *Right palm*

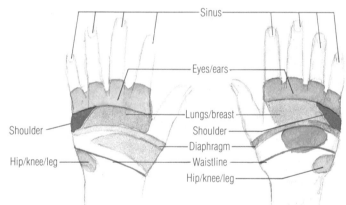

Sinus

Eyes/ears

Lungs/breast
Shoulder — Shoulder
Diaphragm
Hip/knee/leg — Waistline
Hip/knee/leg

Left hand *Right hand*

Hand reflexes chart

The hand reflexes mirror those on the feet in position, but differ in size and shape. They are usually more difficult to locate, for they lie deeper than those on the feet, but they are very convenient for self-treatment.

Relaxation technique

You should begin and end any treatment session with this technique, and return to it after working on any reflexes that are tender.

Hold either side of the foot so that the heels of your palms rest on the soles of the feet, and your fingers are relaxed. Then use one hand to push the side of the foot forward, while pulling back the other side with the other hand. Continue this gentle back and forth movement, keeping up a fairly rapid, steady rhythm.

Thumb technique

This is used to treat the soles and sides of the feet. With one hand wrapped around the toes, use the inside edge of the thumb of the other hand to work on the foot. (Wrap the fingers around the foot.) Bend the working thumb's top joint just slightly and "walk" forward by alternately bending and unbending the joint.

Index finger technique

You use the index finger to work on the top and sides of the foot, once again pressing with the inside edge and making it "creep" forward with the first joint slightly bent. Keep your pressure steady so that the movement is smooth. Use your thumbs on the sole of the foot to provide leverage.

Ailments and remedies

Without proper qualifications, it is unwise to treat specific areas of either hands or feet if someone is unwell. But you can safely use reflexology as an overall relaxing and toning treatment. Study the reflex charts on pp.259-60 to familiarize yourself with the location of the various reflexes. Start with the toes (or fingers) and work down to the heels, then work on the spinal reflexes on the inside edge of the feet (or hands). Pay special attention to areas of tenderness, but don't press too hard, as overworking a sensitive reflex will cause tension. Certain reflexes demand particular techniques, as shown below.

Caution Do not attempt home treatment on people suffering from varicose veins, thrombosis, phlebitis, or ulceration of the feet, or on those who are generally frail or suffering from an acute illness. Instead, consult a qualified practitioner.

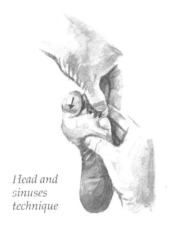

Head and sinuses technique

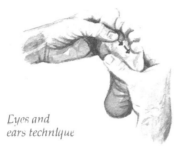

Eyes and ears technique

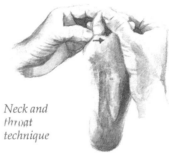

Neck and throat technique

Head and sinuses

Reflexes to the left side of the head are on the left foot and vice versa. The toes will all be sensitive to the touch if someone has congested sinuses, and one particular toe will be painful if a person has toothache.

Support the toes in one hand (right hand for left foot and vice versa) and use the thumb of the other to "walk" down from tip to base of toe, as shown above. Start at the big toe. When you reach the little toe, change hands and "walk" your other thumb along to the big toe.

Eyes and ears

Reflexology can be very effective for eyestrain and other eye problems, since they are often due to tension. The most direct way to treat these reflexes is at the base of the toes, excluding the big toe (where the eye reflexes are hard to locate).

Hold the foot in one hand, using the thumb to pull the skin taut, as shown above. Now "walk" your other thumb along the ridge at the base of the smaller toes. Repeat with the other hand, "walking" along the ridge in the opposite direction.

Neck and throat

The neck, the top of the spine, the tonsils and the thyroid gland are all affected by treating the neck and throat reflex which is located at the base of the big toe.

Use one hand to support the foot and the thumb of the other hand to work across the base of the toe from the side, as shown above. Change hands and work back over the reflex zone, in the opposite direction.

Lung and chest

On the feet you will find the lung and chest reflex between the metatarsal bones and the base of the toes on both the underside and the top of the foot, as shown on p.259.

Work first on the sole, using the inner edge of the thumb to "walk" up between the bones to the base of the toes, holding the toes firmly in the other hand, as shown below left(1). Repeat, changing hands and direction. Then, starting at the big toe, use the inner edge of your index finger to work down between the bones from the base of the toes on the top of the foot, as shown below right(2). Repeat, with the other hand working in the opposite direction.

You can also treat this area with the corresponding reflex on the hands – it lies just above the diaphragm line on the palm and back of the hand. Use one thumb to work down between the metacarpal bones on the palm, using your other hand to flex and stretch the fingers. Turn the hand over and work the reflex on the back of the hand, using the index finger, as shown below.

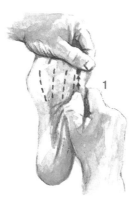
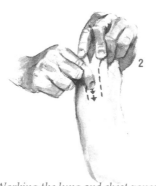
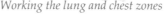
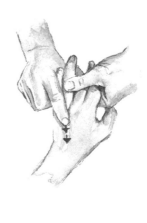

Working the lung and chest zones

Liver and gall bladder

The liver reflex zone is found on the right hand and foot, since the liver is located mainly on the right hand side of the body. The gall bladder reflex is found within the liver zone.

Working on the foot, hold the toes in one hand, as shown right, and "walk" your other thumb systematically over the whole of the reflex area, just below the ball of the foot. Keep the fingers of your "working" hand around the top of the foot, to support it and provide leverage for the thumb. Repeat, changing hands. You can also treat the corresponding hand reflex on both the back and the palm of the right hand. It lies just below the diaphragm line. "Walk" your thumb slowly across the reflex on the palm, while you gently flex and stretch the fingers with your other hand, as shown below right. Use your index finger to treat the reflex on the back of the hand.

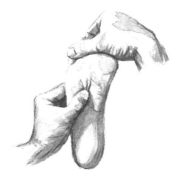
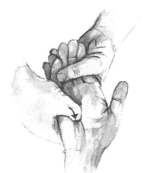

Working the liver and gall bladder zones

Spine

Treating the spinal reflexes, along the inside edges of the feet or hands, is highly effective – not only for backache but for the whole body, since tension in the back impedes the proper functioning of the spinal nerves which "feed" the rest of the body.

On the feet, begin at the inside edge of the heel and "walk" your thumb slowly up toward the big toe. At the start, you give leverage to the thumb by wrapping the fingers of your "working" hand around the heel, as shown below left(1). By the time you reach the lumbar area, you will need to move your "working" hand up, placing the fingers over the instep, as shown below(2). Spend more time on any sensitive spots, and be sure to treat the reflex zones on both feet.

On the hands, the spinal reflexes run up the inner edge of the hand and along the side of the thumb. Unlike many reflexes on the hand, they are easily accessible, and useful for self-treatment, see below. Start at the heel of the hand and "walk" your thumb up to the cervical area. With lower back pain, give extra attention to the lumbar reflex.

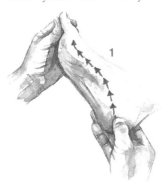
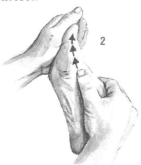
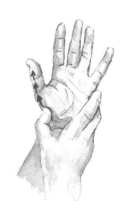

Working the spine zones

Hip/knee/leg

Work on the reflex for these areas is good for backache as well as for hip, knee and leg disorders. The reflex will be very tender if the person has a knee problem.

On the feet, "walk" across the reflex area with your thumb, as shown right, or with your index finger. Make sure that you cover the whole reflex area.

You can also work effectively on this reflex on the backs of the hands. Work over the whole reflex with the index finger of one hand, supporting the receiver's hand with your other hand, as shown far right. Then repeat the treatment, changing the working hand.

Working the hip/knee/leg zones

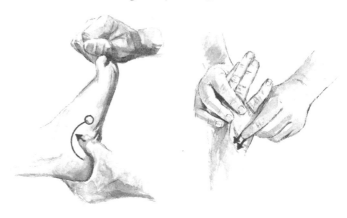

Rolfing

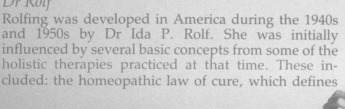

Rolfing is a method of manipulating the connective tissue of the body in order to realign its structure. The goal of the therapy is threefold: to increase the client's range of movement; to improve balance; and to provide greater ease of posture. Though the exact results depend on the initial state of the client, the effects of a course of Rolfing sessions always include more vitality, greater physical stability, relief of chronic structural aches and pains and an enhanced capacity for self-healing. In addition, many clients enjoy beneficial psychological effects. Given that Rolfing produces no adverse reactions, and is cost-effective when compared with other forms of treatment, it is generally well worth trying when stiffness, structural aches and pains, and other types of physical stress are at issue.

Dr Rolf

Rolfing was developed in America during the 1940s and 1950s by Dr Ida P. Rolf. She was initially influenced by several basic concepts from some of the holistic therapies practiced at that time. These included: the homeopathic law of cure, which defines

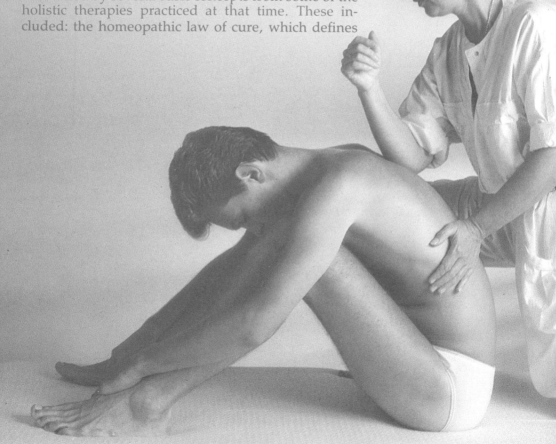

symptoms as the layered residues of earlier illnesses and states that a cure will come from the sequential healing of each residue in turn; the yogic concept of a core line in the body and the lengthening and ease that result when the body is aligned to its core; and the osteopathic approach to well-being, which sees improved bone alignment as an index of improved bodily functioning.

Dr Rolf applied these concepts in her work with the people who came to her for help, augmenting them with concepts of her own. Her main insights were that the earth's gravity exerts a continuous influence on the balance of the human structure and that the body's pliable connective tissues hold the key to its structural re-organization because they are the matrix for all the other components of the body. She called her work "structural integration".

Eventually, Dr Rolf devoted more of her time to her teaching role, and developed her teaching into the ten-session sequence of treatment in practice today. During the 1960s she helped to train chiropractors, osteopaths and other professionals interested in the discipline of Rolfing. At present, there are over 500 Rolfers throughout the world, all certified members of the Rolf Institute in Boulder, Colorado, USA. The Institute functions as a professional organization for Rolfers, and as a research and training center.

Who benefits most?

People from all walks of life find Rolfing helpful. It is particularly popular with those who lead a strenuous lifestyle and with athletes, dancers, musicians and other performers who use it to enhance and maintain their skills. After a course of treatment, some people claim Rolfing has given them a great boost in energy, others that it has changed how they feel or how they see the world. All clients find that Rolfing changes the way they look and move. And the benefits gained frequently last a lifetime.

Clinically, the largest group of people to benefit from Rolfing has some type of chronic myofascial pain (related to the body's soft tissue structure), such as a bad back, bursitis of a joint, non-inflammatory arthritis, or general stiffness. Traumatic injuries, such as the general "shaking-up" from a car accident, also respond well to Rolfing, as do non-traumatic injuries, such as jogger's knee, tennis elbow, and the like.

How Rolfing works

In Rolfing terms, the connective tissue of the body is known as the organ of structure. It is a complex pliable system of tissues of varying density, organized to facilitate movement. The tissue that responds most readily to Rolfing is the fascia – a sheet-like web that wraps around and positions every part of the body.

When we complain of chronic stiffness, soreness, or aches, it is the fascia that is in trouble. It shortens, thickens, and adheres to neighbouring structures and can thus impede freedom of movement. The process of fascial distortion usually starts early in life when, as infants, we fall and twist, distorting the body. In structural terms it all adds up, but it is not until later in life that these distortions become apparent, when we feel a tug-of-war between the movements that we would like to make and our physical restrictions.

What can Rolfing do to help? Primarily it stretches tissue that has contracted. In this way, more space is supplied for the other structures of the body, and it is the space occupied by an organ, nerve, bone or joint that determines its proper functioning to a surprisingly large degree.

Clients often report a sense of widening, lightness, or of opening up and out during a Rolfing session. But much of the benefit also occurs between sessions. This is an after-effect of manipulation, and it can be seen as the influence of gravity on the body as it integrates the changes.

The techniques of Rolfing

Whatever the goals or problems a client brings to Rolfing, the procedure will be more or less the same. Rolfing is a ten-session series of treatments, with sessions generally scheduled about one week apart. The series is designed to release all the components of the body and to integrate them into a balanced whole. Rolfers use their fingers and sometimes an elbow to move the fascia, causing it to stretch and to resume its natural elastic tone and full range of movement. At the beginning and end of the ten sessions, the Rolfer will take photographs of the client to document the course of treatment. The changes gained from Rolfing are ongoing. A few years after the end of a course of sessions, the client will usually look more balanced than immediately after completion of the series.

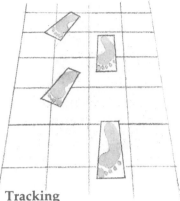

Tracking
One of Ida Rolf's experiments was to take a group of clients to the beach and study the tracks they made, with bare feet, in the sand. Most of them showed a pattern of walking that rotated their ankles outward, restricting and stiffening leg and foot muscles.

Foot and leg muscles
To carry the weight of the body the arched structure of the foot must be strongly supported by muscles within the foot itself and in the lower leg. If they become depleted, or even slightly displaced, the function and metabolism of all the related areas will be affected.

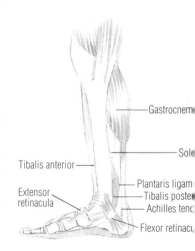

Gastrocnem

Sol

Tibalis anterior

Plantaris ligam

Extensor retinacula

Tibalis poste

Achilles tenc

Flexor retinacu

Rolfing sessions

If you take a course of Rolfing sessions, either to enhance your health in general or to treat chronic pain or a postural problem, you may be surprised how far-reaching its effects can be. In rebalancing the body, painful feelings and memories are often released too, since postural changes are frequently caused by emotional traumas in the first place. Thus the mind and emotions will be freed from their conditioning as well as the body.

Clients often ask for advice on how to maintain a Rolfed body. Dr Rolf once said that a well-balanced body can be kept in tone by simply walking and breathing. For those who exercise regularly, a good rule to remember is that if you treat your exercise as a task by counting laps, meters, etc, it's probably not good for you. Prime examples are push-ups, sit-ups, and set miles of jogging or bicycle riding. If, on the other hand, the exercise you choose gives you pleasure while you are doing it, it's probably doing you good. Pleasure, like pain, is a signal. Pleasure means "this is good"; pain means "pay attention".

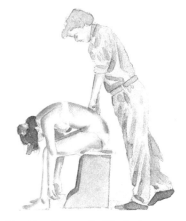

Treating the small of the back during Session 3

The ten sessions

Session 1 The series starts with an introductory session designed to improve your breathing pattern. This first hour allows you to see if the approach is one that you like and wish to pursue.

The Rolfing sessions that follow are focused on different parts of the body:

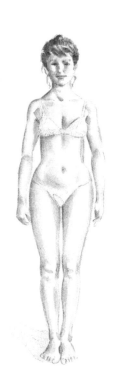

Session 2 the feet and lower legs

Session 3 the sides and the small of the back

Session 4 the inner aspect of the legs

Session 5 the abdomen

Session 6 the back of the legs and the pelvis

Session 7 the head and neck

Sessions 8, 9 and 10 The final sessions are more general, designed to integrate the shoulder and pelvic girdles with the spine and to bring the body together as a whole.

Acupuncture

In the early 1970s, exactly 700 years after Marco Polo's trek to the East, a US presidential visit restored China to a position of prominence in western minds. James Reston, a New York Times columnist accompanying the presidential party, was given acupuncture (literally "needle insertion") treatment to speed his recovery from an emergency appendix operation. Soon afterward, western doctors visiting China were watching in amazement as the anesthesia for major surgery was being successfully performed by the skilled placing of acupuncture needles. Acupuncture became front page news.

Whereas acupuncture had been known in the West only to a select few until that time, now there was an explosion of interest. Patients began to search out acupuncturists and health professionals sought training. Acupressure (p.275), using finger pressure on acupuncture points, also became popular. Today, acupuncture is one of the most popular and effective contemporary healing techniques, practiced in almost every country on the globe. And outside the East, there are now schools or training colleges throughout North America, Europe, and Australia.

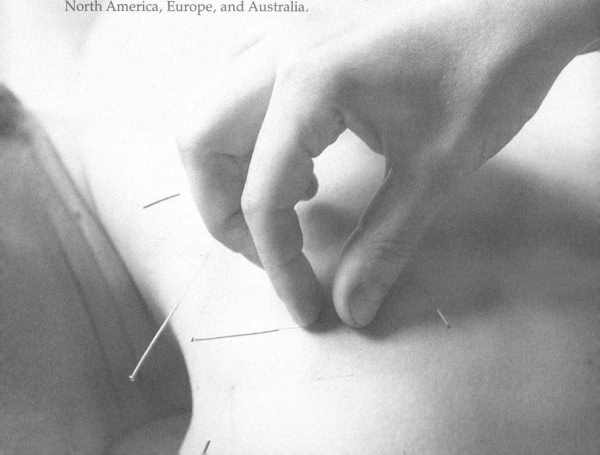

Clinical and scientific evidence

Acupuncture is part of a comprehensive medical system that has survived over millennia. But is it more effective than other traditional or holistic therapies? It is not unique in its holistic treatment of the patient, nor is it in fact unparallelled in the field of anesthesia – pain-free surgery using hypnosis was demonstrated successfully more than a century ago. But as both Chinese and western research has shown, acupuncture provides far more than effective pain relief. Not only is it safe, in the hands of fully-trained practitioners, but its clinical applicability is enormous. The World Health Organization has compiled a huge list of medical conditions that are amenable to treatment with acupuncture, including chronic respiratory problems, such as sinusitis and asthma, neurological and musculoskeletal disorders, such as headaches and low back pain, digestive disorders, such as colitis and gastritis, and chronic menstrual problems. This is apart from the treatment of mental and emotional disturbances and certain behavioral problems, such as addictive habits.

In the last 30 years the Chinese have produced many volumes of evidence demonstrating acupuncture's effectiveness. They have shown that it can affect intestinal peristalsis, vasodilatation and blood pressure, change the heart rate, influence the levels of a wide number of chemicals in the blood, and increase white blood cell counts. Rigorous research in the West began in the 1970s, and since then acupuncture has become one of the most investigated areas in complementary medicine. Much of the research has been concerned with the alleviation of pain. One theory suggests that stimulation from the acupuncture needles "jams" the central nervous system so that other pain signals cannot reach the brain. Another theory proposes that insertion of the needles stimulates the release of endorphins, a class of opiates or potent painkillers naturally produced within the brain.

Oriental cosmology

Acupuncture's history in the Orient goes back at least 3,000 years, perhaps even further to the "legendary" era of Chinese history 5,000 years ago. During the time when philosophical schools such as taoism and Confucianism arose in China, medicine also made new departures. The Chinese sought rational and comprehensible laws and relationships that could explain the dilemma of illness and health. The basic notion was one of balance. They concluded that, just as the universe was sustained by natural energies, so too were human beings. A harmonious interplay of these natural energies resulted in health. A disproportion or imbalance produced illness.

These natural energies are neither material entities nor mythical concepts, but qualities of activity, motivation, sensation, performance, feeling or appearance. They are more like labels or emblems for what might be called fundamental textures, distinctive qualities or vibrations. The basic energies described by the Chinese are called Yin and Yang, the famous complementary opposites of that culture. Yin and Yang are qualities of energy that control a person's entire health. Yin is associated with such qualities as cold, rest, responsiveness, passivity, darkness, interiority, downwardness, inwardness, and nourishment. Yang is associated with heat, stimulation, movement, excitement, light, upwardness, outwardness, and increase. Sometimes health is also seen as a harmonious proportion of another set of emblems, the Five Elements: Fire, Earth, Metal, Water, and Wood. Fire contributes warmth and animation; its motion is upward. Earth provides stability and nourishment; it serves as an anchor. Metal has structure, but can also accept new form when molten. Water softens and moistens; its motion is downward. Wood is the force of growth and flexibility. The interplay of natural forces – whether it is expressed as Yin or Yang or the Five Elements – creates the vital energy of life, what the Chinese call chi (also spelled qi). When this chi is harmonious, health is maintained; when it is disturbed, there is illness. The primary concern of Chinese medicine is the generalized "terrain" of a person's being, the bodily chi. Treatment is directed at this terrain, rather than at any particular part of the body, disease or symptom. The Chinese use this approach of addressing the whole person in every area of human concern.

The challenge to the practitioner is to understand and change the imbalance in the whole terrain. Is it too hot (Yang)? too cold (Yin)? too assertive (Yang)? too passive (Yin)? too damp (a kind of Yin)? too windy (a kind of Yang)? too metallic, too earthy, etc?

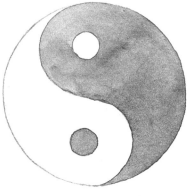

Yin and Yang

Points and meridians

The acupuncturist's principal method of changing disharmony of the bodily chi is by stimulating specific points on the body. These acupuncture points lie along an invisible system of channels or meridians that are thought to link the various energies in the body. There are 14 main meridians that connect the interior of the body with the exterior. Classical theory recognizes about 365 acupuncture points on the surface portions of these channels, but the total number has now risen to at least 2,000.

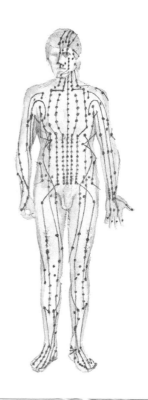

Meridians' associations

The meridian system is made up of 12 regular meridians (see below) that correspond to the vital organs of the body. Together with the Governing and Conception Vessels, these constitute the 14 major meridians. Each of the Five Elements governs a pair of meridians, one Yin and one Yang (except for Fire which has two pairs) and has several different associations.

Mapping the meridians

The pathways of the meridians were first charted many thousands of years ago, but they have since been mapped and measured by modern technological methods. Yin meridians run from the toes upward. Yang meridians run from the head and fingertips down to the toes. As translated for use in the modern therapy "touch for health", they are illustrated on pages 254-5.

MERIDIANS, ELEMENTS, AND THEIR ASSOCIATIONS

Element	Fire	Earth	Metal	Water	Wood
Yin meridian	Heart Heart Constrictor (Pericardium)	Spleen	Lung	Kidney	Liver
Yang meridian	Triple Heater (Triple Burner) Small Intestine	Stomach	Large Intestine	Bladder	Gall Bladder
Tissue	blood vessels	flesh	skin	bone	muscle
Emotion	joy	sympathy	grief	fear	anger
Color	red	yellow/orange orange	white	blue/black	green
Manner in time of change	sadness/ grief/ melancholy/	stubbornness	coughing/ nervous scratching	trembling	control
Sound	laughing	singing	weeping	groaning	shouting
Season	summer	late summer	autumn	winter	spring

Consulting an acupuncturist

Acupuncture is a highly skilled art and is not at all
suited to self-help therapy. After listening to your
complaint, the acupuncturist will concentrate on
trying to locate the disharmony that underlies your
problem. He or she will enquire into every facet of
your life, since the oriental viewpoint sees a person's
physical, mental, emotional, behavioral, social and
spiritual life as intertwined – all are manifestations of
chi, Yin and Yang or the Five Elements (p.270).

Exploring the terrain

In deciding on a course of
treatment, an acupuncturist
looks for signs that may seem
strange to modern western
thinking. Does a hot bath
help? Is the symptom
different in winter? Do you
have a strange taste in your
mouth? Do you feel different
in the evening than you do in
the morning? Who makes
you angry? And what are
your motivations in life?

The acupuncturist will also
examine parts of the body
that other medical systems
may not find important. He
or she may feel your skin or
the palms of your hands, and
look at your tongue – its
texture, color, size, and
moisture level provide a
litmus test of the quality of
your inner terrain.

Finally, all acupuncturists
will feel your pulse at both
wrists, a crucial part of
oriental diagnosis. There are
many different qualities that
can be perceived in the pulse
(wiry, slippery, rough,
leathery, hollow, etc) that give
the therapist valuable
information. Taking all these
findings together the skilled
acupuncturist's ultimate
diagnosis will amount to a
description of the imbalances
in the quality of your chi.

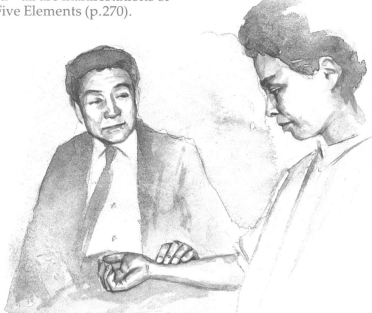

Feeling the pulse

*Treating a stiff or "frozen"
shoulder*

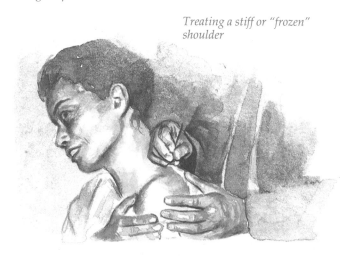

Acupuncture treatment

The main tool for changing the disharmony which causes ill health is the stimulation of specific acupuncture points. Each point has a defined therapeutic action: one can increase a particular kind of Yin in the lungs, for example, while another adds to a particular kind of Yang in the kidneys. The acupuncturist chooses to insert needles at those points that are most appropriate for treating a particular individual's pattern of disharmony.

The depth to which a needle penetrates varies; needles are inserted only one or two millimetres deep at the finger points, for example. Modern needles are made of stainless steel, and are of hairlike thinness. They produce relatively little or no discomfort when inserted correctly. They are sterilized between uses and cannot transmit infections.

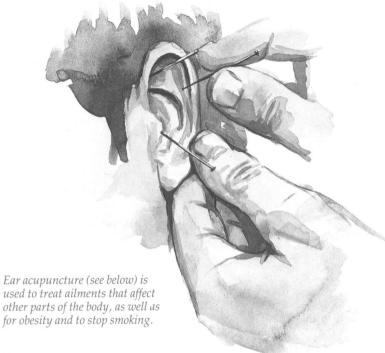

Ear acupuncture (see below) is used to treat ailments that affect other parts of the body, as well as for obesity and to stop smoking.

Ear acupuncture

This is also known as auriculotherapy. Each ear has over a hundred points, with reflex connections to other organs and parts of the body. By inserting needles in points on the outer ear, pain and other disorders elsewhere in the body can be relieved effectively.

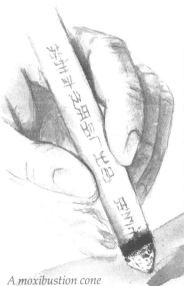

A moxibustion cone

Herbs, heat, and other treatments

While the most common method of stimulating acupuncture points is with needles, acupuncturists may also use other treatments. The application of heat from certain burning substances (usually mugwort, *Artemisia vulgaris*), known as moxibustion, is common. Hand massage techniques (akin to Japanese shiatsu) or "cupping" (applying heated vessels to create a vacuum) can also be used on acupuncture points. And sometimes an acupuncturist may use modern technology, such as electrical or even laser stimulation.

Practitioners with extensive training may also use treatments from other branches of oriental medicine. China's herbal tradition, for example, is very old and complex, and is frequently employed along with acupuncture. Physical exercises or dietary adjustments may also be recommended.

Shiatsu

Shiatsu, which literally means "finger pressure", is a traditional Japanese healing art. It is a form of physical manipulation, but very different from most forms of massage in the West, since there are no kneading, friction, or smooth flowing strokes. Instead, pressure and stretching are used almost exclusively. The practitioner uses the palms, fingers, thumbs, knuckles, elbows, knees, and even the feet to work on the hundreds of tsubos, or acupuncture points, along the body's meridians or energy channels. The technique could be described as "touch communication". In Chinese medicine there is a related therapy, acupressure, (p.275).

Primarily a preventive medicine, shiatsu is simple, safe, and effective, helping to balance an individual's energy flow and to strengthen the vital organs, in order to maintain health and vitality. The therapy encompasses the whole being at the physical, psychological, emotional and spiritual levels, and offers a way of treating each person as an individual, not just the disease or its symptoms. It helps to relieve many kinds of acute and chronic health problems, ranging from everyday ailments to injuries

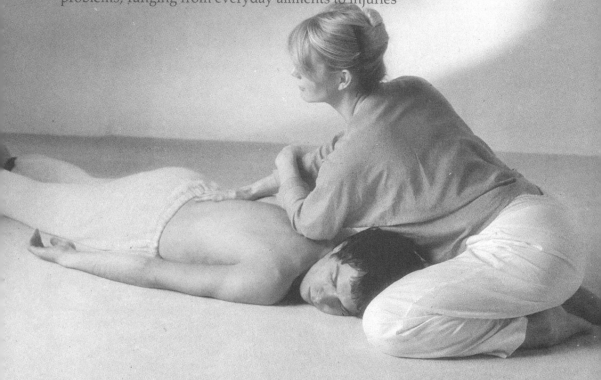

and stress-related disorders. It is also used to reduce pain in childbirth. Today, shiatsu is increasingly popular in the West, and it is now taught in specialist schools in America and Europe.

Origins and philosophy

The roots of shiatsu go back thousands of years, probably to before the beginnings of acupuncture. It is in fact simply an extension of our natural response to pain, of the impulse that makes us "rub it better" when hurt. It developed from the ancient Japanese massage known as amna, which consisted of pressing or rubbing the hands and feet with the fingers and palms of the hands. Amna was mainly practiced by the blind, and it was given more for pleasure than as a therapy.

Shiatsu emerged as an independent therapy at the turn of the century. Originally it used pressure over combinations of acupuncture points to treat specific conditions. But this method was largely replaced by the late Master Shizuto Masunaga who advocated a way of treatment based on the Five Elements theory (p.270) and the "kyo-jitsu" principle (see below) – a method tailored more to individuals than to the problems from which they were suffering.

With acupuncture and traditional Chinese medicine shiatsu shares the view that natural phenomena are different aspects of ki energy (Japanese for chi), and that they are all manifestations of the Five Elements – Fire, Earth, Metal, Water, and Wood. All phenomena are further divided into two complementary energy forces – Yin, or negative, and Yang, or positive (p.270). The human body is viewed as a microcosm of the universe; the meridians and the vital organs are seen as being governed by the Five Elements and by Yin and Yang (see Meridians' associations, p.271). Their function encompasses the whole being, from the physical to the spiritual level. In a healthy person no element is dominant or deficient in relation to the others.

In shiatsu, disease is regarded as the result of energy being blocked or unbalanced, so that it is either depleted (kyo) or over-active (jitsu). The symptom of a disorder is believed to be manifest as jitsu, on the surface, but its cause is believed to lie with the kyo, deep-seated and hidden. The practitioner concentrates on tonifying the kyo or depleted

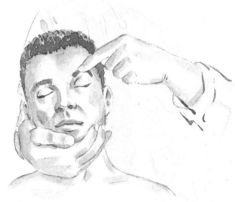

Acupressure
Like shiatsu, acupressure involves pressing specific points on the meridians to stimulate or sedate the flow of vital energy in the body. But whereas shiatsu involves pressure with elbows and knees as well as different parts of the hands, acupressure uses finger pressure only.

meridians and sedating the jitsu or over-active ones, thus enabling the body's natural balance to re-establish itself.

Consulting a shiatsu therapist

A typical shiatsu session lasts between 40 and 60 minutes. In making a diagnosis, the therapist concentrates less on the disease or disorder, more on how it manifests in your daily life, and on how you respond to it. He or she also assesses your ability to return to a state of balance or health. Diagnosis is made through observation (Bo-shin); through sound (Bun-shin); questioning (Mon-shin); and touch (Setsu-shin). The practitioner needs to cultivate skill in seeing, hearing, and sensing what is hidden.

In the past, doctors of oriental medicine are said to have received payment for keeping their clients in good health. Should a client fall ill, the doctor would cease receiving payment – until the client regained good health.

To receive treatment you will be asked to lie on a mat on the floor, wearing loose clothing made of natural fibers. The practitioner will then use his or her whole body – hands, elbows, knees, and feet – to work on balancing your meridians. Applying pressure to the appropriate points corrects the imbalances of energy within the meridian, re-establishing the natural flow of ki in the body. Treatment may also involve muscle stretches designed to correct injuries or structural imbalances. Through touch, there is two-way communication for the benefit of the patient.

In common with many natural therapies, shiatsu treatment works on the whole being, from the physical to the spiritual level. It is also highly individual – two people suffering from the same disorder may well require very different types of treatment. But in both cases, the overall aim will be to increase the body's natural healing power by re-balancing the flow of energy. As a patient you can help the healing process by taking a keen interest in your treatment, and in particular by not eating a heavy meal, drinking any alcohol or taking strenuous activity just before or after a treatment session. After a session you may be given specific corrective exercises, or advice on breathing, relaxation, or diet.

During or after treatment, you can expect to experience a variety of reactions – the release of tears, for example, a slight discomfort from energy shifting in the body, joy, laughter, or stillness. These reactions are nothing to worry about; in fact, they are a good sign, since they indicate that the body is breaking through old energy patterns.

Practicing shiatsu

You can bring relief to a number of everyday disorders at home, using a simplified form of shiatsu therapy. The secret of good shiatsu lies in the quality of the communication between giver and receiver.

It is best to apply pressure as the receiver breathes out as this is the time when he or she will be most relaxed. The safest techniques to use are thumb pressure and palm pressure since these are most easily controlled. When giving shiatsu, always keep both your hands in contact with the receiver – use one hand for applying pressure and place your resting hand near the area you are working on.

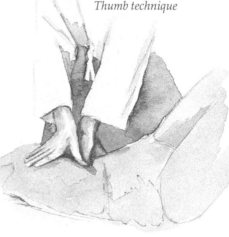

Thumb technique

The importance of posture
For an effective shiatsu treatment, it is essential that both the giver and the receiver are relaxed. As the giver, the correct posture means that at all times you should feel the pressure you apply coming from the hara, the center of energy in your belly, and not from your upper body, shoulders or wrists. It is also important that you are able to press the tsubos from a 90° angle, with your thumb or palm working perpendicular to the body.

Keep your knees apart, to ensure a solid base and to allow you to apply pressure from the hara. If your knees are too close, you will not be able to sustain the pressure. For most ailments, the receiver should be lying on a mat or rug on the floor, as shown right. A few ailments may be treated with the receiver in a chair, if the relevant tsubos are accessible in that position.

Thumb pressure
The thumbs are the basic tools for the beginner, since most of the tsubos are to be found in thumb-sized hollows along the meridians. Pressure is normally applied with one thumb; where the tsubo demands the use of both thumbs, use one on top of the other, as shown above right. Use the pad of the thumb and let the rest of your hand stay in touch with the receiver's body, keeping contact, and helping to support you.

Palm pressure
Palm pressure should be used only to work on the receiver's "hara" or belly. Using your whole palm, not just the heel of the hand, press straight down, at right angles to the receiver's body, as shown below.

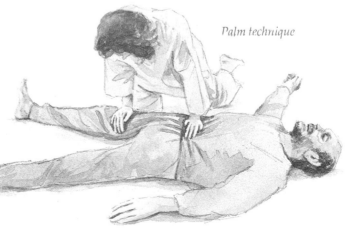

Palm technique

Locating the tsubos

Practicing shiatsu involves learning to locate precise points on the body, along the meridians or energy channels, and pressing them correctly, for the prescribed number of seconds. The duration and strength of pressure vary according to each tsubo's properties. The points are described below in abbreviated form; their names define which meridian they are on. Most of the meridians are bilateral and therefore involve pressing tsubos on *both* sides of the body, legs, arms and so on.

Abbreviations
Lu – Lung
LI – Large Intestine
Sp – Spleen
St – Stomach
K – Kidney
B – Bladder
Liv – Liver
GB – Gall Bladder
CV – Conception Vessel
GV – Governing Vessel

Face and head tsubos: Figure a

In Do Between the eyebrows on the Governing Vessel meridian. Press hard and inward for 7-10 seconds, 3 times, using both thumbs.

Tai Yo One finger's width to the side of the eyebrow, between the end of the eyebrow and the outer edge of the eye. Press with one thumb for 7-10 seconds.

St 3 Lateral to the base of the nose, on a line directly below the pupils when looking straight ahead. Press with one thumb, hard and inward, for 5-7 seconds.

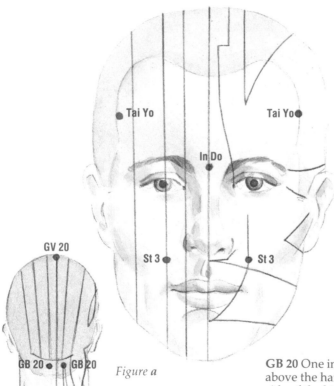

Figure a

GB 20 One inch (2.5 cm) above the hairline, on the side of the big muscle in the neck. Press with one thumb for 7-10 seconds, 3 times.

GV 20 In the middle of the line connecting the upper edge of the two ears (via the crown), at the center of the head. Press hard and downward for 10-15 seconds with both thumbs.

Front of body tsubos:
Figure b
Lu 1 The point between the 1st and 2nd ribs, 1 inch (2.5 cm) below the middle of the clavicle. Press with one thumb for 7-10 seconds.

St 25 Two inches (5 cm) to either side of the navel. Press inward, deeply and gradually, using one thumb or the palm of your hand.

CV 3 On the midline of the abdomen, 4 inches (10 cm) below the navel. Press inward and gradually with the palm of the hand.

CV 6 On the midline of the abdomen, 1 ½ inches (3.8 cm) below the navel. Press inward and gradually with the palm of the hand for 10-15 seconds.

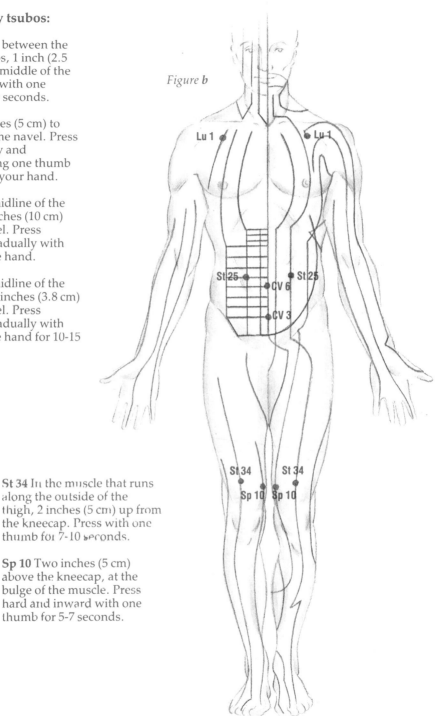

Figure b

St 34 In the muscle that runs along the outside of the thigh, 2 inches (5 cm) up from the kneecap. Press with one thumb for 7-10 seconds.

Sp 10 Two inches (5 cm) above the kneecap, at the bulge of the muscle. Press hard and inward with one thumb for 5-7 seconds.

Side of body tsubos:
Figure c

LI 4 Midway between the two bones of the thumb and index finger in the fleshiest part. Press hard with one thumb for 7-10 seconds.

LI 11 Bend the receiver's elbow at 90°; this point is at the end of the crease on the outside of the arm. Press hard with one thumb for 10-15 seconds.

B 36 At the midpoint of the fold of the buttocks, over the thigh bone. Press for 10-15 seconds, 3 times, using one thumb.

B 57 At the beginning of the bulge of the calf muscle (when the muscle is tensed). Press with one thumb, while the receiver lies on his or her stomach.

B 60 On the ankle, midway between the Achilles tendon and the top of the ankle bone. Press with one thumb for 7-10 seconds, 3 times.

GB 31 To locate (but not to treat) this point, the receiver should stand up, arms at sides, with the hands touching the thighs. GB 31 is to be found on the leg, just below the spot where the tip of the middle finger rests. Press gradually and inward for 10-15 seconds, using both thumbs.

St 36 To find this point, hold the kneecap on either side between index finger and thumb. Place your middle finger on the outside of the shin bone. The tip will rest on St 36. Use both thumbs and press for 7-10 seconds.

Sp 6 To find this point, flex the receiver's foot and put his or her 4 fingers on the inside of the leg, with the little finger resting on top of the ankle bone. Sp 6 is behind the shinbone at the 4th finger. Using both thumbs, press for 7-10 seconds.
Caution Do not press Spleen 6 during pregnancy.

Liv 4 Halfway between the front edge of the ankle bone and the top of the foot. Use one thumb, press for 7-10 seconds, 3 times.

K 1 On the sole of the foot, a third of the distance from the tip of the middle toe to the heel, between the 2nd and 3rd toe joints. Press hard and inward, using both thumbs, for 10-15 seconds.

K 3 On the outside of the ankle bone, halfway between the Achilles tendon and the tip of the ankle bone. Press with one thumb for 7-10 seconds.

Back of body tsubos:
Figure d

GB 21 Draw an imaginary line straight upward from the nipple; the point at which it crosses the shoulder is GB 21. Press firmly but gradually and inward with one thumb for 10-15 seconds.

B 10 Just below the 1st cervical vertebra at the side of the spine. Use one thumb for 7-10 seconds, 3 times.

B 12 Between the 2nd and 3rd thoracic vertebrae, 1½ inches (3.8 cm) to the side of the spine. Press with one thumb for 7-10 seconds, 3 times.

B 18 Between the 9th and 10th thoracic vertebrae, 1½ inches (3.8 cm) to the side. Press with one thumb for 5-7 seconds, 3 times.

B 20 Between the 11th and 12th thoracic vertebrae, 1½ inches (3.8 cm) to the side. Press with one thumb for 5-7 seconds, 3 times.

B 21 Between the 12th thoracic and 1st lumbar vertebrae, 1½ inches (3.8 cm) to the side. Press with one thumb for 5-7 seconds, 3 times.

B 22 Between the 1st and 2nd lumbar vertebrae, 1½ inches (3.8 cm) to the side. Use one thumb for 5-7 seconds, 3 times.

B 23 Between the 2nd and 3rd lumbar vertebrae, 1½ inches (3.8 cm) to the side. Press with one thumb for 5-7 seconds, 3 times.

B 52 Between the 2nd and 3rd lumbar vertebrae, 3 inches (7.6 cm) to the side. Use one thumb for 7-10 seconds.

Ten Shi 3 inches (7.6 cm) from the hip bone, toward the buttocks. Press inward, with one thumb, 10-15 seconds, 3 times.

B 25 Between the 4th and 5th lumbar vertebrae, 1½ inches (3.8 cm) to the side. Press hard and inward with one thumb for 5-7 seconds, 3 times.

B 26 Between the 5th lumbar vertebra and the pelvic bone, 1½ inches (3.8 cm) to the side. Press for 5-7 seconds using one thumb, 3 times.

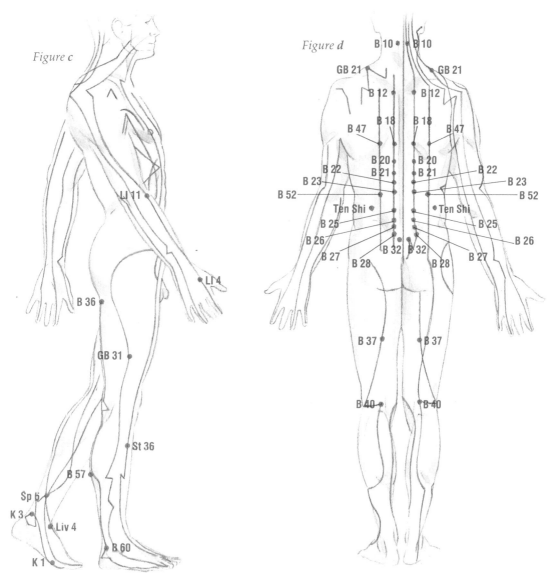

Figure c

Figure d

B 27 In the first pair of hollows or "foramina", in the sacrum, 1½ inches (3.8 cm) to the side of the midline. Press for 5-7 seconds, 3 times, using one thumb.

B 28 In the second foramen in the sacrum, 1½ inches (3.8 cm) to the side of the midline. Press for 5-7 seconds, 3 times, using one thumb.

B 32 3 inches (7.6 cm) to the side of the midline, level with B 28. Press for 5-7 seconds, 3 times, using one thumb.

B 37 On the midline of the back of the thigh, 6 inches (15.2 cm) from the buttocks' fold. Press hard, in, and up for 10-15 seconds, 3 times, using both thumbs.

B 40 On the back of the knee between the tendons on the fold where the knee bends. Press with both thumbs, softly and in, for 7-10 seconds, 3 times.

B 47 Between the 9th and 10th thoracic vertebrae, 3 inches (7.6 cm) to the side. Press with one thumb for 5-7 seconds, 3 times.

Ailments and remedies

You can give shiatsu treatment for a variety of common ailments, using the techniques described on page 277. The tsubos, given here in abbreviated form, are shown on Figures a, b, c, and d on the preceding pages. Whether you practice shiatsu on yourself or on someone else, you should always press the tsubos in the order given below. In general, the pressure you apply should feel comfortable to the receiver; if there is a slight pain it will soon go. If the receiver experiences, sharp, strong, or sudden pain, then stop pressing at once, since this may indicate internal problems. If any ailment persists for more than a few days, or if it returns at regular intervals, seek advice and treatment from a professional therapist.

Caution Do not give shiatsu to anyone who is extremely exhausted or who has a high fever, a contagious skin disease, a slipped disc, broken bones, or to anyone who is taking cortisone.

Respiratory problems

The common cold should not be left untreated or suppressed with drugs. To bring relief use the tsubos: Lu 1 (Fig b); LI 4, 11 (Fig c); St 36 (Fig c); B 10, 12 (Fig d).

For sore throats, use the following tsubos: Lu 1 (Fig b); LI 4 (Fig c).

For sinus congestion, press the tsubos: LI 4 (Fig c); B 20 (Fig d); St 3 (Fig a).

Diarrhea, indigestion

In cases of diarrhea the sufferer must drink plenty of liquids and keep the back and belly warm. For relief, use the following tsubos: Ten Shi (Fig d); St 34 (Fig b); St 36 (Fig c); K 1 (Fig c).

For indigestion press the tsubo St 36 (Fig c) on each leg.

Constipation

A high-fiber diet and exercise help to encourage the elimination of wastes. To bring relief, use the tsubos: CV 6 (Fig b); St 25 (Fig b); St 36 (Fig c); LI 4, 11 (Fig c); B 23, 25, 32 (Fig d). Give gentle massage to the belly, clockwise, starting at the lower left side, to promote circulation and relaxation. During pregnancy, use the tsubos: B 23, 25, 32 (Fig d); LI 4 (Fig c); St 36 (Fig c).

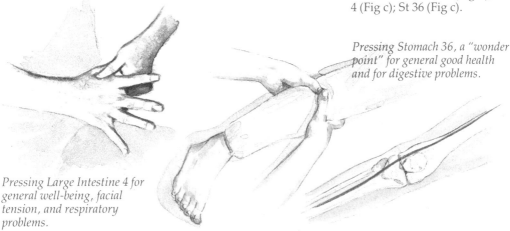

Pressing Stomach 36, a "wonder point" for general good health and for digestive problems.

Pressing Large Intestine 4 for general well-being, facial tension, and respiratory problems.

Stomach cramps

Keep the lower back and belly warm. Rub the hara or belly gently in a clockwise direction, especially around the navel. Use the tsubos: St 25, 34 (Fig b); St 36 (Fig c); B 21, 22 (Fig d).

Hemorrhoids

Constipation, over-eating, and a diet rich in protein and dairy products can cause this complaint. For relief, use the tsubos: CV 3, 6 (Fig b); GV 20 (Fig a); B 18, 23, 25, 26 (Fig d). During pregnancy use the tsubos: GV 20 (Fig a); B 18, 23, 25, 26, 28, 32 (Fig d).

Insomnia

Make sure you get enough exercise during the day. Do some light stretching exercises (pp.54-5) and gently massage the soles of the feet before going to bed. Use the tsubos: Tai Yo, GV 20 (Fig a); B 25 (Fig d); K1 (Fig c).

Backache and sciatica

For backache or sciatica apply hot towels to the lower back to promote the circulation. Give shiatsu first to the side of the back that is not in pain, and then to the painful side.

To relieve back pain use the tsubos: B 25, 26, 27, 28 (Fig d); B 36 (Fig c); B 52 (Fig d); B 60 (Fig c); Ten Shi (Fig d). For backache during pregnancy, use tsubos: Ten Shi (Fig d); B 25, 26 (Fig d); Liv 4 (Fig c).

To relieve the pain of sciatica use the tsubos: B 23, 25, 26, 37, 40, 52 (Fig d); B 57, 60 (Fig c); GB 31 (Fig c); St 36 (Fig c); Ten Shi (Fig d).

Shoulder stiffness

Poor posture and also bad elimination can cause stiff shoulders. Taking more outdoor exercise, such as walking, can relieve the stagnation of energy and strengthen the hara. For relief use the tsubos: B 23, 25, 26 (Fig d); GB 20 (Fig a), GB 21 (Fig d).

Leg cramp

This can be due to lack of exercise, poor circulation or bad digestion. It may be necessary to adjust your diet and take regular exercise. Use the tsubos: B 57 (Fig c); GB 31 (Fig c); St 36 (Fig c).

Headaches

Stress, muscular tension, bad posture, inactivity, or worry can cause headaches. For relief use the tsubos: B 10, 20 (Fig d); B 60 (Fig c); GB 20 (Fig a); GB 21 (Fig d); LI 4, 11; St 36 (Fig c); In Do, Tai Yo (Fig a). For headaches during pregnancy use the tsubos: B 10, 20 (Fig d); K 3 (Fig c); In Do, Tai Yo (Fig a).

Menstrual pain

It is important to take plenty of exercise, to relieve pelvic congestion and promote circulation in the general area of the pelvis. To bring relief, use tsubos: Sp 6 (Fig c); Sp 10 (Fig b); CV 6 (Fig b); K1 (Fig c); B 23, 32 (Fig d).

Menopausal problems

Women going through the menopause can experience a variety of discomforting symptoms. Professional diagnosis is necessary, but you can help the body to normalize itself, using the tsubos: Sp 6 (Fig c); Sp 10 (Fig b); B 23, 47 (Fig d).

Morning sickness

This is due to hormonal changes and the release of toxins, and it usually stops in the fourth month of pregnancy when the placenta is fully formed. Use the tsubos: B 10, 20 (Fig d); GB 20 (Fig a). (For backache, headaches, hemorrhoids, and constipation during pregnancy, refer to the relevant ailment.)

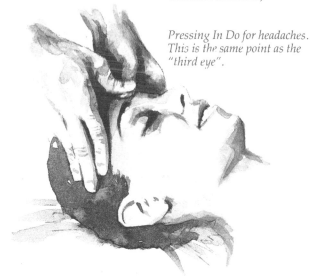

Pressing In Do for headaches. This is the same point as the "third eye".

Yoga

Yoga is a complete science of life which evolved in India over thousands of years. One of the oldest systems of personal development in the world, it deals with every aspect of physical, mental and spiritual health. It is above all a way of health, preventing disease by maintaining harmony and correcting imbalances before they have a chance to become established and cause serious harm. Hatha Yoga – the branch of yoga that is the most widely known outside India – focuses on teaching the physical exercises. As practiced in the West, it consists mainly of simple stretching, breathing and relaxation exercises. The exercises, however, are not just physical workouts – they are psycho-physical, for mental awareness plays a vital part in their practice.

In the philosophy of yoga, the physical body is seen as a vehicle, the mind as the driver, and the soul as our true identity. Action, emotion and intelligence are the three forces that move the body-vehicle. Yoga seeks to balance these three for integrated self-development and, ultimately self-realization – the state of inner peace that we are all consciously or unconsciously seeking. As recently as 20 years ago,

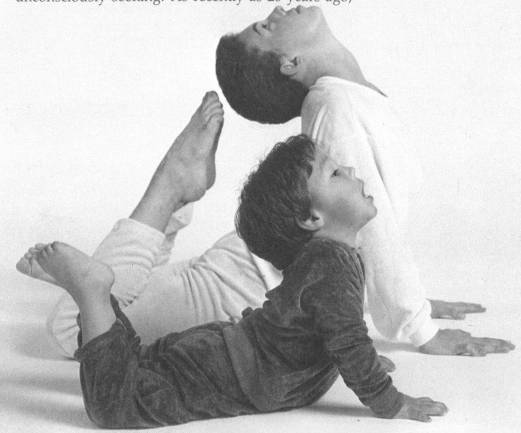

anyone who practiced yoga was considered mildly eccentric, at least to western eyes. Now, however, it is widely taught, both in classes and individually. The growth of interest has been phenomenal, and while at first it was particularly popular among women, as a way of keeping supple and fit, today it is also enjoyed by an increasing number of men, especially as an aid to stress management.

Yoga is universally applicable and can be practiced by people at all ages and stages of life. With its rich therapeutic tradition it can help in the prevention, cure and management of a wide range of disorders (including respiratory, digestive, musculoskeletal, and nervous conditions), in pregnancy and child-birth, in rehabilitation following operations or acci-dents, in caring for the disabled and in the treatment of drug addiction. Psychological problems too are helped, and today many doctors are recommending it as a way to achieve deep relaxation and balance.

"In Yoga, the asanas or postures lubricate the body. They keep the muscles and joints running smoothly, tone all the internal organs, and increase circulation without creating any fatigue. The body is cooled by complete relaxation, whilst pranayama or yogic breathing increases prana, the electric current. Fuel is provided by food, water and the air you breathe. Lastly, you have meditation which stills the mind, the driver of the body."
Swami Vishnu Devananda

The origins and philosophy of yoga

It is not known exactly when yoga first began – but certainly from archaeological evidence it seems its origins date back at least 5,000 years. Mention is first made of it in the collection of scriptures called the Vedas, parts of which date from at least 2,500 BC, but it is in a later portion of the Vedas, the Upanishads, that the main foundation of its teaching is found.

Yoga literally means "union" or joining, and its ultimate goal is self-realization – the joining of the individual soul with the divine or Absolute. In the philosophy of yoga people are regarded as beings in the process of evolution, learning through experience in this world. Yoga sees the world as permeated with a subtle form of energy called prana. There are close analogies between the concepts of prana in yoga, chi in acupuncture (p.270), and healing energy in western healing (pp.298-303). In the human body, prana flows along channels, known as nadis (equiva-lent to the meridians of acupuncture) and is concen-trated in centres of energy called chakras.

Yoga sees ill health as partly due to imbalances and blockages in the flow of prana and seeks to correct these through its practices. The asanas or physical postures and pranayama or breathing exercises that together constitute Hatha Yoga are designed to purify the body so that prana can flow more freely. Some yogis are capable of consciously directing prana to parts of the body, to revitalize and regenerate them.

The asanas or postures work systematically on all parts of the body, stretching and toning muscles, keeping spine and joints flexible and promoting better breathing and circulation. Some asanas improve balance, others develop particular muscles, while the inverted postures such as the headstand and shoulderstand particularly benefit circulation and the endocrine glands. Many of the asanas massage the internal organs and act on trigger points in the body, serving to stimulate your energy in the same way as a session of shiatsu or acupuncture. Deep relaxation, of fundamental importance in yoga, further releases tensions and renews both mind and body. Hatha yoga includes both relaxation and activation exercises, which together result in homeostasis, the balancing of the body's processes and systems. All systems of the body are affected, including the musculoskeletal, nervous, respiratory, circulatory, endocrine, and immunological.

Breathing exercises or pranayama are central to the practice of yoga, because respiration is a key link between the conscious and unconscious processes of the body. Unlike circulation or digestion, we can consciously control our breathing, not only affecting the exchange of oxygen and carbon dioxide but also the muscles and nerve plexuses in the torso. Meditation too is an essential part of serious yoga practice. It acts directly on the brain and nervous system, and leads to heightened awareness, making people more sensitive to the needs of body and mind. While it is clearly linked to Hinduism, the religion of its homeland, yoga is in essence non-sectarian and can be practiced without any religious beliefs or indeed in association with other religions. Various schools of yoga differ in the relative emphasis they lay on asanas, pranayama and meditation, but all three practices are essential for sound health at all levels.

The health benefits of yoga

Critical scientific research has confirmed that advanced yogis have remarkable control over the functioning of their heart, lungs and nervous system. In studies subjects have demonstrated their ability drastically to decrease their heartbeat and respiration rate for hours at a time. Even in lay people simple yoga exercises can have marked physiological effects: Dr Chandra Patel's impressive studies with high blood pressure in London, UK, have shown how patients can influence bodily functions – even those previously thought to be outside conscious control – through the practice of yogic relaxation techniques.

There is a wealth of anecdotal evidence that yoga can provide help for many disorders and research work is starting to confirm this. In a survey of 3,000 yoga students carried out by the Yoga Biomedical Trust (Cambridge, England), many claimed to have fewer minor ailments than before taking up yoga and to be less dependent upon tranquillizers, sleeping pills, and other forms of medication. The respondents reported that they had been helped with every one of the disorders on which they were questioned (see table right). Further analysis revealed that some disorders, such as back pain, improved within a few weeks of taking up yoga, while others, like migraine, took a year or two. Controlled trials have confirmed that yoga promotes vitality and is effective in the management of heart conditions, high blood pressure, asthma, psychological problems and drug addiction. In general yoga leads to reduced medication and normalization of levels of hormones and other body chemicals.

The practice of yoga

The foundations of yoga are best learned from an experienced teacher. Though books, cassettes and videos can all help, there is no substitute for the initial guidance of a skilled instructor in the correct performance of asanas and pranayama. Classes are both economic, enjoyable, and stimulating, since you gain inspiration from observing others. All proper yoga classes follow a basic sequence of postures. Breathing and purification exercises (such as the nasal wash, p.290, and abdominal contraction, p.291) are often integrated into the asana session and meditation too may be included.

To be effective, yoga must be practiced regularly, but the benefits are felt right from the start, long before you reach the "perfect pose". Half an hour a day is sufficient for the average person. For chronic conditions an hour or more a day may be needed, over some months, or even years. However yoga is less time-consuming than you might think since it reduces the time needed for sleep.

Survey of ailments benefited by yoga, 1983-84

Summary of 3,000 responses to the Yoga Biomedical Trust survey.

Ailment	Number of cases reported	% Claiming benefit
Back pain	1,142	98
Arthritis or rheumatism	589	90
Anxiety	838	94
Migraine	464	80
Insomnia	542	82
Nerve or muscle disease	112	96
Premenstrual tension	848	77
Menstrual problems	317	68
Menopause disorders	247	83
Hypertension	150	84
Heart disease	50	94
Asthma or bronchitis	226	88
Duodenal ulcers	40	90
Hemorrhoids	391	88
Obesity	240	74
Diabetes	10	80
Cancer	29	90
Tobacco addiction	219	74
Alcoholism	26	100

Basic yoga exercises

The asanas described below form a short but balanced sequence, good for health maintenance, and for many ailments (pp.290-3). All you need is a light, airy room, a mat or blanket, and loose, light clothing. It is best to practice at the same time each day (at least two hours should have elapsed since your last meal). Ideally you should start with a few rounds of the salute to the sun (pp.54-5), to loosen your body up. Then follow the sequence below, going only as far into each pose as feels comfortable.

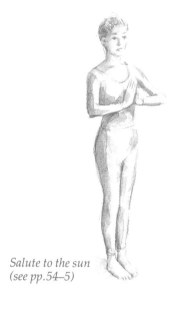

Salute to the sun (see pp.54–5)

1,8 Corpse pose
Always begin and end your practice with a few minutes in the corpse pose (p.63).

2 Shoulderstand
Lie on your back, legs together, hands palms down by your sides. Inhale and, pushing down on your hands, swing your legs up over your head. Now raise your hips up off the floor, and support your upper back with your hands as far down as possible – this is the half shoulderstand. Exhaling, bring your legs up to vertical and straighten your spine, into the full shoulderstand. Breathe slowly and deeply. To release the pose, lower your legs and slowly uncurl. *Caution* Avoid inverted poses if you suffer from high blood pressure.

3 Fish
Lying on your back, legs straight, feet together, put your hands under your thighs, palms down. Inhale, press down on your elbows, and arch your back to bring the very top of your head to rest on the floor. Breathe deeply, then slowly release.

4 Forward bend
Sit up straight, legs together in front of you. Pull the flesh out from under your buttocks to enable you to sit directly on the pelvic bone. Stretch your arms above your head. Now exhale, pulling in the abdomen and, leading with your chest, fold forward. Bring your torso down to your thighs and hold on to whichever part of your legs or feet you can reach comfortably. Breathe deeply, and stretch forward a little further on each exhalation.

5 Cobra
Lie on your front with your forehead resting on the floor and your hands palms down under your shoulders. Inhaling, raise your head up and then your chest, using your back muscles. Slowly straighten your arms and look up and back. Breathe in, then exhale as you slowly release the position.

6 Half spinal twist
Kneel down then sit to the right of your feet. Bend your left leg over your right, placing the left foot against the outside of the right knee. Bring your right arm down on the outside of the left knee to grasp the foot, and place your left hand on the floor behind you. Exhaling, twist to the left. Repeat, reversing the directions.

7 Triangle
Stand up straight, feet well apart (3-4 ft or 1 m), with the left foot pointing to the left and the right turned in slightly. Stretch your arms out to the sides, palms down. Inhale, then as you exhale, bend to the left and slightly forward. Slide your left hand down your leg, grasping the lowest part possible and bring your right arm up vertically. Turn your head to look up at your right hand. After a few full breaths, release the position and repeat on the other side.

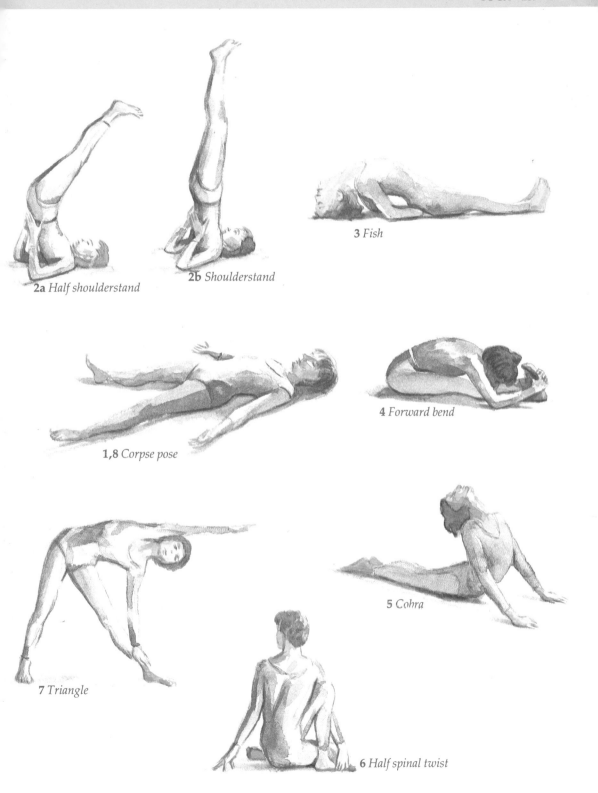

2a *Half shoulderstand*

2b *Shoulderstand*

3 *Fish*

1,8 *Corpse pose*

4 *Forward bend*

5 *Cobra*

7 *Triangle*

6 *Half spinal twist*

Ailments and remedies

Yoga is of great therapeutic benefit for a wide variety of common ailments. Whatever your ailment, however, you should be sure to make a balanced basic sequence the core of your practice (pp.288-9). For difficult chronic conditions, it is advisable to have at least some individual tuition from a skilled yoga teacher in order to work out a suitable daily routine specially tailored to your needs.
Caution Practice yoga only under expert supervision, if you are pregnant, if you have had a recent operation or accident, or if you suffer from any major illness or disorder.

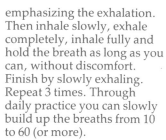

Kapalabhati

Respiratory disorders

Yoga asanas generally help most respiratory disorders, notably colds, coughs, flu, sinusitis, and hay fever. You should keep up your practice of basic asanas and pay attention to deep, rhythmic breathing (see Complete breathing, p.59). Eat a light, cleansing diet (p.193). A period of relaxation in the corpse pose (p.63) is beneficial if you have a temperature. A nasal wash (below) and kapalabhati (above right), a special breathing exercise which clears and stimulates the upper respiratory tract, may also be helpful.

Kapalabhati
Sit cross-legged with a straight back, as shown above right. Breathing through your nose, take 2 normal breaths, then inhale. Now exhale forcefully, contracting the abdomen sharply, and inhale, relaxing your abdomen. (You should consult a yoga teacher on this movement, which some people find difficult to learn.) Repeat this pumping pattern 10 times, keeping a steady rhythm, and each time

emphasizing the exhalation. Then inhale slowly, exhale completely, inhale fully and hold the breath as long as you can, without discomfort. Finish by slowly exhaling. Repeat 3 times. Through daily practice you can slowly build up the breaths from 10 to 60 (or more).

Nasal wash
This is one of the kriyas or purification exercises. Stand in front of a mirror with your head tilted back and to one side. Using a small glass or spouted pot, as shown left, pour lightly salted water into one nostril and out of the other. If the other nostril is blocked the water will flow into the mouth and you can spit it out. After repeating on the other side, blow out any excess water.

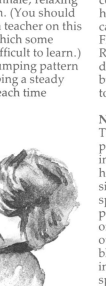

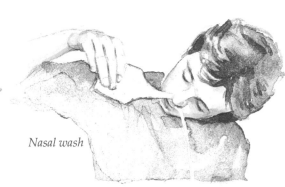

Nasal wash

Asthma and bronchitis

Asthmatics tend to hold the breath in, while slumping the shoulders and constricting the upper chest. Both asthma and bronchitis can be helped by practicing a basic sequence of asanas, including back rolls (p.292), the pelvic lift (p.293), and cobra (p.288), to open the chest and release tension in the back.

Another way of opening the upper chest and releasing tension in the shoulders, is to lie on your back over the end of your bed, arms hanging backward – now move your arms back and forth from side to back positions, feeling the stretch.

Kapalabhati (opposite) and abdominal contraction (above right) are effective for stimulating the lungs. Asanas may be followed by vigorous exercises, such as skipping or push-ups, to strengthen the respiratory and circulatory systems. A daily period of deep relaxation reduces fatigue and the build-up of tensions which lead to asthma attacks. Chanting simple vowel sounds can release tensions in the throat and stimulate lungs and brain by resonance effects.

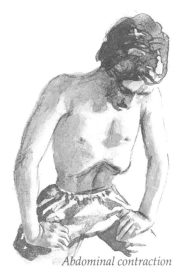

Abdominal contraction

Abdominal contraction
Stand with your knees bent, legs wide apart, hands pressing on thighs, as shown above. As you exhale, pull the abdomen in and up, hold the breath and pump the belly in and out. Stop pumping when you need to inhale, take a normal breath, then exhale and repeat. Aim for about 10 to 18 pumpings at a time.

Digestive disorders

Diet is naturally the first consideration (pp.46-7), but many disorders, such as colitis, ulcers, hemorrhoids, and constipation, are also helped by basic yoga exercises, which reduce stress and relieve tension in the abdomen. Backward and forward bending asanas (p.288) and, more specifically, kapalabhati (opposite) and abdominal contraction (left), massage abdominal organs, increasing circulation and stimulating peristaltic activity.

Obesity and thinness

Attention to diet is crucial (pp.46-7). Regular meals, followed by rest, and the corpse pose (p.63) practiced for 20 minutes daily helps remedy thinness. General yoga practice helps combat obesity by toning muscles and enhancing body awareness and willpower, facilitating a more sensible eating pattern. Leg raises (below) and abdominal contraction (above left) prevent or reduce pot bellies, and lessen the risk of incurring back disorders.

Leg raises
Lying flat on the floor, legs together, arms by your sides, inhale and raise both legs as high as possible. Exhaling, bring them down again. Repeat up to 10 times. If your abdominal or back muscles are weak, you may need to press your palms down as you lift your legs, and slightly bend your knees. Alternatively, try raising one leg at a time, as shown right. Your lower back should remain flat on the floor.

Leg raises for obesity

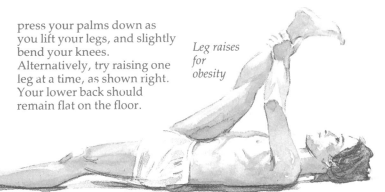

Back problems

Most asanas are excellent therapy for both the prevention and the relief of backache. The asanas stretch and release chronically tense muscles, and work on the muscles of the upper back by promoting proper breathing. For minor back problems, a basic yoga sequence is helpful. You should concentrate on asanas that work on the troublesome parts of your back. But be careful to balance backward with forward bending, and stretch yourself very gently at first. You can also safely do simple tension-releasing exercises, such as the corpse pose (p.63), shoulder rotation (below) and back rolls (above right).
Caution Advice should be sought from a skilled therapist in the case of serious disorders, such as slipped discs.

Shoulder rotation

Rotate your arms, one at a time, from the shoulder. Go forward a few times, then backward. Try it with the arms straight, then bent, as shown below.

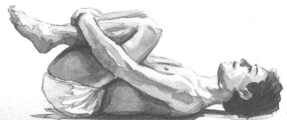
Back rolls

Back rolls

Lie on your back and bend your legs, as shown above. Interlock your hands around your knees and pull them in and down toward your chest. Now rock gently backward and forward or side to side, massaging your spine.

Arthritis

General yoga practice can help in the prevention and management of both rheumatoid and osteo-arthritis, by keeping the joints supple. Shoulder rotation, left, and hand and foot rotation, below, are extremely beneficial, helping to warm and loosen stiff joints.

Hand rotation

Slowly rotate each wrist a few times in a clockwise then counterclockwise direction. Follow this by wriggling your fingers.

Foot rotation

Sit down and put one leg across the other thigh, as shown right. Rotate the foot in each direction using your hands. Then do it without your hands. Wriggle your toes. Repeat with the other foot.

Headaches and migraine

Any form of yoga will help by relieving stress; but asanas that release tension in the upper back, shoulders and neck, such as the shoulderstand, fish and cobra (p.288) are particularly good. If you are a migraine sufferer, cut out fried foods and check your diet for allergies (see Herbalism, p.175).

Insomnia

A regular session of yoga is helpful for reducing tension. The corpse pose (p.63) may help you to fall asleep, or at least provide rest at times of sleeplessness. Back rolls, above, are also soothing, relaxing tension in the spine.

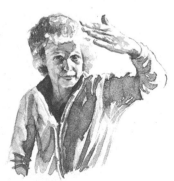
Shoulder rotation

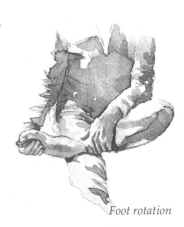
Foot rotation

Depression and anxiety

Yoga allows you to diffuse mental stress by focusing your attention on your body. For anxiety and tiredness, practicing the corpse pose is important (p.63). For depression, concentrate on the more active exercises, such as salute to the sun (pp.54-5), and kapalabhati (p.290). Simple rhythmic breathing through the nose in the ratio of 1:2 is extremely useful for stress relief. Breathe in for a count of 4 and out for a count of 8. Hyper-ventilation or overbreathing is a common problem at times of crisis; it can be overcome by learning relaxed breathing (p.59).

For yoga to help with psychological problems, it is important to complement the asanas with meditation, and perhaps some form of psychotherapy.

Menstrual disorders

Yoga eases all menstrual and premenstrual problems, primarily by relaxing tense muscles and toning the pelvic region. The corpse pose (p.63). practiced in the early stages of premenstrual tension, can reduce its subsequent severity.

Exercises which open and release tension in the lower abdomen are especially helpful – these include the half shoulderstand and the forward bend (p.288), and kapalabhati (p.290), and the pelvic lift, right, which alleviates lower back pain, promotes deep breathing and strengthens the uterus. These poses are also helpful for frigidity and impotence.

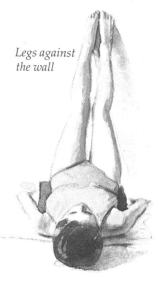

Legs against the wall

Varicose veins

Gentle rhythmic exercises (walking or swimming, for example) are beneficial. Inverted poses, such as the shoulderstand (p.288), help by reducing blood pressure in the legs.

Lying with your legs against the wall, as shown above, is restful. Put your bottom on a cushion, about 18 inches (45 cm) from the wall. Breathe slowly and deeply, and hold the pose for about 5 minutes.
Caution Avoid inverted poses if you suffer from high blood pressure.

Pelvic lift

Kneel down and support yourself with your hands. Now exhale and arch your back upward, as shown right. Hold the position for a count of 5, then inhale and arch your back downward, curving the lower back and stretching your head back. Breathe in this position, then repeat.

High blood pressure

The corpse pose (p.63), practiced for 30-60 minutes a day, after lunch, or perhaps after work, reduces high blood pressure. In addition, you should learn to relax at intervals throughout the day – try those techniques that can be practiced while sitting or even standing, such as meditation (pp.314-17) or autogenics (pp.318-19). Asanas may be practiced with care, but you should avoid holding your breath or doing inverted postures, such as the shoulderstand. The half shoulderstand (p.288) will bring blood pressure down, but should be practiced only under expert supervision. It is also essential to adjust your diet and lifestyle, to reduce undue stress.

Low blood pressure

Practice basic asanas (p.288). You can raise your blood pressure temporarily by a few minutes of inhaling deeply through the nose, then exhaling with a hissing sound.

Fatigue

See Depression and anxiety (above).

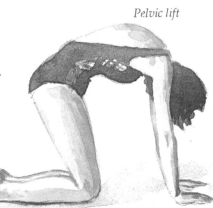

Pelvic lift

Alexander technique

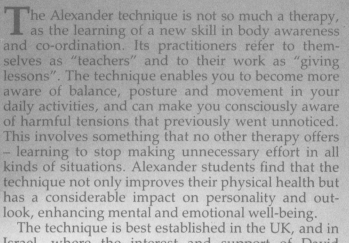

The Alexander technique is not so much a therapy, as the learning of a new skill in body awareness and co-ordination. Its practitioners refer to themselves as "teachers" and to their work as "giving lessons". The technique enables you to become more aware of balance, posture and movement in your daily activities, and can make you consciously aware of harmful tensions that previously went unnoticed. This involves something that no other therapy offers – learning to stop making unnecessary effort in all kinds of situations. Alexander students find that the technique not only improves their physical health but has a considerable impact on personality and outlook, enhancing mental and emotional well-being.

The technique is best established in the UK, and in Israel, where the interest and support of David Ben-Gurion, the first prime minister, encouraged its spread. There are currently about 250 teachers in the UK, another 250 in the rest of Europe, Israel and Australia, and 300 in North America. The technique has a close connection with the performing arts; many of the great academies of music and drama employ Alexander teachers to help their students.

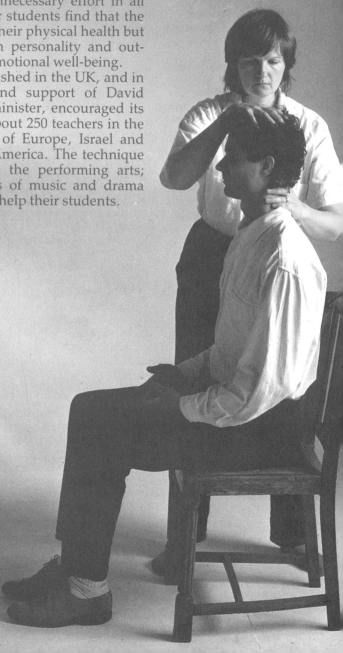

Alexander's discovery

Frederick Matthias Alexander, from whom the technique takes its name, was an Australian actor, born in 1869. Afflicted by recurrent hoarseness and breathing difficulties on stage, he set out on a long and painstaking process of self-observation in order to discover the cause of his problems – a process which was to lead him to unexpectedly far-reaching conclusions. What had at first seemed to be a problem concerning the use of his voice turned out to involve muscular patterns of excessive tension throughout his whole body. In addition, since the very thought of projecting his voice on stage could set off these tensions, he realized that his mental approach, the use of his mind, was also involved. Alexander called the book describing his observations *The Use of the Self*, preferring to include both mind and body in one unit, the "self".

Other actors and public speakers soon came to him for help. Simply telling people how to emulate him proved inadequate, however, and so he developed a unique form of gentle guidance, using his hands to reorganize the muscle patterns in his students' bodies and so help them to a better "use of themselves". This brought about a general improvement in health, as well as in both voice and breathing, and doctors began recommending their patients to him.

In 1900 Alexander arrived in London, where he remained until his death in 1955. Many famous people passed – quite literally – through his hands, including the playwright George Bernard Shaw, the novelist Aldous Huxley, and John Dewey, the American philosopher. After Alexander's death, interest in his work gradually waned, but in the 1970s it revived together with public enthusiasm for the holistic health disciplines.

What was it that Alexander discovered? Basically, that all of us, when making efforts to do even the simplest things, physical or mental, impose on ourselves harmful tensions that restrict our performance. We are all in the habit of interfering with the natural relationship of the head and neck to the trunk. Observe your own reactions in a tense situation – when driving, perhaps, or during a harassing time at work. Tight muscles pull the head down and clench the jaw, the chest is clamped, restricting breathing, and as the upper body is compressed, the

"[The Alexander technique] gives us all the things we have been looking for in a system of physical education – relief from strain ... improvement in physical and mental health ... and along with this a heightening of consciousness on all levels ..."
Aldous Huxley,
Ends and Means

digestive organs or lower back eventually complain. What we popularly call "bad posture" is often the accumulated residue of all those over-tense reactions which have become locked into the body.

Research studies

Controlled experiments of the technique are hard to come by, but some important studies have been undertaken. Between 1955 and 1972 Professor Frank Pierce Jones of Tufts University, Boston, USA, demonstrated changes in movement and muscle tension patterns in patients after Alexander guidance. And a study at the Columbia-Presbyterian Medical Center, New York, in 1983, showed improved breathing functions. Many eminent scientists have found the technique fully in accord with their scientific knowledge, including Sir Charles Sherrington (the great pioneer of neurophysiology), Professor Raymond Dart, and Professor Nikolaas Tinbergen (Nobel prize winner).

Learning the technique

In a series of Alexander lessons, the teacher works with the trainee individually, on a one-to-one basis, using his or her hands gently to feel out hidden tensions and distorted muscle pulls, and then encouraging the muscles into better balance and harmony. Simple, everyday movements are used as tools for teaching you to move with less tension.

This is learning at a non-verbal level, by direct body experience. But the teacher will also, over a number of lessons, explain how you can best help yourself between lessons – by consciously avoiding ("inhibiting" in Alexander jargon) harmful tensions, and encouraging ("directing") more natural posture and movement patterns to emerge. It's a gradual process. Each lesson lasts 30-40 minutes and on average about 25 lessons are needed for results of lasting value.

The Alexander technique is not a therapy for specific ailments. Its primary application is in the field of preventive care and education for positive health and vitality. However, Dr Wilfred Barlow, author of *The Alexander Principle*, has stated that the technique can be helpful in particular for gynecological conditions, digestive disorders, heart and circulation problems, breathing difficulties, neurological and rheumatic disorders, and psycho-neuroses.

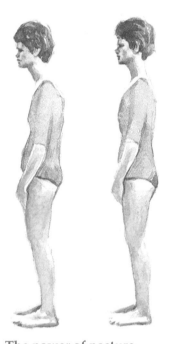

The power of posture
Any distortion to the structure of the spine will affect the way the body works. A hunched posture (above left) will inhibit the natural movement of the head, the shoulders and the ribcage, distort the spine and restrict normal breathing patterns. This sagging stance is associated with constantly anxious and depressed people, and it aggravates their feelings of tension. Correct posture (above right) is a major step toward improving "the use of the self".

Alexander lessons

The Alexander technique is a way of learning to help yourself, which is one of its great attractions. But it is not a do-it-yourself system – at least not until you have completed a course of lessons. This is because we become accustomed to our own muscle pulls and tensions, and what is familiar comes to feel right and even natural. Initially we must rely on a trained teacher's objective feedback. The teacher will focus on your habits of movement to assess how much strain you impose on yourself. Sitting, rising, standing and lying down are important parts of the lessons. The positions shown here are intended as a gentle introduction for your self-observation.

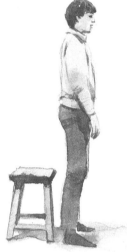

"Poised and free"

If you examine the way that you sit, either in a large mirror, or with the aid of a teacher, you may see that your habitual positions have already pulled the body down, compressing it, distorting the relation of the head and neck to the trunk. The practiced Alexander student will be sitting "poised and free", as shown below. The knees are not crossed since this would twist pelvis and spine.

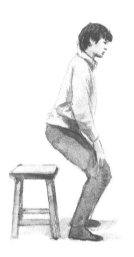

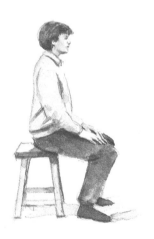

Rising and sitting

When you rise from a sitting position your body follows an automatic procedure. Frequently, the head juts forward and the body folds in the middle before straightening upward. The natural curves of the spine are exaggerated. Similarly, when sitting down the head is often thrown backward, and the lower back is arched. The Alexander student has a simple, easy rising habit, as shown above.

"Forward and up"

Using a full-length mirror, observe yourself standing. The common tendency is to bend the head forward, shortening the neck and rounding the back. The practiced student shown above is upright from head to toe; the head is "forward and up".

Using the teacher's skill

An Alexander teacher's training can help you to feel more accurately what is happening in yourself. Alexander himself said: "Anyone can do what I do if they do what I did". But he went on to say that a skilled teacher can take you in weeks to a point it took him years to reach. Few of us have the patience, insight and genius that he had to do it entirely by ourselves.

Healing

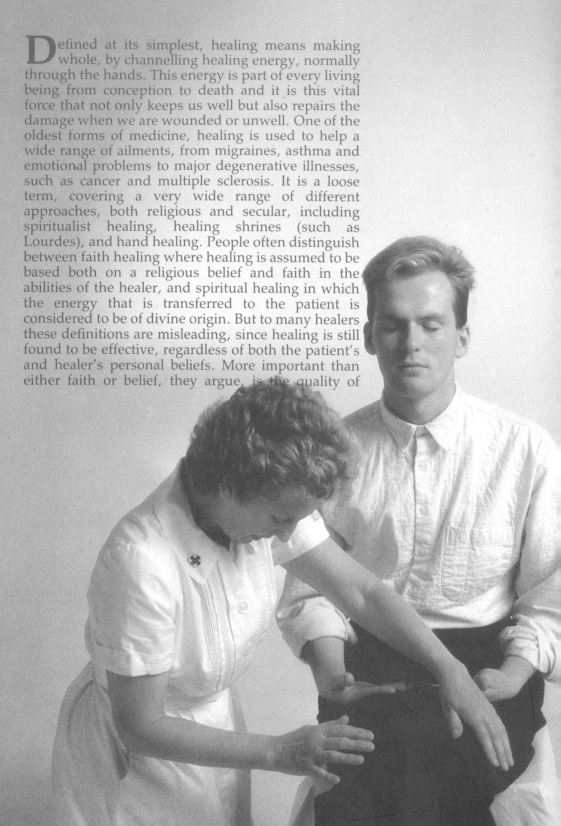

Defined at its simplest, healing means making whole, by channelling healing energy, normally through the hands. This energy is part of every living being from conception to death and it is this vital force that not only keeps us well but also repairs the damage when we are wounded or unwell. One of the oldest forms of medicine, healing is used to help a wide range of ailments, from migraines, asthma and emotional problems to major degenerative illnesses, such as cancer and multiple sclerosis. It is a loose term, covering a very wide range of different approaches, both religious and secular, including spiritualist healing, healing shrines (such as Lourdes), and hand healing. People often distinguish between faith healing where healing is assumed to be based both on a religious belief and faith in the abilities of the healer, and spiritual healing in which the energy that is transferred to the patient is considered to be of divine origin. But to many healers these definitions are misleading, since healing is still found to be effective, regardless of both the patient's and healer's personal beliefs. More important than either faith or belief, they argue, is the quality of communication between the healer and his or her patient, and the patient's receptivity, openness to change and will to be well.

The healing tradition

The roots of healing lie in early religions and in shamanism and magic. Most peoples of the world share a common belief in the power of spirits, gods or saints to influence health and cure sicknesses. The oldest known reference to the healing energies of the gods in western recorded history comes from the ancient civilization of the Egyptians, whose priests presided over healing temples and used their hands to impart healing power to the sick. But there is a continuous tradition of healing in tribal societies that may well predate the Egyptians – the tradition of the shaman, medicine man or witch doctor healers whose ritualized practices are still widespread today.

"Healing is not a science, but the intuitive art of wooing nature."
W.H. Auden

The Christian religion also embraces the concept of a healing God and of His delegates on earth. The Bible contains numerous healing miracles performed by Jesus on both believers and non-believers alike. Over the centuries, however, there has been a divergence of opinion between Christian spiritual healers and the priesthood of the established church. In modern times there have been many famous healers in the West, including the American Edgar Cayce, who made diagnoses while in a trance and the British spiritualist Harry Edwards, a practitioner until the late 1970s, who believed himself a medium from the spirit world.

Research

Since the patient's own self-healing capacity and his or her attitude of mind are crucial to healing, it is difficult to precisely isolate and assess the healer's contribution. Nevertheless a large number of scientific studies have been conducted to try to establish the principles of healing. In one famous experiment the American healers Olga and Ambrose Worrall succeeded in increasing the growth rate of rye grass by sending healing thoughts from their Baltimore home, 600 miles away. The healers visualized the grass being filled with light and energy and, at the pre-arranged time, the strip chart recorder began to register an increase until the growth rate was eight times as fast as before.

Research has also been carried out on the effect of healing on laboratory animals. In a series of experiments at McGill University, Montreal, Dr Bernard Grad demonstrated that the healer Colonel Estebany could accelerate the healing of wounded mice by holding his hands over them for fifteen minutes, twice a day. The biochemist Sister Justa Smith also produced encouraging results, using Estebany to influence the activity of enzymes in a flask – the effect of the healer's hands proved similar to that of a strong electro-magnetic field. In the UK, the healer Matthew Manning recently demonstrated that he could affect cancer cells in a flask, even from several rooms away. His method was to visualize them as surrounded with white light and mentally to tell them to go elsewhere. A medically controlled research program is currently in progress in the UK, to monitor the effects of healing on rheumatoid arthritis, cataracts, neuralgia and other disorders over periods of 6 months to two years. Research trials have also uncovered measurable physical changes in healers themselves while giving healing. The British biofeedback specialists C. Maxwell Cade and Geoffrey Blundell demonstrated that healers share a common pattern of brainwaves while utilizing their healing abilities.

How does healing work?

Healers explain the nature of healing in a variety of ways, depending partly on their beliefs. But whatever their religious convictions, most healers agree on the existence of a source of energy which some people can attune to and channel or transfer to others in order to cure both physical and mental disorders. Some also see themselves as "transformers" who can step down the voltage of energy of a higher frequency in order to make use of it for healing.

In order to understand fully the principles involved in healing you need to set it in the context of natural laws. Everything in the universe is subject to the law of cause and effect – every action creates a reaction. Providing we live and work within the body's capacity, our health is automatically maintained. But prolonged stress, wrong nourishment, an unhappy environment or emotional problems can all disturb the balance of our health. Healing does not work miracles; the healer directs his or her attention to discovering the cause of the patient's own self-healing mechanism.

The ability to relax and center oneself easily is essential to a healer – and in fact an accelerated relaxation response has been observed in healers in tests using biofeedback. The triggers which set healing in motion are compassion and empathy. For healing to be effective, the quality of communication between healer and patient is also of vital importance and the patient's receptivity, openness to change and will to be well. In addition to relieving suffering, the healer's function is to help the patient to understand why the problem has occurred. If the cause cannot be removed, the healer will use counselling skills to help the patient to accept what has happened.

Consulting a healer

Generally, a visit to a healer is a comparatively informal occasion. The approaches of individual healers vary enormously but most begin a session with a brief discussion of your particular needs. Some healers treat people lying down, others treat them sitting down. Some healers lay their hands on the site of the problem, others never touch the body, working solely in the aura. A common approach is for the healer to stand behind you, with his or her hands on your shoulders. Often it is suggested that the two of you start by linking together in thought, in order to help you to relax and open your mind to receive the healing energy. The healer may make use of prayer to ask for help in healing or visualize the diseased part as restored to a state of health. During the session, some healers allow their hands to be intuitively guided to the right place for healing – even if this is seemingly unconnected with the site of the disease.

While being treated, patients report a variety of sensations – many feel heat from the healer's hands, either locally or throughout the body; some experience tingling or an increase of energy; others feel no change at all while healing is taking place, even though they may notice a difference afterward.

Much depends on your attitude to the healer and the process of healing and your own openness or resistance to change. The more receptive you can be, the more you will marshal your own self-healing powers. There is little a healer can do to help if you are unconsciously opposed to the idea of healing.

Caution If you wish to develop your healing powers, it is essential that you train with an experienced healer. Trained healers can give full instruction and advice, teaching you how to "open" yourself to receive healing energy, as well as how to protect yourself while you are "open".

Whether you are learning to heal yourself, or to help others, you must be aware that while you are healing you are also open to external influences. After healing you should give yourself a mental directive to close down.

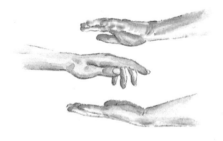

Learning to heal

Everyone possesses the ability to heal, though some people are more gifted than others. You can use healing to soothe all types of injuries, aches and pains, but you should always consult a doctor in cases of serious or unexplained pain.

The best way to develop your own healing powers is through meditation or prayer, using the visualization technique below. But first you must learn to relax physically (p.63), since it is impossible to channel your mental energy if your body is tense. Practice relaxing for a few minutes, at the same time each day. When you have finished healing, you should always seal your energy field (see Caution, p.301). The only time you should avoid giving healing is when you are tired, as healing may deplete your energy further.

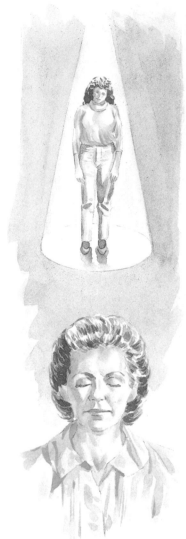

Prayer and affirmations
Prayer in the form of a request for divine intervention can be very powerful, especially when it is combined with the understanding that a change in attitude may be necessary. It has been used since time immemorial by those seeking healing for themselves or for other people.

Affirmations are positive statements or incantations you repeat to yourself in order to reprogramme your beliefs. Like prayer, they are a way of focusing the mind on a problem and opening yourself to the possibility of change. Think of a statement that crystallizes a belief you wish to include in your life – it should be positive, and formulated in the present tense, such as "my body is strong", "I am free of pain". Repeat your affirmation verbally (or write it down) as often as you like, each day.

Visualization and self-healing
This is a powerful tool for increasing concentration and bringing your mind into a state of tranquillity. Sit comfortably and focus on your imagination, forgetting the body altogether. Allow your mind to remember a scene where you felt particularly happy or peaceful – a place in the countryside, perhaps. As you explore the scene, begin to observe the sky, the clouds and the sun. Be aware, especially, of the light, since this will help you to get what you need. Make a conscious decision to open yourself out to receive healing, feeling yourself bathed in light. If you have a specific problem, gently focus the light on it and ask that it may be eased. Practice twice a day, for 10 minutes each time at first, working up to no more than 30 minutes a session.

Absent healing
To send absent healing to others you must first relax yourself, as described above. Visualize the healing light and the person you wish to help. See him or her standing in a pool of light and mentally request that the person receives the healing he or she needs. Keep the person in the light for a few moments, then gently return your attention to your surroundings and open your eyes. Repeat this every day.

Learning to heal others

To heal others directly requires a little practice and preparation. You need to develop your hands as an extension of your mind so that you can pick up sensations from the ill person while healing. Start by learning to sense your own energy field, as shown below, then you can move on to working on others. As you progress you will become more sensitive, and your intuition will become more accurate.

While you are giving healing the reason why the person you are treating is ill may well come in to your mind. If this happens, don't talk about what you think, as this will be seen as a diagnosis. Help the person to uncover the problem for him or herself.

Sensing your energy field

The aura or energy field normally extends up to anything between 9 and 18 inches (22-44 cm) from the physical body. In someone who is ill this field diminishes. To sense your own field, close your eyes and feel the air around you as you gently wave each hand about. Then, starting about 24 inches (60 cm) from your head with the palm facing you, gradually move your hand toward your head. At some point you will feel the atmosphere change - usually it will feel a little warmer and, as you move your hand away again, it will become cooler. This very slight change in sensation signals the edge of the energy field. Don't be disheartened if you don't feel it the first time. You will eventually succeed and, with practice, you will be able to detect areas where the field changes, especially over organs that are distressed.

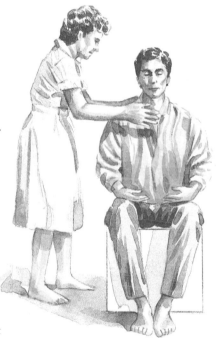

Giving healing

Once you have developed a sense of the changes in your own energy field you can try giving healing to others. Make sure the ill person is warm and comfortable, either sitting or lying down. Then, after centering yourself, start by placing your hands over (not on) the diseased or injured part of the body, sensing the energy field, and ask that healing be given. Leave your hands there for 2-3 minutes or until you instinctively feel ready to move on. Now place your hands directly on the affected part – you may now feel warmth and the receiver may feel your hands to be very hot or cool – a sign that healing is being transferred. When these sensations pass, the session is over. Once you have finished, give yourself a mental directive to "close down". This shuts off the healing energies. Washing your hands in cold water helps to break the mental atunement between healer and receiver. Do not be discouraged if you or the person you are healing felt nothing – the healing will be working anyway.

Therapeutic touch

Therapeutic touch derives from the practice of the laying-on-of-hands (pp.298-303). It is based on the premise that the human body is an open system of energies which are in constant flux, that illness is caused by a deficit or imbalance in these energies, and that the body has a bilateral symmetry.

The therapy was introduced in 1974 by Dr Dolores Krieger, a Professor of Nursing in New York, for use by professionals and non-professionals alike. During the 1960s she had become increasingly uneasy about the neglect of individual needs in institutionalized medicine. After conducting her own research, including an experiment with the healer Oskar Estebany (p.299), she began to train nurses in her own healing methods. In controlled trials, therapeutic touch has proved more effective in improving patients' health than ordinary nursing care.

Therapeutic touch is now taught in health care programs in more than 60 universities in the USA, and in over 35 countries. On the basis of clinical reports, it appears that psychosomatic illnesses respond best, followed by circulatory, lymphatic and musculoskeletal problems.

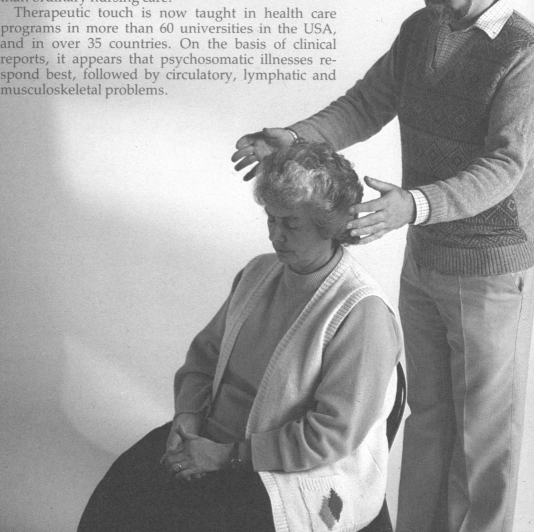

Giving therapeutic touch

Therapeutic touch is not complicated, but it requires practice and is best taught by a trained instructor. The only qualifications you need are compassion and a sense of commitment to others – healing is a natural human potential. The therapy has not only proved effective in treating ailments, but has also been found to enhance the sensitivity and energy of those who practise it. Although it is completely safe, it should not be practised for long, however, and if there are no signs of alleviation, other therapies should be pursued.

Centering
Start by "centering" yourself. Quietly focus your attention within yourself, and sense the depth of your own energies, to the exclusion of stray thoughts and outside disturbances. You will begin to be aware of facets of your own consciousness that can be directed to healing. With practice, you will learn to remain wholly centered throughout a session.

Sensing
The next step is to scan the receiver's energy field. With your hands on either side of the receiver's body, about 3 or 4 inches (7.5-10 cm) from the surface, try to sense whether there are differences in the energy patterns between the two sides.

Sensing the unborn child
Since 1983, clinical studies have observed the effects of the therapy as practiced by husbands on their pregnant wives. While at first many doubted their abilities, after a few moments' practice, they were able to tune in to their wives' energy fields and even detect the energy flow of the unborn baby. For most, the experience gave a new involvement in the pregnancy.

Begin with the head, then move your hands slowly down both sides of the body. You might feel a difference in temperature or density, for example – this indicates imbalances in the receiver's energy flow.

To counteract an imbalance, you need to direct energy through your hands, either into or away from the area, depending on whether you sense a deficiency or an excess of energy.

If your touch is effective, you should notice some reaction from the receiver within a few minutes. Often the first sign will be deeper, slower breathing. The receiver's voice may also drop or you may notice a general flushing in the skin.

The final phase is to reassess the receiver's field. If there are no imbalances you can assume the sides are in balance. If there is no improvement after 5-10 minutes do not continue with therapeutic touch. Give the individual a different remedy or type of treatment, if necessary.

Radionics and radiesthesia

Radionics and radiesthesia are special techniques for diagnosing and healing at a distance. The basic difference between the two is that radiesthetists generally work with only a pendulum and charts, whereas radionic practitioners normally use a variety of instruments for diagnosis and treatment, in addition to the pendulum. These instruments include a radionic "box", designed to identify and measure energy distortions. The success of both techniques, however, depends far more on the skill and sensitivity of the therapist than on the instruments used.

Central to both techniques are certain fundamental principles: that all life forms, both organic and inorganic, exist in and are connected by a vast field of energy; and that all these forms emit energy patterns. Practitioners work by detecting the disharmonies or distortions in patients' energy patterns and directing corrective energy patterns – often over astonishing distances – to treat the basic cause of the disharmony. One of the greatest advantages of the techniques is that they seek out and treat the hidden causes of disease, which may well be completely undetectable by scientific clinical methods.

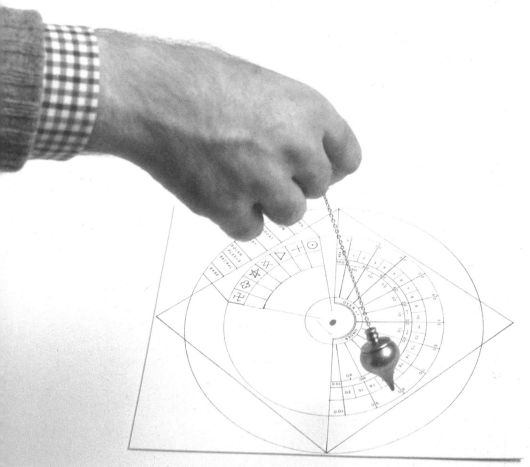

How it all began

The techniques of radiesthesia have been used by tribal societies for thousands of years. Pendulums have been found in ancient Egyptian tombs and shamans are known to use a form of pendulum for healing purposes. However, the term radiesthesia did not emerge until the early 20th century, when a French missionary priest, Abbé Mermet, began to appreciate the potential of the art of dowsing for medical purposes. Mermet's accuracy in pinpointing causes of sickness using the pendulum astonished his contemporaries and brought sudden fame and respectability to his method of distant diagnosis. He published his discoveries in *Principles and Practice of Radiesthesia* (1935) and even received a papal blessing for his achievements.

Scientific trials and experiments

Modern radionics emerged early in this century with the intensive research and fieldwork of Dr Albert Abrams and Ruth Drown of California. Dr Abrams achieved a certain notoriety with his radionic equipment, yet when his claims for the effectiveness of radionics were investigated in 1920 they were substantiated by a committee of top-grade physicists and doctors. Later, the equipment designed by the chiropractor Ruth Drown in the 1930s provoked accusations of fraud, and the medical establishment together with the Food and Drug Administration in the USA saw to it that the therapies were banned in the early 1960s.

In the UK, Dr W. E. Boyd, a homeopathic doctor who used a modification of Abrams' technique, had his work tested in the 1920s by the Horder committee. They confirmed the effectiveness of his work. Since the 1950s, the UK has become the world centre of radionics, but there has been little progress with scientific experimentation, mainly because the subjective nature of the techniques and the subtlety of the energies used make it difficult, if not impossible, to run objective scientific trials. In the 1950s a great deal of research was done at the de la Warr Laboratories in Oxford, England, by George de la Warr and his wife Marjorie. In one experiment a young man was wired up to electronic equipment in the laboratory and his "witness" (a sample of blood or hair) was subjected to radionic color treatment in

New York at a time unknown to him. Within minutes tracings on a strip chart registered his body's response to treatment given around 3,000 miles away.

Radionics and radiesthesia can be used to treat virtually any form of disease, whether physical or psychological. Longstanding conditions such as asthma, hay fever and other allergies often respond particularly well. Both therapies are especially effective where there has been an accumulation of toxins or subtle disease patterns known as "miasms", which are often the legacy of a childhood disease, such as measles. These toxins cannot be easily identified by orthodox clinical means, but radionic therapists and radiesthetists are able to identify and disperse them.

Consulting a professional

If you choose radionic treatment or radiesthesia, you need never meet your therapist. You will be asked to fill in a questionnaire, giving your medical case history, and an outline of your current symptoms. This is sent to the practitioner with a "witness" or "sample" – a spot of your blood on blotting paper or a snip of hair. The therapist places your witness on a diagnostic instrument, mentally tunes in to you, and poses a series of mental questions about your state of health. Most practitioners hold a pendulum over the radionic instrument to indicate the answers. Some may also analyse the state of your chakras, the body's energy centres which play an important role in the science of yoga (pp.284-93).

Once a diagnosis has been made, the treatment is generally purely radionic – healing energies are focused on you from a distance. Some therapists give dietary advice, too, or prescribe homeopathic or Bach flower remedies, exercise, or psychotherapy. A practitioner may also place a phial of an appropriate homeopathic remedy next to the patient's witness on his or her machine, with the intention of increasing the precision of the healing energies and speeding up the patient's response. Color, too, is often used as a therapeutic agent.

The act of diagnosis itself may set up a form of energy exchange between the therapist and the patient. Often, pain that has been intractable for weeks will clear up at the very time that a diagnosis is made – without the patient having any conscious knowledge of the work being done at that time.

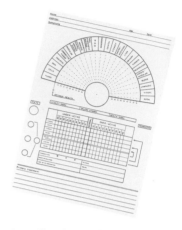

A radionic analysis chart
A completed chart gives a detailed picture of health in terms of energy imbalances at a physical and psychological level. Such data can provide the basis for distance treatment or for counselling.

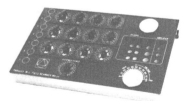

A radionic instrument
This instrument helps the radionic practitioner to determine the state of a patient's health from a distance. The patient's "witness" is placed on the top chrome disc. The instrument is also used to treat at a distance once an analysis has been made.

Using a pendulum

With its use of complex diagnostic charts and boxes, radionics is not a therapy for amateurs. Radiesthesia should also be practiced only by fully-trained, experienced therapists. However, it is perfectly in order to use a pendulum to check simple self-help procedures. Most people are sensitive to the radiations given off by objects to some degree and it is this sensitivity which makes pendulum use, like dowsing, effective.

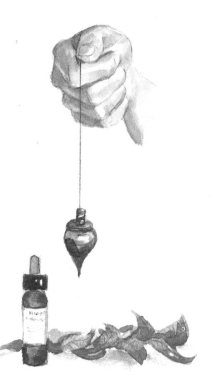

Pendulum diagnosis

You can use a pendulum to check whether certain foods are suitable for you, or to choose an appropriate Bach flower or homeopathic remedy, say, or an aroma-therapy oil for a minor condition, such as a mild cough or cold.

Preparation You should work alone in quiet surroundings, free from any distractions. The process seems to work by a subtle form of resonance, like a sonar echo, and it requires full concentration. Try to put yourself in a receptive and objective frame of mind, a state of passive attentiveness. Any doubts you have about the effectiveness of the procedure, or about your own capabilities, could result in uncertain findings.

Answers Responding to your sensitivity, the pendulum will indicate definite answers with two different types of movement: a clockwise rotation and a counter-clockwise one. For most people the clockwise movement means "yes", and the reverse movement means "no". However, it may operate the other way round. Once you know how your pendulum operates (see Testing, right), proceed to an unsolved question. If the pendulum swings away from and then toward you, it is signalling readiness – you may proceed to a question. If it swings in a roughly left-right-left movement, it means "no answer". In this case you should try rephrasing your question, until you get a definite answer.

Testing a pendulum

To be quite sure which way your pendulum rotates, test it with a question to which you already know the answer. For instance, you could place a remedy which you know is good for you on a convenient surface. Suspend the pendulum over it, and mentally ask yourself whether it is right for you. Your question must not be ambiguous.

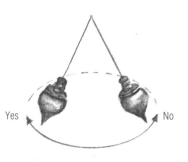

Yes   No

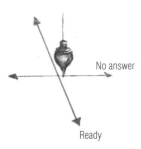

No answer

Ready

Hypnotherapy

Hypnotherapy is a method that uses hypnosis to channel the resources of the unconscious to effect therapeutic change. Hypnosis is defined in different ways by various medical and mental health professionals, but most agree that it essentially involves creating a state of mind in which normal methods of thinking are temporarily suspended and experiences of an unusual nature may take place. In a hypnotic trance the conscious mind is relaxed sufficiently for the therapist to communicate suggestions to the subject's unconscious, without opposition from the subject's conscious mind. A subject's level of relaxation under hypnosis ranges from a very light trance to a much deeper one.

One of the most practical methods of defining hypnosis has come from the influential American psychiatrist, Dr Milton H. Erickson (1901-1980), whose philosophy has had a widespread influence on modern hypnotherapy. Dr Erickson defined hypnosis as a state in which the subject experiences a heightened awareness, concentrating his or her attention on thoughts, beliefs, memories and so on that are beyond normal waking awareness.

The development of hypnotherapy

The use of trance-like states and suggestion has been traced back to Mesopotamia where, centuries before Christ, dream temples were known to exist. Scientific enquiry into these states began relatively recently, however, with the work of the Austrian Anton Mesmer (1734-1815), who discovered a technique which induced convulsions and a loss of mental and physical control in his patients. His followers discovered practical applications for his work and, by the mid and late 19th century, a number of physicians were experimenting with "suggestive therapeutics". Sigmund Freud himself made use of hypnosis while developing his earliest theories of the unconscious.

The approach to hypnosis that Freud used is now known as classical hypnosis. In classical hypnosis trance is induced in a number of ways – with a bright light, pendulum or metronome, or simply with the sound of the hypnotherapist's voice. The patient is passive and compliant and while he or she is in trance the hypnotherapist generally uses direct suggestion, to the effect that a symptom be reduced, for example, or that a pain disappear.

Since the second half of the 20th century, the Ericksonian approach has also been widely practiced, especially in the United States. By contrast with classical hypnosis, this approach does not rely upon an authoritative hypnotherapist and a passive subject. Instead of using direct suggestion to induce a therapeutic trance, the Ericksonian hypnotherapist makes use of subtle indirect suggestions and may even, at times, tell stories that carry a special meaning. This indirect approach allows a greater freedom of response from subjects and from their unconscious minds, reducing the need for resistance. Once their own unconscious problem-solving is stimulated they can begin to apply other resources or capabilities to help resolve their conflicts or problems, and will be guided by the hypnotherapist to direct these resources to solve the real problems out of which their symptoms arise. Ericksonian hypnotherapists feel that most psychological and some physical symptoms result from the way people cope with life's demands. They therefore attempt to affect or treat a far broader area than the presenting symptoms. Most often they bring about a gentle, subtle change, but sometimes it is rapid.

"The hypnotic trance belongs only to the subject – the operator can do no more than learn how to proffer stimuli and suggestions that evoke responsive behavior based upon the subject's own experiential past."
Milton H. Erickson

Hypnotherapy and self-hypnosis are useful for all ailments, such as high blood pressure, asthma, migraine, ulcers or skin diseases, in which anxiety, depression or tension are involved. They also have a wide application for fears, phobias, depressions and medical problems related to stress, tension, attitudes, or health care habits.

Consulting a professional

If you consult an Ericksonian hypnotherapist you should expect your session to begin by simply talking through your problems. You may also be encouraged to relax physically and to focus your attention. In order to induce a trance the therapist will remind you of common experiences related to trance, such as day-dreaming, wondering, "highway hypnosis", or tunnel vision. These types of experience are so different from normal waking consciousness that, when stimulated, they begin to take you into a different state of awareness. The therapist will then use indirect suggestions to encourage you to "retrieve resources", to use aspects of your mental functioning, such as memories of past experiences, as sources of inspiration and guidance on your present problem. This might consist of applying the memory of a childhood feeling of health or joy to recovery from major surgery, for example, or heightening your mechanism of forgetting in order to "unlearn" a sensitivity to pain. Images and ideas from the unconscious can provide a great deal of energy and information that is not normally available.

The unconscious mind can play an extraordinary part in healing body and mind, but it does not necessarily provide a neatly packaged answer that you can identify as such with your normal thinking. One man, for example, who used self-hypnosis to search for a solution to his chronic colitis found that he could think only of lilac trees as he sat quietly waiting for an answer. The unconscious association with lilacs did not at first seem to his conscious mind to provide an answer, but in fact it did. As a child, he had been in the habit of sitting quietly for hours observing the lilacs and smelling their sweet perfume. The lilacs represented a time in his life when, more than any other, he felt relaxed, calm, and carefree. His unconscious was trying to put him in touch with his own powerful associations to relaxation.

Practical applications
As well as being used successfully to treat a wide range of physical ailments, including skin problems and digestive complaints, a course of hypnotherapy is commonly undertaken for speech disorders, such as stammering, and for overeating, smoking, alcoholism and other addictions. Most disorders respond within one to twelve sessions, normally conducted once a week, but the duration of treatment varies according to the severity of the problem and the attitude and mental resources of the subject. Some problems respond very quickly, especially smoking, with an average of three out of every four people giving up after only one session, according to the British Society of Hypnotherapists.

Self-hypnosis

The use of hypnosis at home usually evolves out of professional treatment from a hypnotherapist and involves guidance at the outset. Once a hypno-therapist has helped you to develop a therapeutic trance, as mentioned above, self-hypnosis is a simple matter of using your memory of the trance to regain the condition. Using self-hypnosis, you can aid your own healing by learning to relax, to control emotion-ally based problems or habits and to reduce pain and other medical problems. But even without seeing a hypnotherapist, there are ways you can gain benefit from a type of self-induced trance. Practiced daily, the simple technique outlined below can be used to influence a wide range of problems.

Self-image thinking

Sitting down in a comfortable position, begin by relaxing, following a standard relax-ation routine (p.63), if desired.

Once completely relaxed, let the visual image change under your direction into an image of yourself.

Eventually you will be able to see a visual image of yourself possessing all the qualities you desire to reach your goal. The longer you keep it up, the more clearly you will be able to see this self-image.

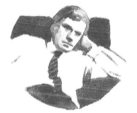

As you let all the tension slip out of your body, form a mental picture of anything that occurs to you.

Spend all the time you need to build the mental image into a person who is healthy and possessed of the qualities you desire such as confidence, calm, etc. Build the desired qualities from your imagination, or recall a time when you experienced that quality and concentrate on the feelings you had at that time in your life.

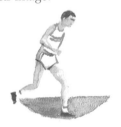

Hold the self-image as long as you experience the feelings it displays. Then let the background scene change slowly, until you see yourself doing things with the new or desired feelings – perhaps playing a game without the pain of arthritis, or sitting at a desk tackling a problem with fresh hope and curiosity.

Meditation

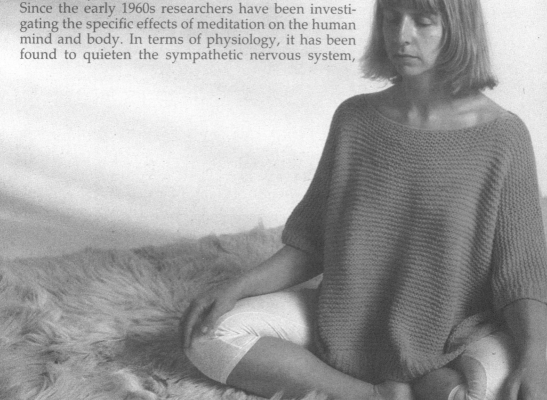

Meditation is not simply a process of reflection or of contemplation, nor is it mere daydreaming or relaxation. It involves training your attention or awareness and bringing your mental processes under voluntary control. It is a structured approach to self-development that has the added benefits of enhancing physical and psychological well-being.

As a spiritual practice, meditation originated over 3,000 years ago. Certain forms of meditation were used by the early Christians, but most of the forms we know today are essentially of eastern origin. It encompasses seated forms such as Zazen or TM (transcendental meditation) and more expressive or active forms. For the yogi it is a means of uniting with Brahman, the Absolute; but for many people in the West today, it is a practical self-help technique for which no particular religious beliefs are necessary.

The scientific evidence

Since the early 1960s researchers have been investigating the specific effects of meditation on the human mind and body. In terms of physiology, it has been found to quieten the sympathetic nervous system, slow down the heartbeat and breathing rate, and lower blood pressure and metabolism. Studies in which meditation was used to treat specific ailments (either alone or in conjunction with other techniques) found that it appears to be most effective in the prevention and treatment of stress-related ailments that have no organic basis. Phobias, nervous tension, high blood pressure, and anxiety, for example, have all been successfully treated with meditation, and some types of headaches, chronic pain, and sleep disturbances have also been improved. It is also used to treat drug and alcohol dependencies.

In research investigating responses to stress, people who meditated were found to respond more rapidly and more appropriately to potential threats, yet their heart activity returned to normal faster than non-meditators once the threat had passed.

Aims and objectives

Precisely how and why meditation works is still a matter of controversy. The ancient meditative traditions insist that we possess a level of being, an inner self, that can provide us with wisdom and guidance. The practice of meditation helps us to quieten the mind, allowing us to gain access to this inner source of strength. Meditation also teaches us to control rather than be controlled by our thoughts and emotions. Ordinarily our minds flit from subject to subject in a string of endless associations, which is possible to detect when we watch ourselves carefully. If a car, for example, cuts us off in traffic, we instantly begin the internal chatter – angrily (usually silently) we tell the other driver what we think, one thought leads to another, and the anger builds up.

"There is an inward centre in ourselves where truth abides in fullness."
Robert Browning

If you allow this type of internal commentary to continue, it can seriously affect your psychological and physical health. But by training your attention with meditation, you can increase your awareness of how the internal process begins, decide whether it is useful and, if it isn't, you can stop it or, at the very least, slow it down considerably.

Meditation also helps to make intentional mental processes, such as planning and problem-solving, more efficient by helping you to focus your mind on a problem without wandering into unproductive reverie. Thus, meditation has been said to be "doing one thing at a time" or "living in the here-and-now".

The meditative process

Meditation takes many forms, some more complex than others. The techniques recommended here are simple, effective, and easily extended into an everyday routine. The type of meditation you practice, however, is less important than that you are regular, consistent, and dedicated in your approach. If you then apply the meditative principles involved to the tasks and challenges of daily life, you will gradually begin to notice subtle but definite changes that will intensify as your practice deepens.

Time and environment

Set aside two periods of 10-20 minutes for meditation each day – one in the morning and one in the evening. Choose a time when you will not be too tired – avoid meditating right after meals or at other times when you may be sleepy. Find a quiet, comfortable spot where you will not be disturbed, and take the phone off the hook, if necessary. Try to establish a habitual time and place – this makes meditation easier and more rewarding.

Preparing for meditation

You can sit on the floor, on a cushion, or on a straight-backed chair, as described below, but avoid overstuffed chairs and sofas, as they tend to induce sleepiness. Your posture should help you stay awake and alert. Experiment with positions until you find one that allows you to sit comfortably erect without undue strain. You are less likely to feel sleepy if your back and head are erect.

Once satisfied, close your eyes and take several slow, deep breaths. Scan your body and gently try to release any tensions or tightness (see Progressive relaxation, p.63). Then survey your mind; if you find that certain thoughts are troubling you, simply draw your attention away from them. Having relaxed and cleared your mind, you are now ready to begin.

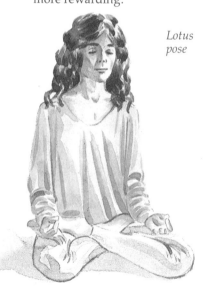

Lotus pose

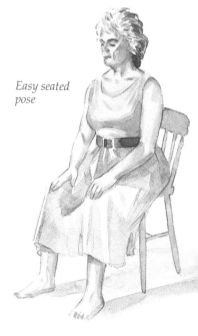

Easy seated pose

Meditation poses The lotus pose makes an ideal steady base. Start by sitting on the floor with your legs spread out in front of you. Then bend one knee and bring the foot up on to the other thigh. Bring the second leg in – either under the opposite thigh (half lotus pose) or over it, as shown left. Beginners may prefer an ordinary cross-legged pose, or easy seated pose.

Focused breathing method

In this technique, you use your breathing as a focal point. Having prepared yourself, as described on p.316, you simply allow your awareness to focus on the rising and falling of your abdomen or on the air flowing through your nostrils. Let your breath come naturally, without any attempt to control or manipulate it. Observe it with the same quiet detachment with which you might watch the gentle breathing of a loved one.

As soon as you become aware that your focus has shifted to any passing thoughts, images, etc, gently but firmly return to your breathing. As you gain experience, your awareness will remain focused for longer periods between distractions, and you will quickly learn to recognize when your attention is first diverted. This exercise can take time to master, so don't be discouraged.

Breath counting method

If you find it difficult to maintain a focus on your breathing, it may be helpful to count each breath silently. Beginning with 1, count each exhalation or inhalation, from 1 to 10, then start again at 1. If you get distracted, simply return your awareness to your breathing and begin again. Counting gives your mind something to concentrate on and it also gives a very clear indication of when your attention has wandered.

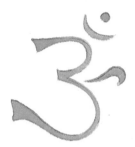

Mantra meditation

This method involves silently repeating a word or phrase that you like or that expresses a deep feeling or belief, with each inhalation or exhalation. Some people use familiar words, such as "peace" or "one", others use a mantra – a Sanskrit word, or a group of words which, when regularly repeated during meditation, help to elevate you to a higher state of consciousness. The original and best-known mantra is "Om", shown above.

Concentrative meditation

Steady gazing, known in the yogic tradition as "tratak", is an excellent method of meditation. All you need to do is focus, without blinking, on a static, relatively small object, then close your eyes and try to visualize the object. Ideally, the target of your gaze should be at eye level, about 3 ft (1 m) away The most commonly used object is a lighted candle. Your gaze should be relaxed, but not vacant – simply look steadily but without straining for about 1 minute before closing your eyes. When the after-image fades, open your eyes and start the process again. In time you will be able to gaze for a longer period.

After meditation

When you have meditated for about 10-20 minutes, gently return your awareness to your surroundings and open your eyes. Slowly begin to move around and stretch, as your awareness refocuses outward on your environment. You should now feel fresh and relaxed, ready to face the tasks before you.

Potential problems

Some people report that meditation makes them feel physically uncomfortable, anxious, agitated, or slightly nauseous, especially during the first few attempts. If you feel any of these sensations, stop meditating for a few minutes, open your eyes, look around, and relax again. Once the feeling has passed, resume meditation.

Another effect sometimes reported occurs when the rational part of the mind is stilled, and thoughts and images from the normally unconscious part of the mind reveal themselves to your awareness. We all have parts of our lives that we would rather not think about, because they are, perhaps, embarrassing, frightening, or unpleasant. Part of the process of meditation involves recognizing these aspects of ourselves, and by accepting them as part of our being and dealing with them appropriately, they gradually lose their emotional impact and fade into the background.

Autogenics

Autogenics is a series of simple mental exercises designed to promote health by inducing deep relaxation and stimulating the body's self-healing mechanisms. Literally, it means "generated from within". In practice it is like a combination of auto-suggestion and meditation. The exercises require no special clothing or difficult postures; and by practicing them for only a few minutes you can achieve a powerful restorative effect. Autogenics cannot, however, be correctly or safely taught by books, tapes or videos. It is a skill, like learning to drive a car, that requires expert tuition.

Stress survival

This therapy is one of the most positive antidotes to stress in modern everyday life. Stress-related health problems are endemic. If you keep turning your thoughts outward, keeping yourself in constant touch with all the sources of stress in your life, you will lose natural resilience. Autogenics helps you to uncouple yourself from the stresses in your life by directing your attention inward, allowing your body to restore itself. You switch off the "fight or flight"

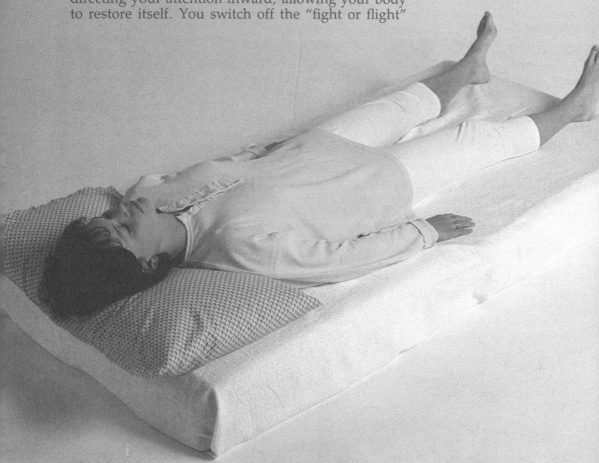

system, and switch on the "rest, relax and restore" system. There is an overall shift in both mind and body from a state of internal war to one of peace. When you use a method of meditation, rather than medication, you learn to help yourself. You can be much more independent and self-reliant when you don't feel you have to run to a doctor for tablets every time you are in an anxiety-provoking situation.

The six standard exercises of autogenic training were developed in Berlin around 1930, by Dr Johannes Schultz. He based his new technique on an extensive knowledge of the physiological changes that occur in deep relaxation, and on eastern meditation techniques (such as Zen and yoga), which can teach voluntary control of the body's involuntary nervous system. Schultz's six exercises were practiced and perfected by his followers, mainly in Europe, for some decades. More recently, the teaching and training of Dr Wolfgang Luthe, now the world's leading expert in autogenics, has made Montreal, Canada, the centre of study, and the therapy has become popular in the USA and in the UK.

Scientific evidence

Internationally, there are now over 3,000 scientific publications which demonstrate the effects of the training – both as a tool of preventive medicine, and as an antidote to stress-related disorders (varying from "mind-made" psychosomatic conditions to general tension, anxiety, insomnia, and addictions).

A recent comparison of the health benefits of autogenic training and physical training showed that while both techniques reduce heart attack risk factors, such as high blood pressure and high blood cholesterol, autogenics produces a greater improvement in mental well-being. It also aids performance, and willpower. Professional athletes who practice autogenics benefit considerably, through the reduction of anxiety associated with intense competition.

Research has revealed another interesting side-effect of both autogenics and meditation – the balancing of the levels of activity on the two sides of the brain. Both techniques stimulate the right side, the imaginative, creative, dreaming, intuitive faculty. They also improve emotional balance. In addition, they often result in better dream recall, and encourage dreaming in color rather than in black and white.

Autogenic training
Autogenics requires expert tuition. You should first check with your doctor that you are suitable for training – especially if you want to reduce, come off, or avoid going on to drugs such as tranquillizers or sleeping pills. The autogenic exercises, taught in individual or group sessions, are introduced progressively. You learn to focus your attention inwardly and passively, and to induce relaxing sensations by mentally repeating standard phrases. There is also a range of advanced techniques for specific disorders and for more deep-rooted anxieties and phobias.

Biofeedback

Biofeedback is a method of monitoring minute changes in bodily function, such as muscle tension or skin temperature, using a variety of machines. It provides a means of consciously influencing processes that were once believed to be beyond voluntary control – functions of the body's autonomic nervous system – and increases awareness of the interaction between mental and physical states. The biofeedback or monitoring device provides information about your state of arousal or relaxation – as reflected in different body functions – by means of a light, sound or meter.

Biofeedback is not a therapy in its own right, but an effective adjunct to therapy, combining well with relaxation techniques, meditation, autogenics, and any form of counselling. Using the biofeedback equipment in conjunction with a physical technique, such as breath control, or a mental one, such as analysis, subjects learn to discover the root causes of their response to stress. In common with other relaxation techniques, biofeedback has found most success in the treatment of stress-related conditions, such as asthma, migraine, insomnia, high blood

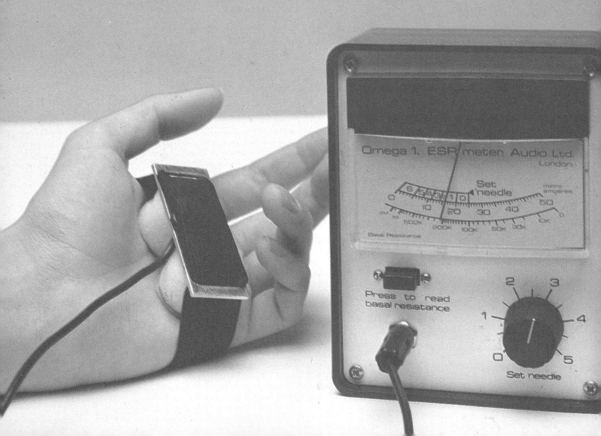

pressure and anxiety. But it can also be used more specifically, since it can bring internal stresses under more precise control than other techniques. Thus, it has been found useful in retraining a function which has been lost due to illness or accident, such as the use of a muscle. There is also some evidence that chronic pain can be relieved with EMG (see below), and alpha brainwave feedback. The technique is popular in the USA and western Europe, and has been introduced in some health services.

The birth of the technique

The technique's origins date back to British scientist W. Grey Walter's research on the electrical rhythms of the brain in the early 1950s. While a subject was listening to a football match on the radio, Grey Walter noticed that his brain's alpha rhythm responded to the fortunes of his favorite team. It was Joe Kamiya, however, working in the USA in 1958, who found that a subject could consciously control his or her own alpha rhythm, when given information about it. Subsequent research showed that animals could learn to make one ear warmer, the other cooler, using biofeedback, and people could learn to voluntarily control their heart rate, muscle tension, stomach acidity and other autonomic responses. US researchers Elmer and Alyce Green later combined Kamiya's research with what they knew of autogenic training, to produce the biofeedback machines and methods that we know today.

Biofeedback training

A course of training is normally given in groups, where group empathy and interaction can aid learning, but it is also available on a one-to-one basis. A typical training course concentrates on teaching you to relax, enabling you to distinguish between mere passivity and the "awake and aware" state of true relaxation, which is shown as a lively response on the monitoring devices. Various machines may be used, from hand temperature meters to electrical skin resistance (ESR) meters, shown right, or electromyographs (EMG), which measure muscular activity. A hand temperature meter shows how temperature varies according to your mental and physical state while an electrical skin resistance meter is designed to detect certain stress-related skin changes in the user.

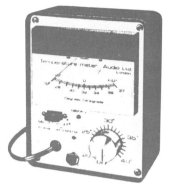

A hand temperature meter

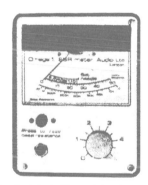

An electrical skin resistance meter (ESR)

CHAPTER SIX

First aid and emergencies

Every adult and every teenage child should learn the basic steps that must be taken in minor and major accidents. Knowing the rudiments of first aid is the best preparation for the unexpected emergency, since most of us are not at our best while trying to deal with a new and possibly threatening situation, or deciding on priorities in a life-or-death crisis. This chapter outlines the essential steps that must be taken, both for day-to-day mishaps, and in those situations which demand immediate action while professional help is being sought. The first section, on minor injuries and aches and pains, includes advice on home remedies for natural first aid.

Everyday first aid

Many minor injuries can be adequately treated without professional help by a sensible person who knows the rudiments of first aid. This chapter gives advice on burns, cuts, sprains, bites, etc, but it also includes basic advice on coping with diarrhea, migraine, stomach ache, earache, and toothache. These conditions may well require that you visit a doctor (or go to your dentist), but you may be able to take some immediate action to alleviate discomfort. First aid also calls for basic nursing equipment and medication such as bandages, scissors, and antiseptics, so it's worth checking that you keep a well-stocked medicine cabinet or first-aid supply closet, at home and at work. At home, make sure that it is out of young children's reach.

When you are choosing medicaments, consider using natural remedies, such as homeopathic Arnica, and distilled witch hazel. Many of these remedies are readily available and widely applicable. Some manufacturers of homeopathic medicines produce ready-made first-aid kits. You may find that some of the natural treatments described here become valued remedies in your household.

Emergency action: golden rules

When a life-threatening event occurs, it is very important to keep as calm and cool-headed as possible. Panicking, though a perfectly natural reaction, doesn't help the injured person and could be positively harmful. It tends to block cool, logical thinking and prompts rash decisions. If you feel panic rising, take a few deep breaths to calm yourself. Then attend to the victim's most essential and immediate needs.

The first general rule is to check that an unconscious person is breathing and that the heart is beating (p.331). Taking immediate action when the breathing or heart has stopped can save a life. The second rule is to get professional help at once. Without medical training you can take prompt action that may save a person's life (by giving the kiss of life, for example), but the chances are that a professional will cope with the situation more effectively. And thirdly, look after yourself. You will only compound the emergency if you injure yourself while trying to help. Take care, for instance, not to give yourself an electric shock by touching someone who is in contact with an electric charge and is "live", and make sure you don't suffer injury yourself when helping others in a road accident.

Once you have carried out life-saving procedures, be careful not to let your eagerness to help run away with you. If you have called for medical assistance, you can leave further treatment to the professionals. Don't try to deal with injuries to eyes or ears, or to remove foreign bodies from wounds (except in the case of a simple splinter or something very easily extracted from a surface wound). Don't pile blankets on an injured person, and don't offer refreshment when someone is dangerously hurt. It is best not to move a casualty unless this is necessary to avoid further danger (as in a fire, or a road accident).

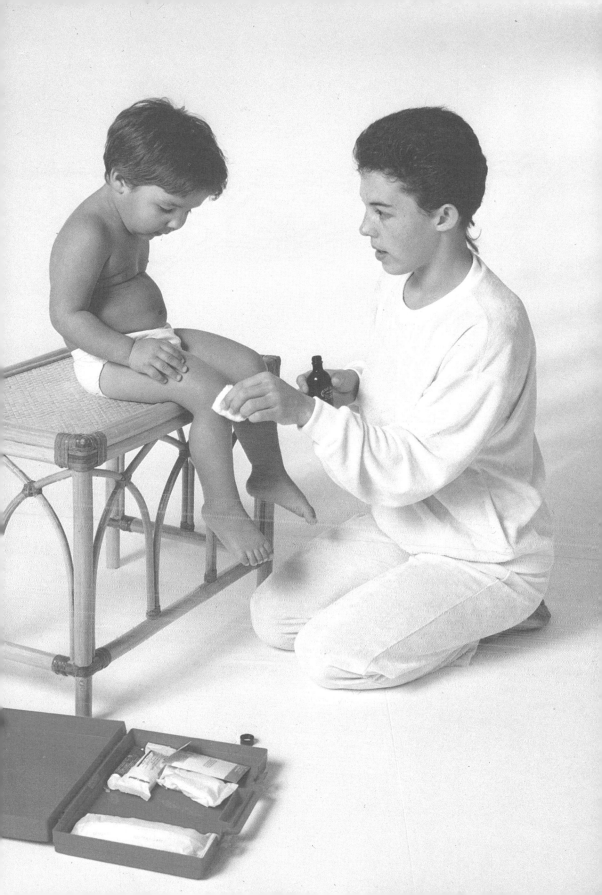

First aid

Follow the commonsense advice listed immediately under the accident or ailment, and then proceed to a natural remedy. If the natural treatment does not improve the problem, discontinue its use, and seek professional advice. For detailed instructions (on dosages, techniques, and applications, for example), in homeopathy, herbalism, aromatherapy, and naturopathy, always consult the relevant section in the Natural Therapies chapter. The recommended potency for homeopathic remedies is 6x (p.146).

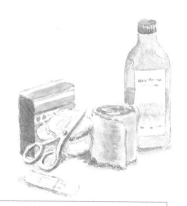

First aid	Natural remedies
Minor burns	
If a burn or scald affects only a small area about 1 inch (2.5 cm) square, and has damaged only the outer layer of skin, it is suitable for home treatment.	**Homeopathy** For the relief of pain and to promote rapid healing of minor burns and scalds take Urtica urens – ointment or tincture. A local dressing moistened with diluted Urtica urens Mother Tincture (10 drops to ½ cup of water) is very soothing. If it is still painful, take Cantharis.
• Remove the source of burning.	**Herbalism** Make a compress by wetting a gauze dressing in distilled witch hazel and gently binding it to the site. Remove the compress when it is dry. This minimizes swelling and prevents infection. An infusion (p.164) of chickweed (*Stellaria media*) also makes a healing compress. Use a healing ointment if necessary, such as marigold (*Calendula*), but try this on unburned skin first, to check that the sufferer is not allergic to the ointment base.
• Cool the affected area by immersing it in cold water, or by applying cold, wet towels for at least 10 minutes, or until the pain is gone.	
• If possible, gently remove any rings, bracelets, etc, from the area.	**Aromatherapy** While the burned skin is healing, apply 4 drops of lavender oil mixed in an eggcup of soya oil.
• Cover loosely with a clean, dry dressing.	**Traditional medicine** Press the cut end of a leek to the burn, or make a soothing compress, using gauze wrapped around grated raw potato, grated raw onion with salt, wet tea leaves, or molasses mixed with flour. Or take a leaf of aloe vera, slit it open, and squeeze its juice on to the burn.
• (*Chemical burns*) Remove any clothing splashed with chemicals and flush the area of skin with running water.	
• (*Electrical burns*) Seek medical advice.	
Caution Do not apply grease, butter, or ice cold water. Do not use a fluffy material to dress the area. Do not puncture blisters. If a burn becomes more painful or infected, get medical help.	

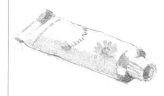

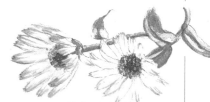

Calendula ointment

First aid	Natural remedies
Minor cuts and lacerations Slight bleeding usually stops of its own accord within a few minutes. If bleeding does not stop after several minutes, call for medical assistance. ● Stop bleeding from cuts by applying pressure for a few minutes. ● Remove any foreign bodies from the wound, if they are clearly visible and not deeply embedded. ● If the edges of the cut gape open, draw them together firmly with finger and thumb and apply strips of surgical tape. ● Cover the wound with a dressing and bandage. If the cut is very minor, it is best left uncovered. ● If you suspect a risk of infection, discuss the advisability of an anti-tetanus injection with your doctor.	**Homeopathy** For all painful cuts and lacerations and to prevent infection, take Hypericum. For puncture wounds, from a nail, needle, thorn, splinter, or similar, take Ledum. If this does not help, follow with Hypericum. Before dressing the wound, clean it with Hypercal (10 drops in ½ cup of water). If it is extremely painful, use a temporary dressing soaked in Hypercal solution (this has antiseptic as well as pain-relieving properties). **Herbalism** Diluted distilled witch hazel is excellent. Applied on cotton wool, it rapidly stops any bleeding, relieves pain and promotes healing. **Aromatherapy** For minor cuts, apply diluted clove oil or lavender oil several times daily. Eucalyptus oil applied neat is a good general antiseptic. **Traditional medicine** Washing a small cut with a solution of sodium bicarbonate is also antiseptic. 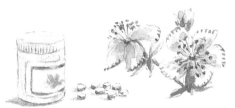 *Hypericum*
Sprains Sprains result from over-stretching or tearing of the ligaments around joints, most commonly the wrists or ankles. ● Make the person comfortable and take any weight off the injured part. ● Apply cold compresses (p.212) to help soothe the pain. ● Support the affected joint with a bandage. ***Caution*** If you suspect a fracture, call for medical assistance.	**Homeopathy** Give Ledum first (especially if the affected part feels cold and feels better with cold applications). Give Arnica first if there is much bruising or shock (then follow with Ledum). Later, give Rhus toxicodendron or Ruta graveolens if the affected part is still painful, and is worse during first movements but better for continued motion. If it continues to be painful during any movement, give Bryonia. **Herbalism** A compress of fresh comfrey (*Symphytum officinale*) makes a wonderful healing remedy for sprains. Soak a gauze bandage in a cooled infusion of the leaves (p.164), and apply to the injured area. **Naturopathy** Apply cold compresses to the area (p.194). Use alternate hot and cold compresses on sprains where there is no swelling. Comfrey in tablet or tea form taken for a limited time will help to heal the ligaments. Give 2 tablets, 3 times a day. **Traditional medicine** A mixture of olive oil and wintergreen, applied on gauze and lightly bound to the sprain, is warming. Tiger Balm is an eastern remedy, ready-made, similarly warming and aromatic.

First aid	Natural remedies
Bruises • Rest and a cold compress (p.194) on the bruise are both helpful. *Caution* Severe bruising, as after a bad fall, may be accompanied by serious internal hemorrhage. Medical assistance is essential.	**Homeopathy** As soon as possible after the injury, take Arnica, several doses at 15-minute to hourly intervals, depending on the severity. This reduces pain, prevents further swelling and promotes speedy healing. If the bruise is very slow to clear, take Ledum. For bruised bones, such as shin bones, take Ruta graveolens. In cases of deep muscular bruising or bruising to the breast, take Bellis perennis. **Herbalism** Distilled witch hazel is strongly antiseptic and reduces swelling. Comfrey used externally is exceptionally healing (see Sprains, above). An infusion of marigold (*Calendula*) applied as a compress also heals bruises. 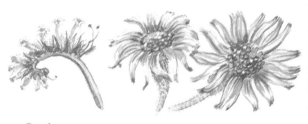 *Comfrey* *Arnica*
Sunburn • Apply a soothing lotion, such as calamine, to the affected areas. • Do not expose the sunburned areas of the skin to the sun for at least a few days. *Caution* Extensive sunburn requires medical attention.	**Homeopathy** Try Belladonna, Ferrum phosphoricum, or Kali carbonicum. If it is severe, with blistering, give Cantharis. **Herbalism** Apply marigold (*Calendula*) ointment, or a compress of an infusion (p.164) of marigold leaves. **Traditional medicine** Bathe the skin gently with a sodium bicarbonate solution, or cool black tea. This can be soothing and healing.
Frostbite • While waiting for medical assistance, keep the person warm, give warm drinks, and raise the feet if they are the affected part. *Caution* Frostbite can be a serious condition that requires urgent medical attention. Do not let the person walk, and do not use direct heat or rub the affected area.	**Homeopathy** Try Agaricus muscarius. **Traditional medicine** Cucumber placed on the affected area may help, if it is not extensive. Peel the cucumber first, dry it and wet it again with warm water. Cold mashed and salted potatoes or raw onion can also be applied directly to the frostbitten skin.

First aid	Natural remedies

Splinters

- Gently wash the area round the splinter with an antiseptic.

- Grasp the projecting end of the splinter with tweezers and gently ease it out.

- If the splinter is just below the skin, sterilize a sewing needle by heating the top in the clear part of a flame, allow it to cool naturally, then use the tip to ease the splinter out.

Caution Don't ignore splinters, since they can go septic. Never dig deeply for a splinter. Large splinters, especially if there is glass, require medical assistance.

Homeopathy First give Ledum, and if this does not help give Hypericum.

Herbalism Slippery elm ointment or a poultice (see below) made with slippery elm powder is excellent.

Traditional medicine A poultice made from kaolin is highly effective and allows even stubborn splinters to be drawn out quickly and easily.

To make a poultice, first heat the poultice paste, or add hot water to the powdered herb. Then apply the mixture either directly to the skin or over a piece of gauze; cover and secure with a bandage. Renew the poultice every few hours until the splinter is drawn out.

Nosebleeds

- Grasp the soft part of the nose firmly between the thumb and index finger. Hold the nose like this for about 10 minutes.

- Once the bleeding has stopped, do not blow or sniff or you could dislodge the blood clot and start the flow again.

Caution Do not throw the head back or lie down. This may cause blood to trickle down the throat, and thus provoke vomiting. Nosebleeds after a blow on the head can be a sign of a fractured skull. Seek medical help at once.

Homeopathy Give either Ferrum phosphoricum or Vipera.

Herbalism Apply distilled witch hazel to the nasal area on cotton wool – this is an effective astringent.

Traditional medicine Soak a plug of cotton wool in the juice of a fresh lemon and insert into the bleeding nostril.

Witch hazel   *Lemon*

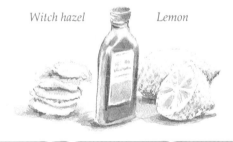

Poison ivy

- Wash affected parts as soon as possible using a strong household soap. Scrub the skin thoroughly.

Caution Do not scratch since this will spread poison.

Traditional medicine Apply the juice of the aloe vera plant, or bathe the area in cider vinegar.

First aid	Natural remedies
Bites and stings ● (*Bee stings*) A bee leaves its barbed sting behind in the flesh. Remove with tweezers, taking care not to grip the poison sac, and gripping the sting near the skin. Alternatively, "wipe" it away with a needle held parallel to the skin. Apply a cold dressing or calamine lotion, or hold the area under cold water to reduce pain. ● (*Wasp stings*) Wasps do not leave their stings in the flesh. Put some lemon juice or vinegar on the affected area. Surgical spirit is also soothing. ***Caution*** Some people are seriously affected by bee and wasp stings. Medical assistance should be sought immediately.	**Homeopathy** (*Bee and wasp stings*) Give Ledum (especially if the part feels cold but feels better for cold application). If there is much swelling and the skin is tight and shiny, give Apis mellifica. To relieve itching, give Urtica urens. **Aromatherapy** (*Wasp stings*) Use cinnamon oil rubbed neat on to the area a few times a day. This will relieve the discomfort. **Traditional medicine** (*Ant and bee stings*) Use sodium bicarbonate, applied as a paste to the site. (*Wasp and mosquito bites*) Apply crushed garlic, lemon juice, witch hazel, vinegar, moistened cornstarch, or crushed plantain leaves. Or apply a sliced onion or some onion juice. 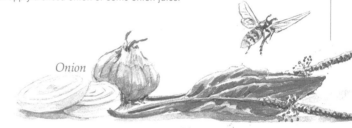 *Onion* *Plantain*
Motion sickness Preventive measures include not reading when you are travelling, not twisting your neck, placing yourself so that you can see the moving horizon, getting plenty of fresh air, and avoiding large, fatty meals before a journey. ***Caution*** If you are driving, avoid proprietary anti-sickness tablets.	**Homeopathy** Try Cocculus or Tabacum. If possible give a few doses before the start of the journey. **Traditional medicine** Before starting a journey, take 3 or 4 teaspoons of brewers' yeast. Ideally, you should start this treatment some time before travelling. Yeast-free vitamin B complex supplements, an alternative for those who are yeast-allergic, may also help. When suffering from motion sickness, suck a lemon or drink fresh lemon juice. Ginger is also of proven value.
Migraines ● Lie down in a darkened room. ● Apply a warm hotwater bottle (or an ice pack, p.212) to the affected side of the head. ***Caution*** Vision is frequently affected, so if you feel the onset of an attack while driving, or operating any machine, stop.	**Homeopathy** See Headaches, p.153. **Herbalism** See Digestive problems, p.168, and Anxiety, p.172. **Naturopathy** See Migraine, Emergency treatment, p.203.

First aid	Natural remedies
Emotional shock, fainting • If someone is feeling faint, encourage him or her to sit down and lower the head between the knees. On recovery, give small sips of water. • If the person has fainted, lift the legs briefly to allow gravity to take blood back to the head. Loosen any tight clothing. Try to ensure that he or she gets maximum fresh air. Place the person in the recovery position (p.335), if they don't come round quickly. ***Caution*** Emotional shock is quite distinct from "medical shock", which may follow a serious injury and requires urgent medical treatment. If a person faints and does not regain consciousness after a few minutes, you should summon medical assistance.	**Homeopathy** If feeling faint is from emotional upset or grief and is accompanied by sighing, then give Ignatia. If it is from fright or anticipation, and there is a weakness, trembling, frequency of urination or diarrhea, give Gelsemium. If from shock or fright, and with great fear and restlessness, give Aconite. If from slight pain, give Hepar sulphuris. If from a hot room, give Pulsatilla. If shock is accompanied by a great desire for air; especially fanning, yet the person feels very cold, then give Carbo vegetabilis. **Bach flower remedies** Take 3-4 drops of Rescue Remedy (p.187) in a little water, in tea, or directly on the tongue. It will help to relieve fear and to restore calm and confidence after a shock or accident. The Grief Mix (p.187) can be taken at times of loss or bereavement. *Star of Bethlehem* *Cherry Plum* *Clematis* *Impatiens* *Rock Rose*
Toothache • For pain associated with a cavity, soak a piece of cotton wool in oil of cloves and apply directly to the site. • For swelling or soreness of the gum over a wisdom tooth, wash your mouth with a solution of salt and water. ***Caution*** Do not take alcohol – this exacerbates the throbbing pain.	**Homeopathy** See p.151. **Herbalism** See p.169. **Aromatherapy** See p.180. **Traditional medicine** See p.221.
Stomach ache ***Caution*** Do not take painkillers. Severe stomach ache requires medical help.	**Homeopathy** See Indigestion, vomiting, p.150. **Naturopathy** See Indigestion, Local treatment, p.199. **Traditional medicine** See Stomach ache, p.220.

First aid	Natural remedies
Earache • Apply a hotwater bottle filled with warm water and wrapped in a cloth to the affected ear. ***Caution*** Earache from a middle ear infection is serious, particularly in children. Seek medical assistance.	**Homeopathy** See p.151. **Naturopathy** See p.201.
Diarrhea • Take plenty of liquid, even during an attack. ***Caution*** A severe attack of diarrhea may cause dehydration, which can be dangerous, especially for a small child or an elderly person. Seek medical advice.	**Homeopathy** See p.150. **Herbalism** See p.168. **Naturopathy** See Diarrhea, Emergency treatment, p.198. **Traditional medicine** See p.220.
Vomiting • Lie flat and don't eat or drink anything for a couple of hours. • After this time, small amounts of iced water or the cool, strained water from boiled rice may settle the stomach. • As soon as you can keep drinks down, drink plenty of water or well-diluted fruit juices to replace lost body fluid. ***Caution*** If vomiting persists over a period of hours, or if you vomit any black or bloody material, if you have a stiff neck, feel dizzy while vomiting, or have a sudden attack of abdominal pain, you should call for medical help.	**Homeopathy** For constant nausea, give Ipecacuanha. For much retching, when sufferer wants to vomit but can't, give Nux vomica. See also p.150. 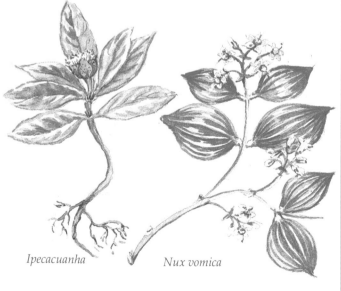 *Ipecacuanha* *Nux vomica*

Life-threatening emergencies

This section features some of the most common life-threatening emergencies. In coping with any such incident it is crucial to act quickly and effectively, while remaining as calm as possible. It helps to be really familiar with the basic emergency procedures, described below, and to know the general rules that apply in all emergencies (see Emergency action: golden rules, p.322). The first rule is to check that the victim is breathing and his or her heart is beating. The second is to seek medical assistance at the earliest opportunity, either at the same time as emergency treatment is being given or immediately afterward.

Unconsciousness

If a person is unconscious (ie, insensible and cannot be roused), perhaps after a heart attack, car accident, drowning, or other emergency, there are two vital points to check for:
1 Check if the person is breathing
2 Check for a heartbeat or pulse.

Checking for breathing
● Put your cheek against the person's mouth and see if you can feel the breath.

● Place a mirror in front of the person's mouth and see if it steams up.

● Check for chest movement.

Checking for heartbeat or pulse
● Feel for the pulse over the carotid artery (as shown below).

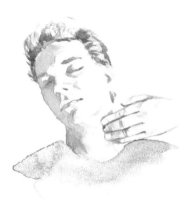

Checking the carotid artery

● Listen or feel for the heartbeat over the heart.

● Check for unnatural pallor. If the heartbeat has stopped, the person will look grayish or blue.

● Check the eyes. If the heartbeat has stopped, the pupils of the eyes will look very large.

Immediate action
If the person is not breathing, but there is a heartbeat, start the kiss of life at once (p.332).

If the heartbeat has stopped, breathing will have stopped too. Heart massage must be performed in conjunction with, or after, the kiss of life (pp.332-3). Don't give heart massage until you have tried 4 mouth-to-mouth breaths of the kiss of life. *Never* give heart massage to someone whose heart is still beating.

The kiss of life

The kiss of life is one of the most essential techniques for saving life.

1 Lie the person on the ground on his or her back. See if there is any object in the mouth, such as false teeth, that could block the passage of air. If there is, remove it. If there is vomit, turn the head to one side, to let it dribble out.

2 Kneel beside the head. Tilt the person's head backward by pulling the chin upward with one hand and pushing the top of the head down with the other hand. (This alone may start the breathing. If it does, get the person into the recovery position.)

3 With the hand that is resting on the forehead, pinch the nose shut. Check that the mouth is open.

4 **Adults** Take a full inhalation. Apply your mouth to the casualty's. Cover it completely, and breathe firmly into it.
    Children Take a shallow breath and breathe gently into the mouth.
    Babies Use only the amount of air you can hold in your cheeks to blow into the mouth.

5 Take your mouth away. The casualty's chest should start to fall.

6 Repeat steps 4 and 5 every 5 or 6 seconds. Continue until the person starts to breathe spontaneously.

Caution While giving the kiss of life, keep checking that the heart hasn't stopped. If it has, begin heart massage.

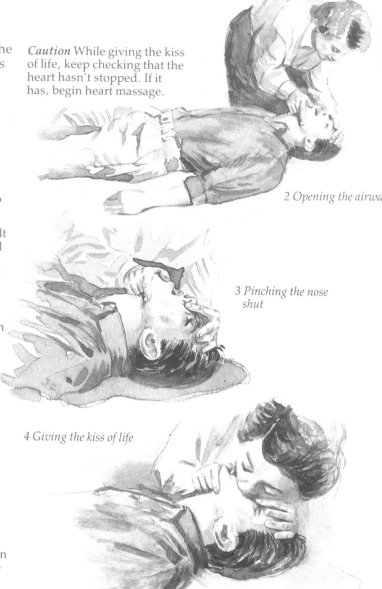

2 Opening the airwa

3 Pinching the nose shut

4 Giving the kiss of life

If you have help ...
One of you can give the kiss of life, while the other gives heart massage (opposite). First, one of you breathes once into the casualty's lungs, then the other does 5 heart compressions. Continue until the person recovers or help arrives.

Recovery If the casualty starts to recover, you must stop giving the kiss of life and get him or her into the recovery position (p.335).

Heart massage

If, after trying 4 breaths of the kiss of life, you still cannot find any heartbeat or pulse, you must try to start the heart at once.

1 Lie the person down flat, and loosen any tight clothing such as a belt or collar. If possible, send someone else for an ambulance or doctor.

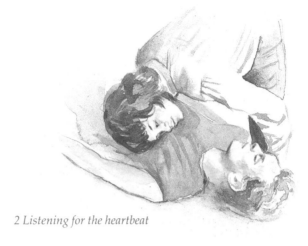

2 Listening for the heartbeat

2 Kneel on the person's right side, facing the head. Check again that you cannot hear or feel the heart beating.

3 Place the heel of one hand over the heart. The rest of your hand should not put any pressure on the chest.

4 Place the heel of the other hand on the back of the first (unless the casualty is a child or baby).

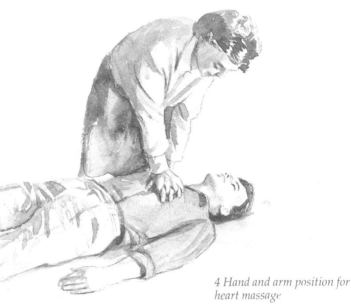

4 Hand and arm position for heart massage

5 Keeping your arms straight, rock your body backward and forward. Don't apply pressure by bending your arms or you'll get exhausted in no time.

6 Adults Depress the chest wall about 2 inches (5 cm) every time you apply pressure. Give about 60 compressions per minute.
　Children Use only one hand, and gently depress the chest wall about 80 times per minute.

Babies *With extreme care* Use only two fingers, and press about 100 times per minute. Press higher up the breastbone to avoid damaging the liver.

7 Continue the heart massage until either the neck pulse returns, or the person begins to look a better color and the pupils reduce to normal size, or the person regains consciousness.

Recovery If the person recovers, put him or her into the recovery position (p.335), even if still unconscious. This ensures that the airway is kept open. Gurgling and snoring noises indicate a blockage.

Caution Don't go on compressing the chest of someone whose heartbeat or pulse has returned.

Choking

If the windpipe is obstructed by any object, such as food (or buttons or sweets, in children), it is an emergency and should be treated immediately. If there is only partial blockage, the person will be able to inhale enough air to cough and this should clear it. A person whose windpipe is totally blocked will be unable to speak, cough, or breathe. He or she may clutch at the throat in panic, and quickly turn blue.

Immediate action

Open the person's mouth and see if you can hook out the obstruction with your fingers. Or slap him or her firmly between the shoulderblades. This usually dislodges the object. If it doesn't, use the Heimlich method, as shown right.

Heimlich method

1 Clasp the person from behind. Clench one of your hands into a fist over the stomach between the navel and the ribcage. Grip the wrist of the clenched hand with the other hand.

Push strongly against the abdominal wall, inward and upward. This sharp pressure drives the air out of the lungs, by compressing the abdomen, and should shoot the obstructing object up through the windpipe.

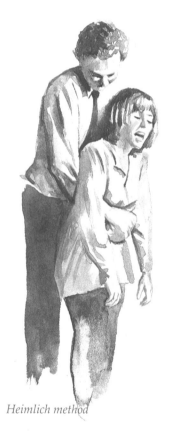

Heimlich method

2 If this procedure fails on the first attempt, repeat 3 times. If the blockage still remains, call for medical help. Should the person lose consciousness, try to give the kiss of life.

Bleeding

The amount of blood lost by an accident victim always looks much more than it is in reality. The average adult in good health can lose up to 1½ pints (0.8 litres) of blood without serious consequences. For children, however, loss of half that amount can be critical. Blood may be flowing so fast it cannot clot and seal the wound. In such cases immediate treatment is essential, and can be life-saving.

Immediate action

1 Get someone else to call an ambulance or doctor. Raise the injured part to reduce blood flow to it.

2 Remove foreign bodies from the wound, but only if they are visible and not deeply embedded. Do not probe around in the wound.

3 Press firmly on the wound (unless it is a head wound) with a clean pad. (Use any clean cloth folded into an appropriate size, or a sterile pad, if available.) If the wound is gaping, pull the edges together and press hard. Maintain the pressure.

4 Bandage the area firmly. If blood seeps through this dressing put more padding over the wound and bandage again. If no proper dressing is available, use a scarf, tie, or any other item of clothing that is to hand.

5 Rest the injured part, elevating it if possible, and stay close to the person. Try to be reassuring. Loss of blood is very distressing and can easily cause panic.

Head wounds Never press hard on a severe head wound; this may result in damage to the tissues around the brain. Lightly cover the area, and bandage.

Signs of internal bleeding
If you notice any of the following signs in a casualty after an accident, call for medical help at once. Don't give the person anything to eat or drink.

● Bruising, especially over a large area or over the trunk

● Dizziness

● Cold, clammy skin

● Difficult breathing and weak, rapid pulse

● Coughing up frothy blood

● Severe abdominal pain

● Signs of fractured bones, such as pain, swelling, bruising, obvious deformity, or loss of use.

Drowning
It is crucial to start resuscitating a drowned person at the earliest possible opportunity. If the person is having great difficulty breathing, or if breathing has actually stopped, you must give the kiss of life. Don't worry about emptying water from the person's lungs. The air you breathe into the lungs will find its way through any water in bubbles, although you may find you have to blow quite hard.

Immediate action
Begin the kiss of life (p.332). Send someone else for an ambulance if possible. Carry on with resuscitation for up to an hour if help has not yet arrived. (Drowned people can be revived after a much longer time than most other unconscious people.)

Once breathing has restarted, put the person into the recovery position and keep him or her warm until medical help arrives.

The recovery position
It is essential to get an injured or unconscious person into this position, as shown below, as soon as possible after giving emergency treatment. The only exception is where there is a possibility of broken bones, in which case the person should not be moved.

1 Turn the person gently onto his or her front, and turn the head to one side.

2 On that side, draw the arm up toward the face, and draw the leg on that side upward, so that the thigh is at right angles to the trunk.

3 Position the other leg so that it is straight, in line with the body. The other arm should lie beside the trunk.

4 Make sure the head is kept on one side, that the airway is open and that clothes are not restricting circulation or breathing. Do not leave the casualty while you are waiting for professional help.

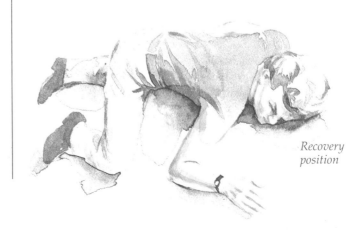

Recovery position

Poisoning

Poisons may be swallowed, inhaled, injected, or absorbed through the skin. Try to discover exactly what the poison is, and keep a specimen if possible, so that an antidote or other appropriate treatment can be identified with the minimum of delay as soon as medical assistance is available.

Immediate action

● If the poison is corrosive (eg, bleach and other cleaning fluids), do not try to make the person vomit. If conscious, he or she should be given milk or water to swallow to dilute the substance and protect the stomach.

● If the poison is definitely not corrosive (eg, an overdose of a medication), try to make the person vomit by thrusting 3 fingers down the back of the throat. Do not give salt water to cause vomiting.

● If the poison has been absorbed through the skin (eg, agricultural chemicals), remove contaminated clothing and wash exposed areas. Wear rubber gloves, if possible, to protect your hands from contamination.

● If the person is unconscious, keep a close eye on their breathing and heartbeat (p.331).

Electric shock

Electricity can kill outright, or produce very serious injury. If a person comes in contact with a high voltage source, anybody nearby must keep well clear, and call for professional help. High voltage electricity can jump gaps.

In the case of electric shock from a household appliance, the person must be "disconnected" from the electric current before anyone touches him or her. As an obvious precaution, never handle electrical appliances with wet hands, and keep all such equipment well away from water.

Immediate action

1 Turn off the current at the socket or give the cord a hard pull so that the plug flies out of the socket.

2 Knock the person away from the source of the current with an insulating object, such as a wooden chair or broom. Until this has been done the person remains *live* and will give an electric shock to anyone who comes into physical contact with him or her.

3 When the person is clear of the current, send someone else to get medical help. Check the casualty's breathing (p.331), and give the kiss of life if necessary. If there is no heartbeat (p.331), give heart massage as well.

Immediate action: breaking the electric current

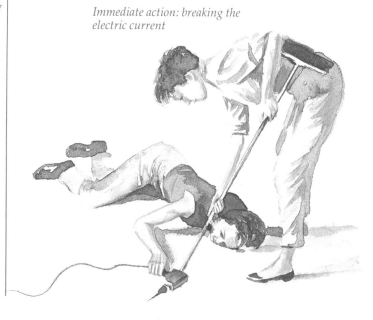

Severe burns

Always treat any burn as severe and get medical help at once if: it involves more than 10 percent of the body; the person is in shock; or if the burn is caused by electricity, chemicals, or molten metal. (For minor burns, see p.324.)

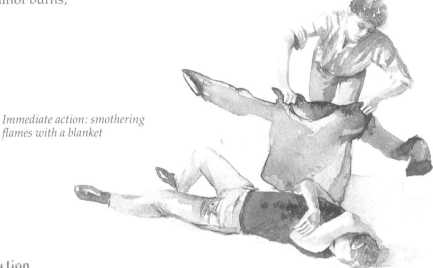

Immediate action: smothering flames with a blanket

Immediate action

• If a person's clothing is on fire, throw him or her to the ground and smother the flames with water, or any thick material to hand. Try to direct the flames away from the person's head.

• If clothing is drenched in boiling fat or chemicals, try to remove it, gently, but take care not to burn yourself in the process. Don't pull off material that is stuck to a burned area of skin.

• If possible, remove anything constricting (such as a ring, belt, or shoes), in or around the burned area.

• Cool the burn by applying towels soaked in cold water. (But never plunge the whole person into a cold bath.)

• Lie the person down, and keep any burned limbs raised.

• If the person is conscious, and not vomiting, try to give frequent, tiny sips of cold water to help replace lost body fluids.

• If the mouth is scalded, give a conscious person ice to suck, to prevent blocking of the airways through swelling.

Glossary
of nutrients and natural remedies

As natural medicines and health foods become increasingly popular, pharmacies and health food stores are stocking more varied and unusual products. This section provides explanations of common nutritional terms, together with descriptions of a number of essential nutrients, foodstuffs of exceptional value, and herbal remedies.

Acerola (*Malpighia goabra*) The West Indian cherry, one of the world's richest sources of vitamin C.

Acidophilus A lactobacillus used for making live yoghurt. Good for constipation and after antibiotic therapy.

Adaptogen A class of remedies that nourish the body to help it cope with disease and "dis-ease". Ginseng is a well-known example.

Agar agar A derivative of the stems of seaweeds of the red algae family. Can be used as a thickening agent.

Alfalfa (*Medicago sativa*) Also known as lucerne. The sprouted seeds make an excellent salad. Its leaves are rich in calcium, vitamins, protein, and trace elements.

Aloe vera Concentrates of the plant's juices are used as a skin tonic, and as an aid to healing minor burns.

Amino acids The 8 essential amino acids – lysine, methionine, valine, tryptophan, threonine, leucine, isoleucine, and phenylalanine – are the main constituents of protein.

Arnica (*Arnica montana*) Also known as mountain daisy, this is used in tablet or ointment form to ease pain and discomfort and shock.

Aspartame A protein-like artificial sweetener, safer than saccharin.

Beta-carotene The yellow color in carrots and other fresh vegetables, thought to be changed by the body into vitamin A. Beta-carotene may be more important than vitamin A itself in preventing degenerative disease.

Biochemic tissue salts The 12 major salts found in the human body. Homeopathic preparations of these salts are used to counter everyday illnesses.

Bioflavonoids Any of a group of biologically active flavonoids (aromatic compounds) which occur naturally in foods containing vitamin C, and which enhance its action.

Brewers' yeast A by-product of the brewing process. It includes a wide spectrum of B group vitamins and helps to control stress and tiredness.

Calcium See p.41.

Calendula Tincture or ointment made from marigold flowers, used to heal cuts and burns, and to stop minor bleeding.

Carob (*Ceratonia siliqua*) A naturally sweet substitute for chocolate. Contains vitamins A and D, and three B group vitamins.

Carrageen A natural extract of several seaweeds, also known as Irish moss. Used to emulsify and thicken foods, and as a remedy for respiratory complaints.

Chelate An organic combination of protein and mineral, easily absorbed by the body.

Choline An alkaline substance found in lecithin, brewers' yeast, and liver; a shortage causes liver problems through fat accumulation.

Chromium An essential trace element (p.41).

Cider vinegar Used as a folk remedy for several common ailments, and as a cleansing drink (a dessertspoon mixed in hot water with a little honey). Research has supported the view that cider vinegar helps some people to slim.

Cobalt A trace element, part of the essential vitamin B12 (p. 41).

Cold-pressed oils Vegetable oils extracted naturally, producing a high biological quality.

Copper An essential trace element (p. 41).

Dandelion coffee A coffee-like caffeine-free drink (best well roasted).

Dextrose Otherwise known as glucose (p.38).

Dolomite A natural mountain fossil earth, available as tablets. High in calcium and magnesium.

Enzyme preparation A commonly used proteolytic enzyme (one that dissolves protein), made from unripe papaya (pawpaw) fruits called papain. Sometimes prescribed for flatulence.

EFAs Essential Fatty Acids or essential fats (p.39).

Epsom salts Chemically known as magnesium sulphate. Used in baths to promote sweating and thus to eliminate toxins.

Evening primrose oil Oil produced from the seeds of *Oenothera biennis*. Research suggests it may be useful in treating many diseases including multiple sclerosis, rheumatoid arthritis and heart disease. It is also used to treat cramp.

Eyebright *(Euphrasia officinalis)* Herb used to prepare an eye lotion; excellent for eye inflammations.

Fiber See p.38.

Fish oils Oils from fatty fish, containing special fatty acids. Available in the concentrated form MAXepa. A diet including 1 or 2 fish dishes a week has been shown to help protect against coronary heart disease.

Friars' balsam Preparation containing benzoin, used as an inhalant to relieve sore throats and colds.

Fructose Fruit sugar, a permitted natural sweetener, suitable for diabetics (p.38). It is twice as sweet as ordinary sugar.

Gamma linolenic acid (GLA) The body should be able to produce its own GLA, a substance used to control certain cell functions, but it may be inhibited by alcohol consumption, the Pill and hardened fat. Evening primrose oil contains GLA.

Ginseng The root of the Asiatic variety *Panax ginseng* contains a stimulant and a stress reducer. American ginseng (*P. quinque-folium*) and Siberian ginseng (*Eleuthoroccus senticosus*) have similar properties.

Glucomannan The purified active ingredient of the Japanese konjac root, used as an appetite reducer and as a substitute for cereal fiber.

Gluconates An organic combination of minerals with gluconic acid, easily absorbed into the blood and in the correct amounts.

Glucose See Dextrose.

Gluten The elastic part of wheat and rye flour, a useful source of protein, but must be completely avoided by those with coeliac disease. It is best avoided by all babies until at least after the fourth month.

Green-lipped mussel *(Perna caniculata)* There are many reports that an extract from this large New Zealand mussel can bring relief from arthritic and rheumatic pain and stiffness.

Guar A gum extracted from the seeds of *Cyamopsis tetragonolobus* or *C. psoraloides*. It is used as a thickening agent, an emulsion stabilizer, and to help diabetics control blood sugar levels, reduce cholesterol and gain control of excess weight.

Hydrogenation Many margarines are more or less hydrogenated (ie, treated with hydrogen), a process that produces trans-fatty acids which are thought to block several bodily processes. Hydrogenated products are best avoided.

Inositol This substance helps to prevent an excessive amount of fats being deposited in the liver and to keep cholesterol levels stable.

International Unit (IU) A system of expressing vitamin values. (Current nutritional guidelines favour the elimination of IUs.)

Iodine An essential trace element (p.41).

Irish moss See Carrageen.

Iron An essential trace element mineral (p.41).

Jojoba The oil from the kernels of jojoba nuts is used as a conditioner for hair and skin. It can also be beneficial for arthritis and constipation.

Kelp *(Fucus vesiculosus)* A common seaweed, rich in minerals, especially iodine, and trace elements. Available as a food supplement.

Kuzu A white starch extracted from the roots of the wild kuzu vine, used for thickening. Aids digestion.

Lecithin A complex mixture of choline, inositol, fatty acids, and phosphorus, which is present in all living cells. It has been used experimentally to treat some of the problems associated with old age. Found in egg yolk and soya. Available as a food supplement.

Macrobiotic Describes a diet based on the Chinese energy forces, Yin and Yang (p.270). In theory, macrobiotic foods grow well in the area where the consumer lives; in practice many high-quality oriental ingredients are used.

Magnesium An essential mineral, important in heart disease (p.41).

Manganese An essential trace element (p.41).

Margarine Often produced from processed vegetable oils (see Hydrogenation). Those containing over 45% of polyunsaturates are best.

Marigold See Calendula.

MAXepa See Fish oils.

Minerals Metallic and non-metallic substances which are needed in quantities of at least 100 mg per day. The metallic elements are calcium, magnesium, and potassium; the non-metallic elements are carbon, phosphorus, and sulphur (p.41). Minerals needed in smaller amounts are classed as trace elements.

Molasses Heavy syrup from which cane sugar is extracted.It is rich in B vitamins and contains significant magnesium, calcium, and potassium.

Monosodium glutamate (MSG) Flavor enhancer introduced to many processed foods, occurs naturally in soy sauce and some other soya products. A high intake can cause severe headaches, heart palpitations, and other ailments, but moderate use seems safe.

Multi-mineral supplements Tablets or capsules that contain at least half of the recommended daily amounts of calcium, iodine, and iron, and may contain other minerals.

Multi-vitamin supplements Tablets or capsules that contain at least half of the recommended daily amounts of vitamins A, B1, B2, B3, B12, folic acid, C, and D, and may also contain vitamins B5, B6, biotin, E, and K.

Octacosanol A substance found in wheatgerm, said to be effective in increasing stamina and vitality after middle age.

Olbas oil A traditional Swiss remedy used for colds, catarrh, rheumatic pains, and lumbago. It contains a mixture of essential oils from several aromatic plants (p.220).

Organic In terms of diet, foods that are grown under ecologically desirable conditions, ie, without artificial fertilizers, pesticides, and herbicides, added hormones, etc. Organic crops also depend on a lack of local environmental pollution, such as major roads or large industrial complexes.

Orotates Combinations of minerals with orotic acid. Mineral orotates are normally well absorbed and tolerated by the body.

Paba Para-amino benzoic acids related to the B complex vitamins and normally synthesized in the intestines by healthy bacteria. Paba is prescribed when bacteria have been destroyed by sulpha drugs. It is also a natural sun-screening agent when taken orally. Natural sources are liver, eggs, molasses, brewers' yeast, and wheatgerm.

Papain See Enzyme preparation.

Pectin A substance found in quantity in such food as apples and plums. It is used as a setting agent when making jams, but it is also an excellent source of dietary fiber.

Phospholipids Describes fats containing phosphorus, which are a major component of the body's fat. Used experimentally for circulatory and nervous problems in senile dementia. Lecithin, see above, is a major nutritional source.

Pollen The male element of a flower contains over 95 identified micronutrients, vitamins, minerals, and enzymes. Pollen has been identified as an adaptogen.

Polyunsaturates See p.39.

Potassium See p.41.

Propolis The black resin used by bees to line their hives has marked anti-bacterial and anti-viral properties.

RDA Recommended daily amount (or allowance) of various nutrients, varies according to different ages and sexes. The RDA is based on a factor that should prevent or cure deficiency in the majority of the population. There is widespread variation between countries.

Royal jelly A highly nutritious substance secreted by honeybees and fed to queen larvae. Research has shown that it supports the body's immune system. It has been classed as an adaptogen.

Rutin The active ingredient of buckwheat, a bioflavonoid which strengthens the blood capillaries.

Salt substitutes These fall into two forms. First, those that contain a mixture of sodium chloride and potassium chloride (low in sodium). Second, those that are even lower in sodium and can be used in certain special diets. They are not recommended for patients with kidney problems.

Slippery elm food The bark of the slippery elm *(Ulmus fulva)*, when used as a powder and taken in milk-based drinks, coats the gastric lining with a layer of mucilage, which helps to promote the healing of ulcers and aids digestion.

Sodium See p.41.

Soya products The only generally available single source of complete plant protein. Soya proteins have been shown to help reduce cholesterol levels.

Spirulina A blue-green algae that grows in certain alkaline lakes. Contains valuable vitamins and minerals.

Tahini Sesame seed paste, an excellent source of calcium, phosphorus, and iron.

Tea tree oil Oil extracted from the Australian shrub *Melaleuca alternifolia*. An antiseptic and germicide used for healing wounds, and for treating urinogenital and other infections.

Textured Vegetable Protein (TVP) Meat substitute made from spun soya bean protein.

Tiger Balm A preparation of aromatic ingredients invented by the Haw Par brothers in Singapore. It is effective for minor injuries and sprains.

Tofu Soya bean curd, a good source of unsaturated fat and protein. Tofu is a staple part of macrobiotic and Chinese cooking.

Trace elements Mineral substances that are needed by the body in extremely small amounts (less than 100 mg daily), and include iron, copper, manganese, zinc, iodine, cobalt, selenium, molybdenum, fluorine, silicon, chromium, vanadium, nickel, tin, and arsenic.

Tryptophan An essential amino acid, used to help sleep and combat stress.

Umeboshi plum Salt-pickled plums from Japan, rich in enzymes and lactic acid. Thought to aid digestion.

Vitamins Micronutrients that are essential for health. New vitamins are being discovered and their roles redefined. They are divided into 2 groups – fat-soluble, stored by the body, and water-soluble (those that need to be replaced every day). (See p.40.)

Wheatgerm The embryo of the wheat kernel that is present in wholemeal flour. It is rich in vitamins B and E.

Wheatmeal A flour from which a proportion of the bran has been extracted.

Wholemeal Flour that contains 100% of the edible portion of the wheat grain with no additives.

Witch hazel *(Hamamelis virginiana)* The distilled herb is an excellent healing astringent.

Yeast extract A very rich source of vitamin B.

Yoghurt Live yoghurt provides bacteria which help maintain a healthy intestinal environment.

Yucca South-western American plant used successfully to treat conditions such as rheumatoid arthritis and varicose veins. Recent research suggests that an extract of the flowers can reduce cancerous tumor.

Zinc See p.41.

Resources

The list that follows includes addresses of organizations concerned with preventive or general health care; major national institutes of complementary medicine; and associations or individuals representing each of the natural therapies covered in Chapter 5.

General health care organizations

Alcoholics Anonymous
175 Fifth Avenue
New York, N.Y. 10010

American Health Foundation
320 East 43rd Street
New York, N.Y. 10017

Center for Medical Consumers
and Health Care Information
237 Thompson Street
New York, N.Y. 10012

National Health Council
70 West 40th Street
New York, N.Y. 10018

Planned Parenthood
380 Second Avenue
New York, N.Y. 10010

Diet Research Institute
1365 York Avenue
New York, N.Y. 10028

Living Tao Foundation
507 West Oregon Street
Urbana, Illinois 61801

Stress Management and
Counseling Center
110 East 36th Street
New York, N.Y. 10016

Tai Chi Society
1047 Amsterdam Avenue
NewYork, N.Y. 10025

American College of
Nurse-Midwives
1000 Vermont Avenue N.W.
Washington, D.C. 20005

International Childbirth
Education Association
P.O. Box 20852
Milwaukee, Wisconsin 53220

American Mental Health
Foundation
2 East 86th Street
New York, N.Y. 10024

Association for Humanistic
Psychology
325 Ninth Street
San Francisco, California 90025

Family Planning International
810 Seventh Avenue
New York, N.Y. 10019

Natural therapies organizations

American Holistic Medical
Association
2727 Fairview Avenue East
Seattle, Washington 98102

American Holistic Nurses
Association
205 St. Louis Street
Springfield, Missouri 65806

Association for Holistic Health
P.O. Box 9532, San Diego,
California 92109

Omega Institute
P.O. Box 571
Lebanon Springs, New York
12114

Homeopathy

Homeopathic Education Services
5916 Chabot Crest
Oakland, California 94618

International Foundation for
Homeopathy
1141 N.W. Market Street
Seattle, Washington 98107

National Center for Homeopathy
1500 Massachusetts Avenue
Washington, D.C. 20005

Bach flower remedies

Bach Center Seminars
457 Rockaway Avenue
Valley Stream, N.Y. 11580

Naturopathy

National Association of
Naturopathic Physicians
609 Sherman Avenue
Coeur D'Alene, Idaho 83814

Osteopathy

North American Academy of
Manipulative Therapy
12238 113th Avenue, Suite 106
Youngtown, Arizona 85363

American Academy of
Osteopathy
2630 Airport Road
Colorado Springs, Colorado
80910

American Osteopathic
Association
212 East Ohio Street
Chicago, Illinois 60611

Chiropractic

American Chiropractic
Association
2200 Grand Avenue
Des Moines, Iowa 50312

International Chiropractors
Association
741 Brady Street
Davenport, Iowa 52808

Massage

American Massage and Therapy
Association
152 West Wisconsin Avenue
Milwaukee, Wisconsin 53203

Boulder School of Massage
Therapy
2855 Walnut Street
Boulder, Colorado 80301

Esalen Institute
Big Sur, California 93920

The Swedish Institute
875 Avenue of the Americas
New York, N.Y. 10001

Applied Kinesiology and touch for health

Thie Chiropractic Corporation
1192 North Lake Avenue
Pasadena
California 91104

International College of Applied
Kinesiology
542 Michigan Building
Detroit, Michigan 48226

Reflexology
International Institute of
Reflexology
P.O. Box 12642
St. Petersburg
Florida 33733

Reflexology Center
1307 Avenue J
Brooklyn, N.Y. 11230

Rolfing
Rolf Institute
Box 1868
Boulder
Colorado 80306

Acupuncture
National Commission for the
Certification of Acupuncturists
1424 16th Street N.W.
Washington, D.C. 20036

National Council of Acupuncture
Schools and Colleges
Box 954
Columbia, Maryland 20144

Traditional Acupuncture
Foundation
The American City Building
Columbia, Maryland 21044

Acupuncture Research Project
Lincoln Hospital
349 East 140th Street
Bronx, New York 10434

Shiatsu
Shiatsu Education Center
52 West 55th Street
New York, N.Y. 10019

The Toronto Shiatsu Center
177 College Street
Toronto, Ontario, Canada

Therapeutic touch
Nurse Healers/Professional
Associates
175 Fifth Avenue, Suite 3399
New York, N.Y. 10019

Pumpkin Hollow Farm
Box 135 RR1
Craryville, N.Y. 12521

Radionics and radiesthesia
American Society of Dowsers
Danville, Vermont 05828

Hypnotherapy
The American Society of Clinical
Hypnosis
2400 East Devon Avenue
Des Plaines, Illinois 60018

Associate Trainers in Clinical
Hypnosis
567 Split Rock Road
Syosset, N.Y. 11791

Milton H. Erickson Foundation
3606 N. 24th Street
Phoenix, Arizona 85016

International Society of
Hypnosis
111 North 49th Street
Box 144
Philadelphia, Pennsylvania 19139

Meditation
Transcendental Meditation
Program
200 East 23rd Street
New York, N.Y. 10010

Healing
Consciousness Research and
Training Project
315 East 68th Street
Box 90
New York, N.Y. 10021

Yoga
Integral Yoga Institute
227 West 13th Street
New York, N.Y. 10011

International Sivananda Yoga
Community
8157 Sunset Blvd.
Los Angeles
California 90046

Alexander technique
The American Center for the
Alexander Technique, Inc.
142 West End Avenue
New York, N.Y. 10023
and
931 Elizabeth Street
San Francisco, California 94114

Biofeedback
Biofeedback Society of America
4301 Owens Street
Wheat Ridge, Colorado 80030

Recommended reading

General works on the natural therapies are followed by books on individual therapies in the order in which they occur in Chapter 5.

Carroll, D. *The Complete Book of Natural Medicine*, Summit Books, 1980, New York

Fulder, Stephen *The Handbook of Complementary Medicine*, Coronet Books (Hodder & Stoughton), 1984, UK

Grossman, Richard *The Other Medicines*, Doubleday, 1985, New York, and Pan, 1986, London

Inglis, Brian, and West, Ruth *The Alternative Health Guide*, Michael Joseph, 1983, London

Stanway, Dr Andrew *Alternative Medicine*, Macdonald and Janes, 1979, London, and Penguin, 1986, London, and Penguin, 1982, New York

Panos, M. and Heimlich, J. *Homeopathic Medicine at Home*, Corgi, Transworld Publ., 1984, London, and Tarcher, 1981, Los Angeles

Coulter, Harris L. *Homeopathic Science and Modern Medicine*, N. Atlantic Books, 1981, USA

Vithoulkas, G. *Homeopathy, Medicine of the New Man*, Thorsons, 1985, Wellingborough, UK, and Arco, 1979, USA

Coulter, Catherine R. *Portraits of Homeopathic Medicines: Psychophysical Analyses of Selected Constitutional Types*, Wehawken Book Co., 1986, USA

Griggs, Barbara *Home Herbal*, Pan, 1983, London

Buchman, D. *Herbal Medicine*, Rider, 1983, London

Hoffman, D. *Holistic Herbal*, Findhorn Press, 1984, Forres, UK

Wright, B. *Natural Healing with Herbal Combinations*, Green Press, 1984, Burwash, Suffolk, UK

Ryman, Daniele *The Aromatherapy Handbook*, Century Hutchinson, 1984, London

Tisserand, R. *The Art of Aromatherapy*, C. W. Daniel, 1985, Saffron Walden, UK

Hyne Jones, T. W. *Dictionary of the Bach Flower Remedies*, C. W. Daniel, 1985, Saffron Walden, UK

Chancellor, P. *Handbook of Bach Flower Remedies*, C. W. Daniel, 1985, Saffron Waldon, UK, and Keats, 1980, USA

Newman Turner, Roger *Naturopathic Medicine*, Thorsons, 1984, Wellingborough, UK

Lindlahr, H. *Philosophy of Natural Therapeutics*, Maidstone Osteopathic Clinic, 1975, Maidstone, UK

Lindlahr, H. *Practise of Natural Therapeutics*, Maidstone Osteopathic Clinic, 1975, Maidstone, UK

Leibold, G. *Practical Hydrotherapy*, Thorsons, 1980, Wellingborough, UK

Clark, Linda *Handbook of Natural Remedies for Common Ailments*, Pocket Books, 1976, New York

Jarvis, D. C. *Folk medicine*, Pan, 1961, London, and Fawcett, 1985, USA

Powell, Eric *The Natural Home Physician*, C. W. Daniel, 1975, Saffron Walden, UK

Chaitow, Leon *Osteopathy*, Thorsons, 1982, Wellingborough, UK, and Thorsons, 1985, New York

Stoddard, Dr Alan *The Back: Relief from Pain*, Dunitz, 1979, London

Dintenfass, J. *Chiropractic: a Modern Way to Health*, Harcourt Brace Jovanovich, 1971, New York

Scofield, A. G. *Chiropractic*, Thorsons, 1982, Wellingborough, UK

Tappan, Frances M. *Healing Massage Techniques – a study of Eastern and Western methods*, Prentice Hall, 1978, Reston, Virginia, USA

Lidell, Lucy *The Book of Massage*, Ebury Press, 1984, London, and Simon & Schuster, 1984, New York

Valentine, T. and C. *Applied Kinesiology*, Thorsons, 1985, Wellingborough, UK, Thorsons, 1985, New York

Thie, John F. *Touch for Health, a practical guide to natural health*, De Vorss and Co., 1979, Princeton, USA

Bayly, Doreen *Reflexology Today*, Thorsons, 1984, Wellingborough, UK, and Thorsons, 1984, New York

Byers, Dwight C. *Better Health with Foot Reflexology*, Ingham Publishing, 1983

Rolf, Ida *Rolfing, The Integration of Human Structures*, Harper & Row, 1977, New York

Kaptchuk, Ted *Chinese Medicine, The Web That Has No Weaver*, Rider, 1986, London, and Congdon and Weed, 1984, New York

Ohashi, Wataru *Do-it-yourself Shiatsu*, Allen and Unwin, 1979, London and E. P. Dutton, 1976, New York

Connelly, Dianne *Traditional Acupuncture: The Law of the Five Elements*, Centre for Traditional Acupuncture Inc., 1979, USA

Acknowledgments

Lidell, Lucy *The Book of Yoga*, Ebury Press, 1983, London, and *Sivananda Companion to Yoga*, Simon & Schuster, 1983, USA

Iyengar, B. K. S. *Light on Yoga*, Allen and Unwin, 1985, London, and Schocken, 1977, New York

Barlow, Dr W. *The Alexander Technique*, Arrow, 1979, London, and Warner Books, 1980, USA

Gelb , Michael *Body Learning*, Aurum Press, 1985, London, and Delilah Books, 1981, USA

MacManaway, Bruce, and Turcan, Johanna *Healing*, Thorsons, 1985, Wellingborough, UK, and New York

Gordon, Richard *Your Healing Hands*, Wingbow Press, 1978, Berkeley, USA

Krieger, Dolores *Therapeutic Touch*, Prentice Hall, 1979, New York

Lankton, Stephen R. (ed.) *Elements and Dimensions of an Ericksonian Approach*, Brunner-Matzel, 1985, New York

Le Shan, Lawrence *How to Meditate*, Thorsons, 1985, Wellingborough, UK, and Bantam, 1975, New York

Goldstein, J. *The Experience of Insight*, Wildwood House, 1981, London, and Shambhala Publications, 1983, USA

Poteliakhoff, Max, and Carruthers, M. *Real health: ill effects of stress and their prevention* Davis-Poynter, 1981, London

Brown, Barbara *Stress and the Art of Biofeedback*, Bantam, 1978, USA

Cade, C. Maxwell, and Coxhead, Nona *The Awakened Mind*, Element Books, 1986, UK

Green, Elmer and Alyce *Beyond Biofeedback*, Dell Publishing Co., 1977, New York

Dr Andrew Stanway would like to acknowledge the help of all the contributors and the editorial staff of Gaia, particularly Lucy Lidell and Ros Mair.

Photographic credits All photographs in this book were taken by Fausto Dorelli, except for p.11, Sally & Richard Greenhill, and p.119, David Pearson.

Gaia would like to extend particular thanks to Lesley Gilbert for copy preparation, to Phil Wilkinson and to Kate Poole for editorial and design assistance, and to the following practitioners and individuals who gave much invaluable help: Ann Golland (hydrotherapy); Simon Fielding (osteopathy); Michael Durtnall, Ian Hutchinson (chiropractic); Geoffrey Hardy (massage); Brian Butler (touch for health); A. J. Porter (reflexology); Tom Myers, Pru Rankin Smith (Rolfing); Frances Newman (acupuncture); Peter Walker (yoga); Lynn Nicholls (Alexander technique); Betty Barney (healing); David Tansley (radionics); John Butler (hypnotherapy), Geoffrey Blundell, Isobel Cade (biofeedback); and Rachel Osorio for helping to prepare the traditional medicine section.

For photographic modelling we would like to thank: Geraldine and Harry; Judy Baillie; Peter Barney; Jerry Burman; Georgiana and Joseph Carter; Teruko, Alyusha Mamiko and Nicholas Chagrin; Douglas Cosgrove; Dejon; Demian Dorelli; Fausto Dorelli; Des Hayes and Jean Higgs; Robin Hayfield; Lucy Joplin-Waters; Anna Kruger; Lucy Lidell; Susan McKeever; Erik Ness; Alison Nicholls; Lucy Oliver; Julia Parr; Cassandra Pearson; David and Joss Pearson; Michele, Steve and Alexander Pendleton; Kees Ritsema van Eck; Graeme Shawe; Fiona, Jason and Mimi Walker; and Peter Warren.

The following organizations and businesses provided information and assistance: AcuMedic Centre (Benny Mei); Ainsworth's Homeopathic Pharmacy; Alfa Electronics (Ross Mackelvie); ASH (Action on Smoking and Health); Dr Edward Bach Centre (Nickie Murray); Faculty of Homeopathy; Four Counties Foods; the Health Education Council; the Institute of Complementary Medicine; International Planned Parenthood Federation; The Koestler Foundation; Ministry of Agriculture, Food and Fisheries; A. Nelson and Co.; Odyssey Bookshop; St John Ambulance Association; Tyringham Clinic; and the World Health Organization.

The diagrammatic illustrations shown in the Touch for Health, Shiatsu, and Reflexology sections are reproduced with permission from, respectively *Touch for Health, a practical guide to natural health* by John F. Thie; *Do-it-yourself Shiatsu* by Wataru Ohashi; and *Better Health with Foot Reflexology* by Dwight C. Byers. The Shiatsu illustrations on p.227 are based on photographs by David West, Norton Canon, Hereford.

The diagrams on pp.44, 45 and 57, illustrate statistics in the *Statistical Abstract of the US*, 1985.

Illustrators
Gill Tomblin
Joe Robinson
Peter Mennim

Index